Dr Sandra Cabot
Women's Health

Pan Books
London, Sydney and Auckland

This book
is dedicated to my father,
Ronald Charles McRae
and my mother
Jacqueline Mary.

First published 1987 by Pan Books (Australia) Pty Ltd

This edition published 1990 by Pan Books Ltd,
Cavaye Place, London SW10 9PG

9 8 7 6 5 4 3 2 1

ISBN 0 330 30597 2

Photoset by Parker Typesetting Service, Leicester
Printed and bound in Great Britain by
Richard Clay Ltd, Bungay, Suffolk

Contents

16 Obesity and eating disorders   407

Your desirable weight; the causes of obesity – inherited fatness, disorders of the hormonal glands, medical drugs, disorders of the brain; the risks of being obese; eating disorders – bulimia, anorexia nervosa; dieting, fasting and exercise; the use of drugs to stimulate weight reduction; surgical procedures for weight loss – intestinal bypass operations, wiring of the jaws, liposuction, the stomach bubble; treatments for obesity that will not work; 300-calorie menus; a calorie counter.

Acknowledgements

I would like to acknowledge the kindness of Dr Andrew Child, MB, BS, MRCOG, FRACOG, Director of Obstetrics and Gynaecology at King George V Memorial Hospital, Dr Oscar Horky, MB, BS, MRCOG, DGO (Paris), FRACOG, obstetrician and gynaecologist, and Dr Anthony Helman, MB, BS, DRCOG, for their time in checking the manuscript and for their valuable suggestions.

I would also like to thank Barbara McAllister who spent many long nights typing and arranging the manuscript and Egidio Cianciosi for his assistance in compiling the tables.

Finally, I would like to thank my sister, Madeleine Koren, for her autobiographical anecdotes on pregnancy and motherhood, and also the thousands of women whose enquiring spirits and heartfelt needs inspired me to put pen to paper.

Foreword

A number of very significant changes have occurred in the practice of medicine over the past ten to twenty years. It is not so long ago that the family general practitioner was regarded as the major authoritative source of medical information in the community and his or her advice and recommendations were accepted without question. The flood of medical information now debated frankly and explicitly in glossy magazines, on television and as part of the school curriculum, has resulted in a heightened awareness in the lay general public regarding their own health. Gynaecological topics are by far the most popular subjects to come under the media spotlights.

The modern woman is expected to accept a certain degree of responsibility for her own gynaecological health. In order to do this she needs an adequate knowledge of her own anatomy and normal functioning, she needs a clear, concise and understandable source of information regarding abnormal and disease processes and then she needs to be aware of all the available options for management of these conditions. Unfortunately, much of the literature available through the lay press does not satisfy these criteria. Some publications are based solely on personal observations, some are biased by radical authors trying to promote their own theories and some are biased in the interests of entrepreneurial, commercial endeavours.

It is therefore encouraging and refreshing to know that this book is written by a doctor who has listened sympathetically to her patients over a number of years, who has exhaustively researched her topics and who is not afraid to discuss the orthodox and the naturopathic methods for managing some of the more controversial problems. More importantly, the fact that this book is written by a woman gives it an aura of uncontradictable authority.

Dr Andrew Child, MB, BS, MRCOG, FRACOG
Director of Obstetrics and Gynaecology,
King George V Memorial Hospital

The information contained in this book is intended to be a general guide for people seeking to improve their health. Anyone suffering from a physical disorder should only follow guidelines contained in this book under their own doctor's supervision.

Preface

Here I am, a doctor from the 'Land Down Under', having written a book for my sisters all over the world. For you and me the cultural barriers are merely superficial and we are united in our common desire to achieve physical, mental and spiritual well-being. To my English sisters I wish the 'best of British luck' in realizing these common goals that are finally accessible to the twentieth-century woman.

For many years I have been talking to women via radio, TV and newspapers with the aim of communicating new and exciting advances in the areas of their health disorders. As a result of this, I have received thousands of letters from women in Australia, New Guinea and America, as well as talking to many women by means of talk-back radio.

This experience has been very revealing for me and I think sometimes even more so for some of the male hosts of the pro-grammes, who would say to me during commercial breaks 'I thought these issues were kept behind closed doors'. However, radio switchboards were chock-a-block with calls from enthusias-tic women and television mail departments were plagued with enquiries for weeks.

This is a testimony to the fact that women are hungry for knowledge concerning their bodies and they are no longer ashamed to ask for it, even in front of embarrassed or cynical males. For too long now, such prevalent disorders as the premen-strual syndrome (PMS), menopause (MP) and sexual disorders have been treated as a 'Pandora's Box'. However, we now realize that they have huge psychological and economic implications for all societies and are worthy of public scrutiny.

I would like to encourage and congratulate those women who

openly and courageously search for a more complete knowledge of well-being, whether physical, mental or spiritual. Free discussion of these issues can only help our more timid sisters to vent their fears and needs.

I read many letters revealing to me that in this so-called modern age we live in, women are still subjected to the doctor who, when faced with their probing questions, responds 'I suggest you stop reading women's magazines' or 'suffering in the menopause is all imagination and your body will keep making sufficient hormones all by itself'. It is incredible, but it is happening out there somewhere, right now.

It is the individual attitudes of the doctor and the woman which are important, because every doctor is different, as is every woman. One must have the patience, sense of humour and optimism to experiment a little. If the first treatment one tries does not succeed then try another. One thing which is certain is that with modern medicine, good nutrition, naturopathy and life-style modification, there will be very few women unable to find some measure of relief.

1 Introduction

I have decided to devote this first chapter to telling you a little about myself and my medical philosophies. I feel that this will enable you to see my views against a particular background when I deal with specific health disorders in later chapters – and hopefully give you some confidence! I do not want to be a faceless technical author with whom my reader has no personal empathy. Perhaps I am being a little optimistic in assuming that I will not achieve the contrary with a few of you, but I do sincerely hope that we will be friends and confidantes by the end of the book.

My first introduction to medicine came from my mother, Jacqueline Mary, a strong beautiful liberated woman who was a schoolteacher by profession. She would often expound the virtues of naturopathy and she also successfully used the homoeopathic remedy 'phosphorus' for my chronic infantile tonsillitis, after all the antibiotics available had failed. She took me to the only naturopath in Adelaide on several occasions and I was always annoyed to find the queue of people waiting stretching out onto the footpath. And I never enjoyed the way in which the naturopath would rather obviously divert my attention and then abruptly manipulate my cervical vertebrae in or out of place, depending upon the inclination of my unsuspecting neck at the moment of attack.

My mother cured the neighbourhood's piles (haemorrhoids) with apple cider vinegar and raw bran during an epoch in which natural healing was not trendy. There were a few who regarded her as slightly deranged, but all up she proved to be a remarkable saleswoman for these ghastly tasting remedies. Alas, she had no entrepreneurial skills and never made a cent out of her efforts. My mother was also a sensible person and whenever I was really sick she would unhesitatingly call the local GP, Dr Odlum. I must say I was more impressed by Dr Odlum than by the naturopath, as to my innocent eyes, Dr Odlum seemed to have an air of enormous, if not infallible, wisdom; such are childhood impressions which are incredibly powerful and remain buried in the subconscious mind for ever.

Then there was my delightfully eccentric grandmother, Suzanna Berlow, whose life was narrowly snatched from the jaws of the mortal 'Bright's Disease'. This was the name given to inflammation and failure of the kidneys in the days before renal transplants and dialysis. The hero was her husband, a hospital dietician and chef. He had taken her away from the hospital with a prognosis of no hope and immediately began his dietary treatment of a raw juice every hour on the hour, made alternately from a vegetable under and above the ground. He was definitely not a man to romanticize or embellish a tale and he told me quite categorically, on several occasions, that he had saved her life.

Thus, by the time I was an adolescent, naturopathic healing was no longer alternative to me. At the age of seventeen, I enrolled in the School of Veterinary Science at Sydney University but discovered to my horror that I was terrified of large dogs and became bored by the prospect that my future patients would be mute. This led to a rather sudden but profound inspiration to become a medical doctor and I entered the Medical Faculty at Adelaide University.

As always, my mother was right behind me and she adapted well to keeping a fermented human brain in a bucket in the bathroom and finding the odd mislaid bone of a human skeleton buried in the couch. On occasions she would stay up late with me the night before exams and I would read aloud to her the symptoms of various diseases. It was then that I discovered she had a slight tendency to be a hypochondriac, as she would question me anxiously after every third symptom, fearing she had the relevant disease. These pre-exam collaborations proved to be immensely amusing to me but unfortunately anxiety-provoking for my mother and thus were short-lived!

As I approached the fourth year of my six-year medical degree, I began to see certain imperfections in the perspective of hospital medicine in treating many chronic diseases, which is really the bread and butter of general practice. My main objections were:

1 The cause of too many diseases was considered 'idiopathic', meaning unknown. Thus one was not able to treat the cause in, for example, many cases of arthritis, high blood pressure, allergies, eczema, dementia and headaches, just to name a few.

2 Doctors assigned to patients very stereotyped diagnoses. As a result the same standard drugs were used for all cases of arthritis or eczema or asthma, and so on.

3 The majority of treatments were suppressive drugs and there was not enough emphasis on removing possible causes and aggravating factors or increasing the body's resistance to disease.

4 Education in nutrition only dealt with gross deficiencies and nutritional medicine was not given enough credence.

I felt these flaws could act like blinkers and inhibit my investigating spirit. Take, for example, Mrs Bloggs who has rheumatoid arthritis, the cause of which is idiopathic, meaning that the cause is unknown. If one accepts that in her case, as in all cases of rheumatoid arthritis, it is impossible to find the cause, this could inhibit deeper inquiry and encourage the use of suppressive drugs at a premature stage.

Please don't think I was anti modern medicine or anti drugs. They can be life saving and indispensable. But I felt that the perspective was unbalanced towards suppressing, too quickly, physical and psychological symptoms before taking time to look at all possible causal factors. This was partly politically and economically motivated, as powerful multinational drug companies were coming out every day with some new drug which was supposed to work like a magic bullet. An official handwritten prescription is the exclusive preserve of doctors and carries prestige and mystery, whereas anyone can give you a written or spoken recommendation to take something as banal as a vitamin or mineral. Thus there was no incentive for doctors to use naturopathic medicine and, indeed, there was disincentive.

Out of a sense of frustration and intuition I began to spend my extracurricular hours with various well-known acupuncturists, naturopaths and homoeopaths. I was thought a little strange by my colleagues because in the early 1970s such types of treatment were considered to be of historical interest only. These days medical journals and doctors' magazines abound with advertisements for doctors' courses in these areas.

I was impressed with the results obtained by a well-known South Australian naturopath using raw foods, juices, vitamins and herbs. He would often read signs in the coloured ring around the patient's pupils (iris diagnosis) and his patients were fascinated when he pointed out signs of acidity, toxicity and chronic weaknesses in the photos of their irises. His patients were often difficult cases who had not achieved success with conventional medicine. I spent many sessions with him over several years and saw him relieve a variety of chronic painful symptoms. His treatments took some time to take effect and on occasion even provoked unpleasant elimination reactions, but the patients kept on coming back because deep down they were feeling better and their vitality was increasing.

To me his total faith in iris diagnosis was not always scientific, for how could one see the state of an internal organ by merely observing superficial marks in the iris, and yet I saw his judgements vindicated on many occasions. I concluded that iris diagnosis could be used as a helpful addition if conventional blood tests, X-rays and so on did not reveal a cause for the symptoms. Iris diagnosis was not just a figment of someone's imagination but had been developed by observation after a young man noticed striking changes in the large irises of his pet owl after it had fractured bones in its legs. As the fractured bones healed, white criss-crosses appeared over the original mark of injury in the iris.

I was also fortunate to spend many clinical sessions with Australia's most famous homoeopath, who was also a medical doctor. He was a man of great charisma and reputation and attracted patients from all over the world. I was full of enthusiasm to understand the mysterious art of homoeopathic medicine and spent many months studying the thousands of remedies in the homoeopathic bible known as the *Materia Medica*. Homoeopathy was almost the opposite of conventional medicine in that every patient was treated as an individual and their disease was not seen to be the most important clue in choosing the correct remedy. The homoeopathic doctor did not categorize his patients into stereotypes of diseases, for example arthritis, asthma, migraine and so on, but rather gave huge importance to their individual peculiarities such as fondness for spicy foods and hot climates, emotional tendencies and the times of the day during which they felt worst. After such a history had been painstakingly compiled a homoeopathic remedy which most exactly fitted the symptoms was chosen. This I thought must be the most difficult branch of healing to practise, as there were literally hundreds of thousands of possible remedies to choose from and, to be really spot-on each time, a computer would be necessary. The remedies were always given in very diluted form, the original substances often being diluted one thousand or one million times.

Nevertheless, I saw many patients respond to treatments by this famous doctor. However, I felt that the patients' faith in him may have played an important role in his success rate. This curing of a patient merely by faith and the passing of time is largely psychological and is known as the placebo effect. My famous homoeopathic doctor was a man of great presence and force of character and he sat in a rather dark surgery that was full of huge books and impressive antique furniture which all added up to create an atmosphere of wisdom and mystery. Add this to his long experience and reputation and no wonder his mere suggestion carried an enormous placebo effect.

Over the years I have kept an open mind to homoeopathy and have used it with benefit to treat childhood illnesses. However, in a really sick patient I would never rely solely on its powers of cure.

After a three-year residency in obstetric, general and paediatric hospitals, I went into private practice in Sydney and took over the care of all the pregnant patients in the practice who were planning a home birth. Thus I found myself driving around a strange city at night, street directory and torch in hand, and a home birth kit in the boot. Fortunately, all the mothers and their babies did well and I had more trouble catching the fainting fathers. However, I eventually decided that 'home births' are better done in a birthing unit situated in close proximity to a fully equipped hospital. One can never be 100 per cent sure, even in an apparently normal birth, that distress of the infant or a massive haemorrhage will not occur, so why not have the best of both worlds?

Private practice was good for my creative spirit. I kept my approach flexible, treating patients with a combination of orthodox drugs and naturopathic medicines. I found by using dietary modifications, vitamins, minerals, enzymes and herbs, I could in many cases reduce the dosage of drugs, or avoid their use entirely. Most patients were very gratified to be given something natural and safe, although I never forced the issue as I feel the patient should always be given a well-informed and democratic choice, otherwise they may not follow the instructions.

My patients were not always easy cases as they had often consulted several doctors before without success, and thus there was an ever present challenge. I became aware of the enormous gap between practitioners of conventional medicine and naturopathy which resulted in patients being prejudiced and too paranoid to seek both opinions. I met some patients who literally feared doctors and for years sought only the advice of naturopaths and health food stores. Unfortunately, it is always the poor old patient who becomes the meat in the sandwich and I saw several cases of nasty infections and cancers that had been missed and mistreated under the exclusive supervision of alternative practitioners. I was also horrified to hear from several severely diabetic patients that their naturopaths intended to wean them off their insulin injections and control their blood sugar by fasting!

My own philosophy is that these dangerous and potentially lethal situations can be avoided by educating patients to use a balanced approach. It may be very worthwhile to see a naturopath but always check with your own doctor over serious matters. If your doctor is hostile to your desire to try natural medicines and you are the courageous type, you may be able to open up his or her mind to their possible benefit or at least encourage a little democratic tolerance. You should feel free to assert your needs and ask all your questions, as it is to yourself that you should feel loyal, not to any particular doctor or naturopath.

Getting back to my own private practice, life went smoothly until 1982, when I began to suffer from the dreaded premenstrual syndrome (PMS). This made me aware of the devastating effect PMS can have upon physical and mental well-being. What's more, not only was I a victim of PMS, but so were a good percentage of my female patients. This drove me to an extensive research of the scientific literature existing on PMS and I discovered that among the experts there were many differing opinions and much uncertainty. However, the work of the English doctor, Katharina Dalton, appeared like a lighthouse in the storm and her idea of hormonal imbalance was close to my own concept of the cause of PMS. The hormone therapy which she recommends is certainly effective in severe cases. However, various nutritional studies made of PMS sufferers are indicative that nutrition and naturopathy can also serve as a basic treatment foundation. Over four years I have treated hundreds of PMS sufferers with dietary changes, vitamins, minerals and herbal medicines and have achieved an excellent success rate and these treatments have been free from side effects. In very severe cases of PMS it is necessary to add hormonal therapy but this must be administered very carefully.

Once I had solved the problem of PMS, including my own, I continued in my medical practice with renewed vigour and discovered there were other hormonal problems to conquer. In particular, I became very interested in menopausal women, as it seemed to me that women over the age of forty-five were a sadly neglected group in society. Many of these women were not as liberated psychologically as women of my generation and were often reticent and afraid to express their needs. Many breakthroughs in the treatment of menopausal symptoms had occurred in the last five years, but many women remained ignorant of them despite their devastating menopausal symptoms. I thought to myself 'how many long and worthwhile marriages could be saved if women going through the menopause really understood how to cope and come through it smiling'. We will talk in depth on this subject in a later chapter as there is so much for you to know.

I have not only interested myself in Australian women. In 1984, I spent time in France working with a French psychiatrist who specialized in the depressive illnesses of women. This was fascinating as I learned that even though European women are superficially more sophisticated than Australian or American women, deep down in the subconscious mind females have the same fears and needs.

While I was in France there was a renaissance of public and government interest in naturopathic medicine and the female minister for social affairs established an institute for research into the mechanism of the action of herbal medicines. Europeans are the people who originated naturopathy and they have been using it for centuries. Now at last they are studying scientifically how and why these remedies work.

French women are well versed in the virtues of herbal and nutritional remedies and many use them as a first choice for their everyday complaints. However, I was a little shocked to see the generally unhealthy life-style of many Parisian women. They tend to be heavy smokers and drinkers and live in polluted air and cramped spaces. The typical scene at a French swimming pool is that of women of every age group sunbaking topless and smoking, while languidly regarding the pool water as a pleasant backdrop to a lazy day, not as a medium to limber up one's body.

There are very few health food stores in France as virtually all of the French pharmacies stock and prescribe naturopathic medicines. There is also a greater acceptance of homoeopathy by French doctors and seven per cent of them use it regularly. Homoeopathy is officially recognized as part of the medical system by the French government and this is reflected in payment of health insurance rebates for the cost of homoeopathic consultations and medicines.

In England, although you can have homoeopathic treatment on the NHS, it's not yet a standard alternative. There are several homoeopathic hospitals and clinics within the NHS and there are GPs who practise homoeopathy in addition to orthodox medicine but if you have an orthodox GP and you want homoeopathic treatment, you may need to go privately to another GP who can offer it.

In Germany, the use of semi- and completely herbal mixtures for general medical conditions is quite popular, including within the medical profession.

However, what distinguishes the European health scene is not so much that the majority of doctors embrace alternative medicine in their own practices, but rather the acceptance of it by the public and within European culture. This in turn has provided the necessary liberal attitude in the law makers, which has encouraged the development of professional standards and some role for naturopathic medicine within government-funded health insurance. I feel that such acceptance within a disciplined framework does more to protect patients from the excesses of unqualified fanatics than an attitude of hostile denial.

After my sojourn in Europe I travelled to India where I worked in a large Christian missionary hospital in the Himalayan foothills. I travelled alone and was motivated by a longing for adventure and a desire to work with women in the underdeveloped world. My desires were fulfilled as the hospital was situated on a crossroads for several different ethnic states and was a place every anthropologist would dream of visiting.

The hospital was called the Leyman Hospital by the locals after its missionary founder, the English aristocrat and eye specialist, Dr Geoffrey Leyman. I arrived at the hospital with two large suitcases, one full of new toys for the children and the other packed with medical equipment and sundry clothes.

I began working in the female wards, looking after obstetric and gynaecological cases, many with tuberculosis infections.

I was shocked by the high mortality rate of Indian women which was partly a result of their low self-esteem and inferior position in a rural society. These women had been taught to put their men and families first and only came to hospital when things went seriously wrong, often after long delays. They were very stoical and could endure enormous suffering and debility while continuing to work hard, keep their families together and produce large numbers of children to satisfy the paternal desires and future security of their husbands.

Two thirds of rural Indian women are illiterate and this, combined with a virtual non-existence of social security provision in the country, means that they can never escape from their impoverished and downtrodden position. A lack of family planning and contraceptive facilities results in an annual population increase of 2.1 per cent (this equals an increase of fifteen million people per year) and this high birth-rate contributes to the high mortality rate of Indian women. In the area where I was, good obstetric care was not always available and unqualified midwives not only did most of the deliveries but also performed backyard abortions using dangerous and primitive methods. Once complications ensued these women would often come to the Leyman Hospital, but they were then usually already in a serious condition.

Such obstetric complications often required an urgent blood transfusion and in most instances it was necessary to extract blood from the relatives, as no on-site blood bank was available. Trying to persuade the male relatives of some of these critically ill women to give a few pints of blood was a very frustrating experience. They were often childish and cowardly, believing that if they gave blood their virility would diminish, and I chased several of them around the hospital grounds yelling in my broken Hindi, only to be greeted with the reply 'if she dies, it is God's will and I will find another wife to bear the children'. It was really brought home to me how cultural taboos can be entirely resistant to scientific logic or human compassion.

I found working at the Leyman Hospital fascinating. I saw physical signs of diseases that a Western doctor rarely ever sees outside the pages of a textbook and became proficient at diagnosing the tropical and infectious diseases of Northern India. I was a little nervous of contracting tuberculosis from the patients, as 35 per cent of them had an active infection and I had several chest X-rays and skin tests done while in India, all of which thankfully proved negative.

Ward rounds at night provided many amusing opportunities to test my skills of diagnosis and improvisation. As I walked through the wards around seven o'clock each night, I would find that the hospital beds contained not only the patient, but also numerous visiting relatives, as well as bowls of chapati, rice and vegetables, which had been prepared by the visitors. I suppose my greatest diagnostic dilemma was deciding who was the sick patient and who were the visiting relatives. Once this mystery was solved, I would ask all the unwilling relatives to leave so that I could examine the often squashed patient. They would stand on tiptoes, peering through the windows, anxious not to miss a trick while I examined their next of kin.

There were regular instances of power failure at the Leyman Hospital and we would often have to continue operating or do the ward rounds by candlelight. On these occasions we would sing Christmas carols to make the waiting time for generator repairs go faster.

Although the problems of the Indian women are predominantly due to physical disease, there is still a significant amount of psychiatric illness in India. This usually presents itself to the doctor as physical symptoms of stress and rarely as neurotic symptoms such as depression or anxiety. To treat their vague symptoms of psychiatric illness, Indian women often turn to their religion or the traditional herbal medicines which are part of the ancient system of medicine known as ayurvedic healing. Thus, the abuse of sedatives, alcohol and anti-depressant drugs is far less prevalent than in the Western world.

After five months in India, I returned to Australia in 1985 and founded the Sydney-based 'Women's Health Advisory Service' (WHAS) with the objective of giving information about holistic medical treatments to women with difficult health problems. I felt that if women had a balanced and up-to-date perspective on these problems, this would help them to ask useful questions, use self-help methods and participate with their doctor in decisions concerning their own bodies. The WHAS provides such information through the post and, since its inception in June, 1985, it has received many thousands of letters from women all over Australia, in New Guinea and the United States.

You may well ask how I managed to spread the news of the WHAS so far and wide. Believe me, it took many months of talking on local and national media and I am still doing it. Some radio stations such as the ABC transmit on high frequency waves which enabled me to talk to outback farmers and bring them up-to-date information normally restricted to city areas.

In 1986 I took the WHAS to Phoenix, Arizona, as this is the most rapidly growing city in America. I toured the USA telling women about holistic medicine and I had the opportunity to appear on national TV with several famous American film and music stars. On one show I even interviewed the petite Gladys Knight of the famous Pips group and listened to her problems with low blood sugar and weight gain. For a shy and private person like myself, I had to learn that nervous apprehension was a waste of time and that women all over the world want to hear the same basic truths.

On my return to Australia, I became interested in the nutritional treatment of the many chronic painful conditions which afflict women. Of course, many of these same conditions afflict men and the principles of treatment can be applied equally to both sexes. In particular, such conditions as recurrent headaches, arthritis, backache and other painful musculoskeletal symptoms can be gradually and surely reduced by dietary modification and special nutritional and naturopathic supplements. I have developed several programmes for these conditions and in many patients they have proved to be successful and often enabled dosages of anti-inflammatory painkilling drugs to be reduced. This will be discussed in another chapter, as will many other exciting and fascinating topics.

As you can see, I have travelled extensively and observed women and medicine in many different cultures. This, plus the thousands of letters I have received from women, has made me aware of the type of information that women are searching for: complete, balanced, up-to-date, practical, simple and combining the best of both worlds. I have endeavoured to provide that in the following chapters and I sincerely hope you enjoy my book.

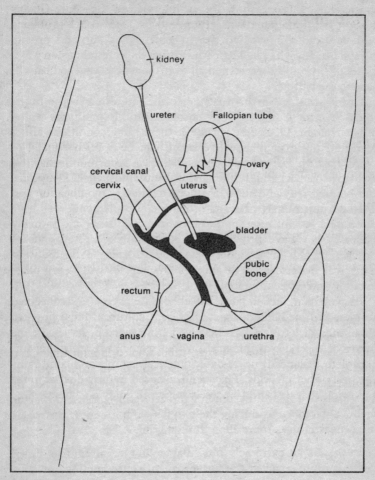

Figure 1

2 Understanding what makes you a woman

There are two aspects to the female physiology, namely physical structures and hormonal chemicals, and these serve to make you the feminine, sexual and physically beautiful creature that you are.

The physical structures

The pelvic bones provide a bowl-shaped bony cavity which houses and protects the ovaries, the uterus and its tubes (Fallopian tubes) and the cervix and vagina. The bladder sits in front of the uterus and vagina, and the lower bowel (rectum) sits behind these structures. See Figure 1.

The two ovaries are a greyish-yellow colour and resemble two large stewed prunes in their size, shape and wrinkly surface. They rest inside the curve of the Fallopian tubes and, although they have several supporting ligaments, they can still move around quite a lot in relation to the uterus. Each ovary contains hundreds of thousands of eggs at the time of puberty and is also a powerful chemical factory, producing the two female hormones, oestrogen and progesterone – more about this later on.

The uterus is an extremely muscular hollow organ and its inner cavity is quite small in the non-pregnant state, holding approximately one teaspoon of liquid. Its inner cavity communicates freely with the inner canal of the cervix and the two small openings of the Fallopian tubes which are attached to its sides.

The lining (endometrium) of the inner cavity is made up of special cells which are under the control of the two female hormones. During menstruation the endometrium is shed in the form of menstrual blood and it is important to understand that the ovaries and Fallopian tubes do not contribute to the menstrual blood. The average size of the uterus is that of a small pear; however, it can expand up to the size of a giant watermelon during pregnancy. The uterus rests in the anteverted position in most women, meaning that it is tilted forward in relation to the vagina and thus rests on the top of the bladder. However, in around twenty per cent of normal women the uterus rests in the retroverted position, meaning that it is tilted backward in relation to the vagina and rests against the bowel. See Figure 2.

By itself a retroverted uterus will not reduce your chances of falling pregnant and will not cause pain or malfunction. It is only when the uterus is tightly fixed backwards by scar tissue and disease that pain and malfunction can occur.

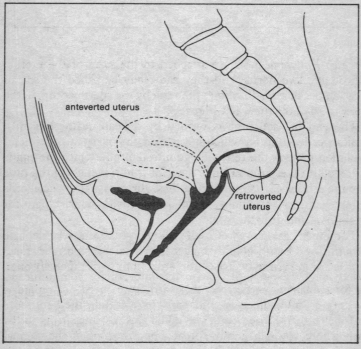

Figure 2

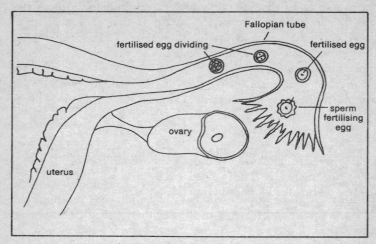

Figure 3

The two Fallopian tubes are attached to the sides of the uterus, almost like two horns, and they can really be called the site of creation because fertilization of the egg by the sperm occurs in the outer third of the tube. See Figure 3.

The end of each tube is formed by delicate featherlike projections called fimbria which hover over the ovary at the time of ovulation to suck the released egg into the tube. Once the egg is fertilized it takes around three days for it to travel along the tube into the uterine cavity and during these three days the special cells lining the inner passageway of the tube provide nourishment for its survival and growth.

The inner passageway of each Fallopian tube is a very delicate structure and is only slightly bigger than a hairbrush bristle. Each tube is around ten to twelve centimetres (four to five inches) long.

As for *the vagina* and *cervix*, these structures need not remain a mystery as any woman is quite capable of feeling their contours with her fingers. The easiest way to do this is while sitting in the bath where you can gently spread open the lips of the vaginal opening (labia) and slowly insert two fingers into the vagina. Your fingers will feel the soft warm muscular walls of the vagina and if you sweep your fingers around you will feel how pliant and stretchable they are. Insert your fingers as far as they will go and you will find that the upper roof of the vagina is closed by the cervix which feels like a large round button with a small hole in its centre. This hole is called the cervical os and it produces mucus to help the sperm swim through it on their way to the Fallopian tubes. In the non-pregnant state the os remains closed and is only one or two millimetres in size. However, during childbirth it dilates to accommodate the baby's head.

The consistency of the cervix is quite firm and similar to that of your nose. The cervix projects down about two centimetres (an inch or so) into the upper vagina and is continuous with the uterine muscle. In women who have had a total hysterectomy the cervix is absent and the roof of the vagina is closed by a surgical scar.

With your fingers deep in the vagina press upwards and forwards and this will probably give you the sensation of wanting to pass urine. This is because your fingers in this position are pushing on the bladder with its contained urine. See Figure 1 on page 13.

The most sexy parts of a woman are contained in *the vulva*. The vulva can be easily explored by yourself if you sit down on a bed, bend your knees and spread your legs apart, while holding a mirror in front of the area between your upper thighs. Make sure you have good illumination, and take your time!

The vulva is fully exposed to the outside world, unlike all the other genital organs we have just described and consists of the area contained between the ends of the upper thighs, extending upwards to the pubic bone and downwards to the anus. See Figure 4.

The various parts found on the vulva are known as the external genitalia and are endowed with a rich nerve and blood supply, making them extremely sensitive and erotic.

Just as your face has lips, so has your vulva, and indeed it has two sets which surround the vaginal opening. The larger external lips are called the 'labia majora' and the smaller inside lips are called the 'labia minora'. The outside lips are covered with pubic

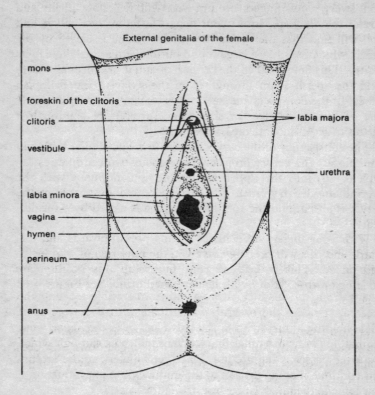

Figure 4

hair and form two protective fatty cushions which protect the inner sanctum of the vaginal opening. Conversely, the inner lips are thin, hairless and much more sexy as they contain glands which secrete oil with an amorous odour. Although the inner lips are thin, they can vary in size between women, and may be long enough to protrude beyond the outer lips. Their colour varies from pale pink to dark brown, and the texture from silky smooth to very wrinkled

If you follow the inner lips up towards the pubic bone, you will see that they join together just above the clitoris, and they partly surround the clitoris to form its hood or foreskin. To find the most exquisite part of your sexual anatomy, trace the inner lips to the place where they meet together just below the pubic bone. Here you should see the clitoris protruding like a small pink knob from beneath its little hood. Touch the clitoris gently and you will find it to be exquisitely sensitive and perhaps erotic. Remember where it is situated, because during love-making it may require stimulation before you can achieve an orgasm. Some women think that their most erotic parts are found deep inside the vagina, around the cervix, and some call this area the elusive 'G Spot'. However, for most women their most erotic zone is not so elusive and is simply the clitoral area. Inside the inner lips is a deeper area known as the vestibule. Within the vestibule you will see two openings – the larger one is the vaginal opening and the smaller one the opening of the urinary tract (urethra). See Figure 4.

To find your urethra, place your index finger on the clitoris and move it downwards, trying to stay in the centre of the vestibule. The first dimple that you feel is the urethra, which allows urine to escape from the bladder. If you still have trouble locating the urethra, stand in the bathtub and urinate with your legs apart while holding a mirror up to the vulva and spreading apart your vaginal lips with the other hand. The small hole through which the urine passes is the urethra. Place your fingers on the urethra and continue moving it back in the midline of the vestibule until you come to the much larger opening of the vagina.

All women have some soft membranous tissue around their vaginal opening and this is called the hymen. In some virgins the hymen is almost completely intact, meaning that it covers nearly the entire opening to the vagina, whereas in other virgins only small pieces of the hymen will be found. A virgin does not necessarily have an intact hymen. Some women who have had children may find that their hymen has become ragged or torn looking, especially across the lower portion of the vaginal opening. Such ragged areas are of no medical significance and should not be confused with warts or growths.

Some young girls believe that the first episode of sexual inter-course will be quite painful because of the myth that the penis must forcibly tear the hymen. Normally in sexually mature girls, the hymen only partially covers the vaginal opening and is very stretchable, so that the first episode of intercourse is not painful.

Very rarely the hymen may fully cover and block the vaginal opening and this unlikely condition is called an 'imperforate hymen'. This will prevent normal sexual intercourse and will also prevent menstrual blood from escaping from the vagina, so that the first menstrual period is delayed. In this situation the hymen can be easily divided by a scalpel under a general anaesthetic and thereafter all will proceed normally.

The area of skin between the vagina and the anus is called the perineum. It is this which sometimes tears or is cut (called an episiotomy) during childbirth.

Physiology of the female hormones

Let us leave behind the discovery of your physical structures and delve into the mystery of the hormonal chemicals that wield so much power over your mind and body.

The hormonal glands that are concerned with the production of the two female hormones, oestrogen and progesterone, are the pituitary gland and the ovaries.

The 'master controller' of all these glands is the primitive part of the brain called the hypothalamus which regulates not only sexual function, but also hunger, thirst and body temperature. See Figure 5.

The hypothalamus has intimate nervous connections to the emotional and higher centres of the brain and thus its function can be affected by our thoughts, feelings and environmental stress, which all feed down to it from the higher brain.

The pituitary gland resembles a mushroom on a stalk growing down from the base of the hypothalamus. Through this stalk the hypothalamus sends chemical and nervous messages to control the pituitary gland. See Figure 5.

It is easy, then, to see how emotional problems and stress can upset the hypothalamus and therefore the pituitary gland, causing problems with menstruation and hormonal imbalances.

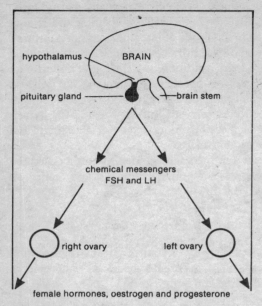

Figure 5

How does this pituitary gland communicate with the ovaries?

Nature has provided a very sensitive system of chemical messengers which are manufactured in the pituitary gland under the control of the hypothalamus and then secreted into the bloodstream which carries them to the ovaries. These chemical messengers are called follicle stimulating hormone (FSH) and luteinizing hormone (LH). See Figure 5.

What do the chemical messengers, FSH and LH, do when they reach the ovaries?

FSH stimulates the growth and development of egg follicles in the ovaries which mature and secrete the female hormone oestrogen. See Figure 6.

Oestrogen stimulates the endometrium (lining) of the uterus to grow or proliferate. For this reason, the phase of the menstrual cycle occurring prior to ovulation is known as the 'proliferative phase'. See Figure 7.

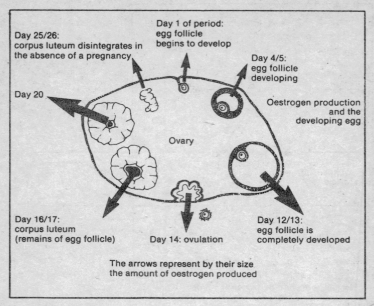

Day 25/26:
corpus luteum disintegrates in
the absence of a pregnancy

Day 1 of period:
egg follicle
begins to develop

Day 4/5:
egg follicle
developing

Oestrogen production
and the
developing egg

Day 20

Ovary

Day 16/17:
corpus luteum
(remains of egg follicle)

Day 14: ovulation

Day 12/13:
egg follicle is
completely developed

The arrows represent by their size
the amount of oestrogen produced

Figure 6

Oestrogen also causes the cervix to secrete increasing quantities of thin clear mucus which is detected by you at the vaginal opening.

Out of all the follicles stimulated in any one cycle by FSH, usually only one becomes dominant and produces a mature egg. See Figure 6. Ovulation will occur from this mature egg, normally twelve to sixteen days before the onset of the next menstrual bleeding. See Figure 7. If you study Figure 7 carefully you will see that the oestrogen level is very high just before ovulation.

What causes ovulation?

There is a two-way communication between the ovaries and the pituitary gland. As the ovaries produce more and more oestrogen, this travels back to the pituitary gland, via the circulation, and stimulates the pituitary gland to secrete another chemical messenger called luteinizing hormone (LH). The LH travels back to the

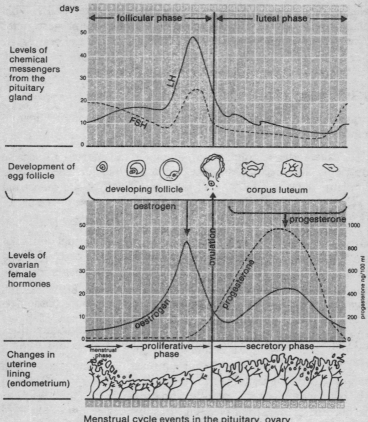

Menstrual cycle events in the pituitary, ovary
and uterus in the ideal situation

Figure 7

ovaries via the blood and causes the egg to be released from the
follicle – this is the process of ovulation. See Figures 6 and 7.

In Figure 7 you will notice a very high peak in LH just before
ovulation.

What happens in the ovary after ovulation?

The dominant follicle which has just lost its egg is not wasted and its remaining cells develop into a remarkable circular yellowish gland called the 'corpus luteum' (CL). See Figures 6 and 7. This gland now begins to secrete another hormone called progesterone, as well as continuing to secrete a significant amount of oestrogen. See Figure 7.

Progesterone has several effects:

1 It increases body temperature.

2 It changes the cervical mucus into a thicker more opaque mucus and decreases its amount.

3 It causes the endometrium (lining of the uterus) to secrete nutrients and become suitable for a possible fertilized egg to implant. That is why we call the second half of the menstrual cycle, occurring after ovulation, the secretory phase of the cycle. See Figure 7.

After ovulation, if the egg is not fertilized, the normal course of events is that the corpus luteum stops secreting oestrogen and progesterone, usually twelve to sixteen days after ovulation. See Figure 7. Without oestrogen and progesterone, the growth of the uterine lining cannot be maintained, and this lining (endometrium) begins to break up and is shed in the form of blood (menstruation). Without progesterone the body temperature returns to the level it was before ovulation.

This cycle is self-perpetuating up until the menopause, when no more egg follicles remain. It is self-perpetuating because when the ovarian hormones, oestrogen and progesterone fall to very low levels during menstrual bleeding, this feeds back to the pituitary gland causing the release of FSH, which sets the cycle in motion again.

When does a woman become hormonally active?

Any time after nine years of age the hypothalamus gland begins to stir and awaken, secreting chemical messengers to awaken the pituitary gland, which in turn awakens the childlike ovaries, via its own chemical messengers. Eventually the ovaries will produce enough oestrogen to stimulate the growth of the uterine lining and a menstrual bleed will follow.

The first menstrual bleed of puberty is called the 'menarche' and normally occurs between nine and sixteen years of age. If a menstrual bleed has not occurred by the age of seventeen years a medical opinion should be obtained. It is interesting to note that the average age of the menarche has become younger and is now thirteen years as compared with fifteen years one hundred years ago. The reasons for this are better nutrition and an environment which is more sexually stimulating. In the first four years after the menarche the production of the female hormones from the immature and sluggish ovaries tends to be erratic because the ovaries find it difficult to respond in synchrony with the pituitary messengers. In a mature ovary a normal response results in a mature egg being released approximately every twenty-eight days, giving a regular menstrual cycle. In the case of the adolescent, ovulation usually occurs every second or third month and this can result in menstrual irregularity and heavy painful bleeding. It is not unusual for there to be a gap of one or two years between the menarche and the next menstrual bleed.

With this delay of the period, symptoms of PMS (for example, tension, irritability, depression, sore breasts, acne and headaches) are more likely to be exaggerated and can have devastating effects on school performance and family, social and romantic relationships. Where these symptoms are severe they may need medical treatment or psychological counselling because if they are neglected they may result in serious emotional instability and personality disorders.

Treatments need to be tailor-made for the adolescent female as her metabolism is still evolving and maturing and the growth spurt is in full swing. Heavy-handed drug therapy can interfere with the natural development of the menstrual cycles and the attainment of optimal physical and mental potential.

However, the typical menstrual irregularity of adolescence is nothing to worry about and treatment is not needed, apart from reassurance that within four to six years of the menarche, menstruation usually becomes regular by itself.

During adolescence, if the period is very heavy and painful time and time again, this can sometimes be prevented with the hormone progesterone and the most natural one available that can be taken in tablet form is 'dydrogesterone' which is given twice daily from day five to twenty-five of each menstrual cycle. Dydrogesterone is safe and gentle and usually free from any side effects; however, it will not suppress ovulation and thus does not act as a contraceptive.

Many adolescents become obsessed with themselves, particularly if their newfound hormonal fluctuations produce acne or weight problems. These problems may be pushed aside and ignored by the doctor and the family who may be unaware of the extreme degree of psychological suffering locked within the adolescent's mind.

Often there is a very poor self-image and lack of self-esteem and monthly hormonal changes may bring these to the surface. There is a great need for friends and parents to act as 'ego boosters' during these times, giving praise, compliments, encouragement and reasssurance that these turbulent times lead on to calmer waters.

Menstrual irregularity

The length of the menstrual cycle is calculated as the number of days between the first day of bleeding to the first day of bleeding of the next menstrual period. Not every woman has a cycle of exactly twenty-eight days and the normal menstrual cycle length can vary from twenty-one to thirty-five days.

Abnormal lack of menstruation (amenorrhoea)

The absence of menstrual bleeding is called amenorrhoea, and it is diagnosed when a woman who previously had regular cycles fails to menstruate for over three months. It is a quite common event and 20 to 30 per cent of women experience episodes of amenorrhoea at some time during their reproductive life.

What are the causes of amenorrhoea?

In the vast majority of cases, a hormonal imbalance resulting in failure to ovulate is the culprit, but disorders of the uterus and blockage of the cervix or vagina must also be checked for.

Hormonal imbalances can result from upsets in the sensitive hypothalamus–pituitary–ovarian communication link. Such things as weight loss, excessive exercise, obesity or emotional stress may upset the hypothalamus and pituitary, resulting in failure to stimulate the ovaries with resultant failure of normal female hormonal production and menstruation.

The pituitary gland may have a tumour growing in it, causing excessive amounts of the hormone prolactin to be produced which turns off the ovaries. Women with a pituitary tumour may also have secretion of milk from the breasts although they are not breastfeeding.

A small percentage of women fail to menstruate spontaneously after they stop taking the oral contraceptive pill and will need treatment with drugs to stimulate ovulation.

The ovaries may be affected by various diseases which reduce their capacity to manufacture the two female hormones and this can eventually result in a failure of menstruation. One of the most common diseases affecting the ovaries is multiple cysts which gradually destroy the normal ovarian tissue. The ovaries may also be destroyed by endometriosis, infection or cancer. See Chapter Seven for more information on these diseases.

Some women stop menstruating in their thirties and early forties because of a premature failure of the ovaries – this is called a premature menopause and the only treatment available is hormone replacement therapy. We do not know the cause of premature menopause or why the ovaries stop functioning so early but perhaps in the future ovarian transplants will provide a cure.

Abnormally small amount of menstrual blood loss

When menstrual bleeding is extremely light and perhaps no more than slight spotting for a day or so the diagnosis of 'hypomenorrhoea' is made.

Common causes of hypomenorrhoea are advancing age, weight loss, heavy athletic training or imbalances in other hormonal glands, such as the thyroid situated in the neck or the adrenal glands which sit on top of the kidneys.

Menstrual bleeding that is totally irregular and excessive in amount

This type of bleeding is called 'menorrhagia' and is commonly due to the hormonal imbalances and lack of regular ovulation that occur during the adolescent and premenopausal years – in other words at the beginning and end of the reproductive life span.

Whenever there is heavy and delayed bleeding, a miscarriage or ectopic pregnancy must be checked for by doing a pregnancy test.

Menorrhagia can have a serious underlying cause such as cancer of the uterus or cervix, pelvic infection or endometriosis, and thus a thorough pelvic examination and curette is always necessary. See Chapters Seven and Nine for further information on these diseases.

The internal examination – a mere necessity

All sexually active women should have a routine internal examination by a doctor every twelve months, whether they have problems or not. Some women dread this examination and find it a demeaning and painful experience. However, if the doctor is gentle and reasonably quick and experienced it should not be a traumatic event. If you are a virgin and in need of an internal examination, it can be helpful to insert two fingers into your vagina while in the bath for five to ten minutes each night for three weeks gently to stretch the vaginal opening backwards – this will prepare you for the vaginal examination.

What will happen during an internal examination?

Firstly, the doctor will take a look inside the vagina by inserting a metal or plastic speculum into the vagina and gently opening up its blades. See Figure 8.

This is necessary as the walls inside the vagina are collapsed like an empty balloon and the speculum blades hold them apart. Using a bright light the doctor will check the appearance of the vaginal walls and cervix. The next step is to rotate a wooden or metal spatula (flat spoon) around the hole in the cervix to check for cancer cells growing on the cervix. See Figure 9. This simple and painless screening test for cancer is called a Pap smear of the cervix and only takes a few seconds.

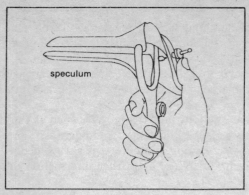

speculum

Figure 8

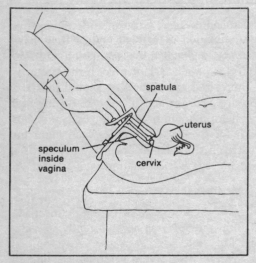

spatula

uterus

speculum
inside
vagina

cervix

Figure 9

Finally, the speculum will be removed and the doctor will insert two fingers inside your vagina and the other hand over the lower abdomen in order to feel the size and consistency of your ovaries, tubes and uterus. The doctor will check for abnormal tenderness, lumps or thickening in these organs which are often a sign of disease. See Figure 10.

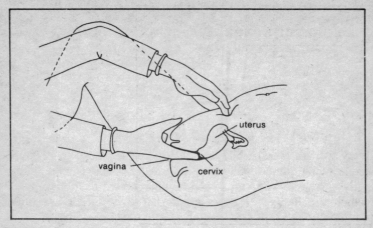

Figure 10

Voilà, the internal examination completed and your mind at rest for another year, in the knowledge that prevention is better than cure.

3 Exploring sexuality

Every woman is a deeply sensual being with a need to be loved intellectually, emotionally and physically. This is not always easily achieved and, after communicating with thousands of women of all ages, I have learnt that these needs are often unfulfilled, with resultant mental and physical imbalances.

There are many obstacles to a happy love life and in trying to overcome these a woman needs to have a good sense of humour, patience, confidence, assertiveness and a willingness to explore and experiment.

There will be times when your love life is fantastic and other times when sex seems highly overrated and so it is most important to have plenty of other exciting challenges in your life. When your sexuality seems to fly out of the window, you can try to redirect your sexual energies into the development of intellectual, professional or spiritual pursuits; in this way frustration can be avoided.

Members of the Women's Health Advisory Service (WHAS) receive a questionnaire in which there is a section on sexual frustration and poor libido. About 50 per cent of women answer yes to these problems and many of them have resigned themselves to a life of zero sexual inspiration or satisfaction.

I will not deny that to some women, particularly in the older age bracket, a healthy sex life is not important. However, for many of those who have given up hope, a deep disappointment and frustration is buried in the subconscious mind. A woman who is being loved deeply and sensitively usually appears happy, radiant and relaxed.

Before we delve into the many factors which can hamper sexual satisfaction, it is important to understand the normal physiology of a woman's sexual response.

A woman's sexual responsiveness changes from day to day and depends on her mood, time of the menstrual cycle, hormone levels, general health and the art and technique of her lover. If we examine the experience of a *complete sexual response*, it will be seen to have four different stages:

1 Excitement stage.

2 Plateau stage.

3 Orgasmic stage.

4 Resolution stage.

If a sexual response is incomplete, it will finish at the excitement or plateau stage.

1 The excitement stage

As a woman first becomes sexually stimulated, whether it be from a sexy movie, kissing or manual stimulation, the blood circulation to the vagina increases and this results in the secretion of a fluid-type mucus from the vaginal walls. After approximately thirty seconds of sensual stimulation, the vagina and vulva will be bathed in this lubricating fluid. For vaginal lubrication the only prerequisite is an increase in vaginal blood circulation and it does not require the presence of a uterus or cervix. Older menopausal women can also still experience adequate vaginal lubrication; it just takes longer to achieve.

As sexual excitement increases, pelvic blood supply continues to increase so that the lips of the vaginal opening (labia majora and labia minora) become congested with venous blood, the clitoris enlarges and the vaginal lips move outwards and upwards to expose the vaginal opening.

2 The plateau stage

During this stage the inner deeper part of the vagina begins to enlarge upwards and also in a sideways direction so that the cervix and uterus become elevated higher into the pelvis and congested with blood. The lower vagina becomes tighter, thus enabling a firmer grip of the penis and the clitoris begins to shrink. The labia minora change in colour from a light pink, to a bright red, to a deep burgundy colour.

There is a general stimulation of the body with an increase in pulse rate, blood pressure and respiratory rate, dilation of the pupils and a flushing of the skin. The breasts enlarge and the nipples become erect.

3 The orgasmic stage

This is the climax of the plateau and is an intensely pleasurable experience with involuntary muscular contractions of the vagina, uterus and surrounding muscles. The average orgasm lasts ten to fifteen seconds, but a very strong orgasm may produce up to fifteen separate pelvic muscular contractions. There may be a desire to pass urine associated with these contractions.

The orgasm is associated with deep sighing respirations or grunting, a release of tension and fulfilment of desire.

4 The resolution stage

When the muscular contractions of the orgasm stop, the resolution stage begins and continues until the congestion of the pelvic organs with blood has been reversed, so that the pelvic organs return to their pre-excitement state. This decongestion may take up to half an hour, but if orgasm has not occurred, complete resolution may not occur.

Orgasm – a closer look

This is only one aspect of the total experience of love-making and it assumes a different significance in individual women. I feel it is important that a woman experiences an orgasm at least occasionally; however, it is not necessary that *every* episode of sexual intercourse end in orgasm for a happy satisfying sex life. Surveys of married women have shown that 22 to 75 per cent usually experience orgasm during intercourse, 30 to 45 per cent experience it occasionally and 5 to 22 per cent have never experienced it during standard sexual intercourse.

Some women need to reach a certain level of sexual maturity and relaxation before their first true orgasm can occur and others never find a sufficiently caring lover capable of inducing orgasm in them. I have spoken with women in their fourth and fifth decade of life who have never known what it is like to have an orgasm.

It is necessary to understand that it is often not as easy for a woman to have an orgasm during standard sexual intercourse as it is for a man. Some men think that the simple unembellished act of thrusting an erect penis in and out of the vagina is sufficient to bring all women to orgasm. However, it has been shown that the length of time devoted to romantic foreplay, especially stimulation of the clitoris, is the most important factor in inducing an orgasm. The size of the penis and the positions adopted by the couple do not play as big a part in achieving orgasm as does appropriate stimulation of the clitoris.

Do all women have a normal clitoris?

All women are born with a clitoris and this undergoes a small degree of growth during sexual maturation. The clitoris has no other physiological role, apart from its function as a source of sexual stimulation and pleasure.

In the occasional woman, in whom a small or underdeveloped clitoris seems to contribute to lack of orgasm, the local application of a male hormone cream to the clitoris may increase its responsiveness. For example, testosterone cream, if applied for some weeks, can increase the size and vascularity of the clitoris which may heighten its sensitivity to stimulation. Testosterone cream is not available on the market in the UK but pharmacists do make one up themselves. This would only be done with a prescription and, as it's quite a powerful sex hormone, you'd only get this if your doctor considered you needed it. The same result can be achieved by taking male hormone pills, but at the price of inducing masculine side effects such as increased facial hair, acne, weight gain and voice deepening.

For some women the achievement of orgasm is psychologically difficult even though deep down inside they desire to have one. Often they are too scared or inhibited to help themselves, although these days many liberated women's magazines describe techniques of sexual assertiveness. Some of the ideas given are very practical and help to peel away the many myths and taboos which surround the subject of achieving sexual satisfaction.

In particular, women can now find out what brings them to orgasm and ask their partner to aid them in the process. Twenty years ago, many women would have been embarrassed to ask a man to modify or embellish his sexual technique so that orgasm and satisfaction could be mutual. The man was seen to be the director and producer of the show and the woman would often feign orgasm so that his masculine ego would not be ruffled.

Thankfully, these days it has become acceptable for the woman to be co-director and co-producer of the show. This should be encouraged, as how can a man read the mind of his female partner when every woman is an individual needing different ingredients in her love-making. He can only guess and blunder on hoping for the best or, worse still, not really caring whether his partner is satisfied. These is nothing wrong in expressing your sexual fantasies and exploring new dimensions in your sexuality with the man you love.

For those women who do not have a partner, self-masturbation or the use of a vibrator can bring sexual release and for some women this is a physical and emotional necessity. Whatever you do, do not feel guilty or that you are abnormal, as the expression of adult sexual fantasy is quite healthy; there is nothing good or bad about it, only conditioning makes it so.

If you are ignorant of the position of your clitoris in relation to your vaginal opening, you can visit a family planning clinic doctor who will demonstrate your anatomy and erogenous zones to you with a mirror. Alternatively you can find it for yourself by using a mirror and following the instructions in the previous chapter in the section on the *vulva*. See page 17.

The section which follows here on masturbation could also be a great help to you in finding out exactly what turns you on. Equipped with this knowledge you can then show your partner what to do.

Can orgasm ever be dangerous?

In a pregnant woman who is close to the due date of delivery, an orgasm can stimulate uterine contractions and if her cervix is ripe (thin and slightly dilated) this may be enough to induce labour. If the woman is six weeks or more before term, this can result in a premature labour and birth of a premature infant, particularly if the waters are ruptured by the uterine contractions.

Therefore all women who have a ripe cervix, six weeks or more before term, should be warned against any type of sexual stimulation that could induce orgasm.

Masturbation

Masturbation is the technique of stimulating the genital organs, with the fingers, a vibrator or whatever object pleases the fancy, with the aim of producing sexual arousal and hopefully a satisfying orgasm.

Masturbation used to be considered a shameful pastime and if adolescent boys and girls were caught in the act by their parents they were chastised and made to feel guilty. Times have changed and nowadays it is accepted that women, as well as men, enjoy giving pleasure to themselves.

Indeed, if a woman really wants to take responsibility for her own sexual satisfaction and be able to achieve an orgasm regularly, she may need to learn to masturbate effectively. Many women would never have experienced an orgasm if they had not discovered how to stimulate their clitoris effectively through masturbation, and a significant percentage of women have their first orgasm between the ages of thirty and forty by masturbation alone, although they have been married for some years and have several children.

Masturbation can also be useful for the single woman who needs regular sexual release and yet wants to avoid casual heterosexual intercourse with its attendant risk of sexually transmitted diseases.

Some women want to wait until 'Mr Right' comes along and in the meantime masturbation can be a useful means of avoiding sexual frustration.

The art of masturbation is sometimes discovered by surprise, when a woman accidentally or casually plays with her clitoris, and this may occur normally any time from childhood right up until the fifth decade! Other women are introduced to masturbation by their partners, who encourage it during mutual sexual play so as to ensure an orgasm for the woman.

Conversely, 70 per cent of women do not tell their partners that they achieve sexual pleasure through self-masturbation, for fear of provoking jealousy or making their partner feel sexually inadequate. Some men take the fact that their partner masturbates as an outright rejection of their own sexual abilities. Unfortunately, many men do not realize that sexually, women are very different from men. Some women who masturbate like to keep it as a secret, private thing which has nothing to do with their partner.

There is no one way that a woman should treat masturbation, as every woman is an individual. Some women have easy orgasms and will never feel a need to masturbate, others may prefer to do it and keep it a secret, while others may unabashedly show their partners how to help. Some women like to embellish self-manipulation of the clitoris with sexual fantasies or dressing up. So it's really up to you, take control, make a personal decision and feel good about enjoying your female body which is the gift of Mother Nature.

Homosexuality in women

This is probably an appropriate time to mention the subject of homosexuality in women or 'lesbianism', as mutual masturbation often plays a large part in the physical aspect of such a relationship. There is no doubt that some women are sexually attracted to other women from an early age, while other women turn to women for sexual and emotional fulfilment after men have disappointed them. Experimenting with or becoming a homosexual woman is a personal decision. It often stems from a strong and genuine desire and is not something to feel guilty about. Homosexual women are no different from heterosexual women in their genetic make-up or biological functions. Homosexual women do not have an increased risk of AIDS, as do homosexual men, because they do not practise anal intercourse. However, they can transmit herpes, venereal warts, gonorrhoea and syphilis to each other, so care should still be taken.

Physical factors that affect the female sex life

Hysterectomy

The surgical removal of the uterus will not in itself reduce the capacity of a woman to achieve the four stages of the sexual response. Vaginal length, lubrication and ability to expand is not affected by carefully performed abdominal or vaginal hysterectomy. Some women may notice a slight increase in vaginal length after an abdominal hysterectomy.

A significant percentage of women become depressed and anxious after a hysterectomy, mainly because of imagined fears, and these emotional problems can reduce libido and the capacity to achieve orgasm. Such emotional problems are usually only temporary, especially if your doctor takes the time to explain that a hysterectomy will not make you any less of a woman and lover.

Surgical removal of the ovaries

If the ovaries are removed prior to the natural menopause a woman will experience a premature menopause and oestrogen deficiency. This will cause a loss of muscular tone in the vagina and increased fragility of the vaginal walls. Vaginal lubrication will take longer and orgasm may be less intense in its physical aspects. All these problems can be overcome by early hormone replacement therapy.

A vaginal opening that is too small or tight

This is quite rare as, with repeated stimulation, the vagina will lubricate and expand to accept deep penetration by a penis of any size.

The membrane which covers the vaginal opening is called the hymen. In some virgins this membrane is still intact and it may tear and bleed a little during the first occurrence of sexual intercourse. This is a once-only experience but it can be avoided. Virgins who think they have a narrow vaginal opening should visit their gynaecologist and if necessary the hymen can be opened. They can also practise gentle self-dilatation of their vaginal opening as described in the following paragraphs.

In some anxious women, deep psychosexual conflicts can produce excessive contraction and spasm in the muscles which encircle the vaginal opening. This painful muscular spasm is called 'vaginismus' and it can be so strong that the penis is unable to enter the vagina. This gives a false impression of a 'small' vaginal opening although, in reality, women with vaginismus have a normal anatomy and suffer only from a psychological fear of sex.

In all cases of a tight vaginal opening, including vaginismus, the woman can improve it by using a set of graduated vaginal dilators. She begins with a very small dilator (pencil size) and gradually increases up to an erect penis size dilator. If she has a caring sexual partner he can help her with these exercises, but sexual intercourse should be avoided until the largest size vaginal dilator can be easily and confidently inserted.

Some women may be wondering if their vaginal opening is too small for comfortable sexual intercourse the first time. A good way of finding out is to see if you can place the ends of your middle and index fingers into the vagina and then separate them half a centimetre (a quarter of an inch) or more, without pain – if you can, your vaginal opening should be sufficient for intercourse. If, however, this test causes pain, a course of vaginal dilators to be used at home is worthwhile. If you don't like the idea of plastic dilators, you can use your fingers gently to dilate your vagina. To do this, sit in a warm bath and with one or two fingers in the vagina, press backwards towards the back passage (rectum) until you can feel the vaginal opening stretching. Only five to ten minutes a day of these exercises for about four weeks will bring normal stretch and elasticity to your vaginal opening.

A vagina that is too large and relaxed

Some women find that after having several children their vagina becomes excessively stretched and loses tone. These women may notice that the penis seems lost inside their large vagina and that the vaginal muscles are unable to grip the shaft of the penis firmly. A too relaxed vaginal opening may also reduce the ability of the penis to stimulate the clitoris during intercourse. These things all serve to reduce sexual enjoyment and satisfaction.

Some couples find that changing position during intercourse helps to overcome this problem. For example, the woman can close her legs after the penis has been introduced or she can sit astride the man to increase direct clitoral contact during penile penetration.

A more satisfactory method of improving and bringing back

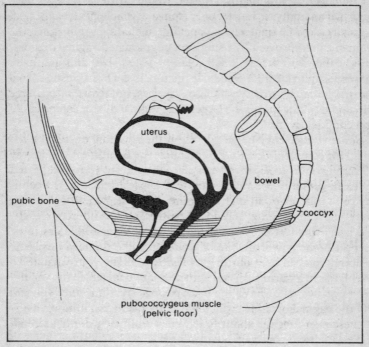

Figure 11

muscle tone to your vagina is to exercise the muscle known as the 'pelvic floor' or 'pubococcygeus muscle'. This muscle is like a sling and stretches from the pubic bone back to the tail bone (coccyx). See Figure 11.

The pelvic floor or pubococcygeus muscle forms the floor of the pelvis and encircles and supports the base of the bladder, the middle third of the vagina and the rectum. Thus it not only increases vaginal tone but also aids control of the bladder and bowels. If this muscle is exercised regularly great benefit can result in minimizing sagging pelvic organs and strengthening vaginal muscular tone.

How do you exercise your pelvic floor?

Firstly, you must be able to *feel* which muscle it is, as you cannot see it or touch it. The best way to sense its contractions are by:

1 Placing one or two fingers in the vagina and tightening the vaginal walls around them.

2 While passing urine, intermittently stop the flow by voluntarily contracting this muscle.

You will find that these movements give you the sensation of lifting the vagina and bowel upwards and that there is no need to contract any other muscle in the process. In particular, there is no need to contract the muscles of the abdomen or buttocks. Avoid pushing down as if straining to have a bowel action, because this will worsen a tendency to sagging of the pelvic organs. Also, avoid constipation by eating a high fibre diet and unprocessed bran regularly.

If you really want to see good results with this exercise, you will need to contract your pelvic floor at least 200 times a day, trying to make each contraction last for three seconds. Get into a rhythm, contract for three seconds and relax for three seconds and keep going for as long as you can. You can do it while you are doing the housework or sitting at work. No one will notice a thing. You can even practise it while making love and surprise your partner with your newfound vaginal fitness. Over a period of several months, with regular daily contractions, you will find that your loose and flabby vagina becomes tighter, longer and more capable of partici-pating actively in sex.

Exercising the pelvic floor also improves the circulation of blood to the pelvic organs and you may notice that premenstrual syn-drome, hormonal imbalances, painful periods, haemorrhoids and dull pelvic pains are greatly improved. Having a fit set of pelvic floor muscles also aids bladder control and reduces your chances of prolapse of the pelvic organs during the menopausal years.

If stretching of the vagina has progressed to an advanced stage, especially if sagging (prolapse) of its walls has occurred, vaginal plastic surgery, known as a 'vaginal repair', may be necessary. When the front wall of the vagina becomes stretched the bladder will often sag downwards into the loose vagina, resulting in bladder

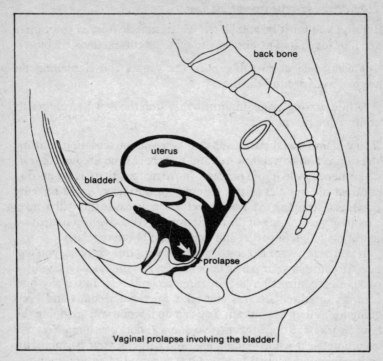

Vaginal prolapse involving the bladder

Figure 12

infections or urinary frequency and irritation. See Figure 12.

When the back wall of the vagina is excessively loose and stretched, the lower bowel (rectum) often sags forward into the lower part of the vagina. This may result in recurrent vaginal infections and a feeling of incomplete emptying of the bowel. See Figure 13.

In these severe cases of vaginal wall sagging, the surgeon's knife can yield spectacular results. The sagging bladder and bowel will be stitched back into place and the vaginal walls reduced to form a smaller and firmer vaginal opening.

Pain during sexual intercourse

If pain is experienced at the vaginal opening during penetration by the penis, this may be due to a small vaginal opening, a vaginal

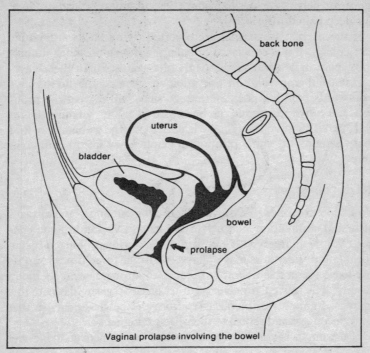

Vaginal prolapse involving the bowel

Figure 13

infection or scar tissue from a recent episiotomy cut. If the woman has not been sufficiently excited sexually, vaginal lubrication may be insufficient for a smooth penile entry and excessive friction on the vaginal walls may produce a burning sensation.

Occasionally a burning sensation follows ejaculation of sperm into the vagina and this may be caused by an infection in the prostate gland of your partner or on rare occasions by an allergic reaction to your partner's sperm.

If a *deep pelvic pain* is produced by full penile penetration and thrusting, the woman may have a pelvic infection, ovarian cyst or endometriosis. See Chapters Seven and Nine for more information on these conditions. Previous pelvic irradiation for cancer or pelvic scar tissue from pelvic surgery may also produce this deep pain during sex.

If the uterus is extremely retroverted (lying backwards) and, particularly, if it is congested or enlarged from a hormonal imbalance, pain may occur as the penis hits against it. In these cases hormonal therapy and an operation to suspend the uterus in a frontwards pointing position (anteversion) will correct the problem. Excessive scar tissue can be helped by taking vitamins E and C. If pelvic pain on intercourse is persistent, the woman may find that changing the coital position to penile entry from behind will help.

Pelvic congestion

You will remember that during the excitement and plateau stages of sexual stimulation, the pelvic organs and vagina become congested and engorged with blood. Indeed, during prolonged sexual stimulation the uterus may enlarge by two or three times from its pre-excitement stage, simply because of an increase in its blood supply. The muscular pelvic contractions of orgasm dissipate this increased amount of blood away from the pelvic organs so that they decongest and return to their pre-excitement size.

If a woman is continually stimulated to the plateau stage, yet never has an orgasm, the pelvic organs will remain congested with blood. Decongestion and a return to normal size of the pelvic organs may take many hours without the muscular contractions of orgasm, and a condition known as 'chronic pelvic congestion' can occur. This means that a large amount of stagnant blood remains pooled in the pelvic blood vessels and organs. Chronic pelvic congestion can result in unpleasant physical symptoms such as:

1 Vague abdominal pains.

2 Low backache.

3 Dull heavy dragging feelings in the lower abdomen and upper thighs.

4 Vaginal discharge.

5 Anxiety, irritability and insomnia.

What can be done to relieve chronic pelvic congestion?

1 Yoga and swimming will be of great benefit.

2 Vitamin E with pectin, 250 milligrams daily, and vitamin C, 2000 milligrams daily.

3 A herbal tablet containing beta-hydroxy-rutosides 100mg, nicotinic acid 10mg, bioflavonoids 100mg, calcium ascorbate 150mg and the herbs ruscus aculeatus 50mg, aesculus 20mg, hamamelis 20mg, ranunculaceae 10mg. Dosage: two tablets three times daily. Ask a reputable naturopathic practitioner to make this up for you.

4 Pelvic floor exercises (see page 41).

5 The attainment of orgasm by self-masturbation may be necessary if you do not have an understanding partner. However, if possible, it would be better to communicate your needs to your partner and try new sexual techniques. For some women, oral genital sex is the most effective method of achieving orgasm. Surveys have shown that 60 per cent of all college-educated heterosexual couples practise oral genital sex. Oral sex is not dangerous and the only prerequisite is to wash the genitals thoroughly before commencing.

Anal sex

This is the type of intercourse practised by male homosexuals, although it is sometimes also practised by heterosexuals. The use of anal sex as a regular method of sexual intercourse can lead to problems because the rectum was never designed to be a receptacle for the erect penis. Lubrication is a problem and for many women the anus is too tight which causes great discomfort on penile insertion. The mucosa of the anus is fairly fragile and local anal problems such as infection, haemorrhoids or fissures can result from anal sex.

The practice of anal intercourse followed by vaginal intercourse is quite dangerous as the penis can introduce unwanted bacteria, including gonorrhoea, from the rectum into the vagina. If anal intercourse is practised regularly, over a long period of time, stretching of the sphincter muscles around the anus can occur, which may result in a constant anal discharge and leaking of faeces.

Libido

Many women write to me about the problem of lack of sexual desire and a total loss of interest in sexual activities. In extreme cases, this can lead to frigidity in which the woman is totally turned off and repulsed by sex.

What can destroy sexual desire?

1 *Stress* from business worries, family conflicts, legal wrangles and so on will preoccupy the emotional centre of the brain and not allow relaxed sensual feelings to take effect.

2 *Fatigue and insomnia* caused by overwork, poor general health and exhaustion will make an individual more concerned with getting enough sleep than with sexual matters. A woman with a large family or newborn baby may be totally exhausted at the end of the day and need her sleep as a precious restorer. She may become angry at repeated attempts to arouse her sexually when all she wants is a deep sleep.

3 *Fear of impotence* A fear of poor sexual performance can put a dampener on desire. It may be easier to say 'not tonight, darling, I have a migraine' than to face the anxiety of disappointing a sexual partner and feeling inadequate.

4 *Boredom and routine* may have crept into a relationship, particularly if the male is ignorant of how really to please a woman. If a man is only interested in a quick 'in and out type' exercise, to give himself an orgasm, it is easy to understand why a woman may find the TV soapies a more romantic choice.

5 *Excessive food and alcohol* These are strong desire and performance killers and should be avoided on a night of planned love-making.

6 *Various medications* There are many medications which can transform a tarzan into a mouse. Take the example of George, a

forty-three-year-old aggressive business manager. Despite normal ups and downs in their thirteen years of marriage, he and his wife had never had sexual problems until George accepted drug treatment for his ulcer pains. He still has strong desires but is discouraged to find that his erections no longer last.

Or take the case of Jane who has started tricyclic anti-depressant medication for her intermittent depression. She finds that her mood and libido have returned to normal during treatment and yet she is frustrated by an inability to achieve orgasm.

It is now increasingly recognized that situations such as those of George and Jane are common. A wide range of drugs may affect sexual function, causing loss of libido, arousal difficulties, orgasmic dysfunction or reproductive impairment.

Various groups of drugs which may impair sexual function are:

Appetite suppressants.
Some muscle relaxants.
Some drugs to combat epilepsy.
Ketoconazole, which is a tablet taken for vaginal thrush.
Some drugs used to prevent migraine headaches.
Some drugs used to treat high blood pressure.
Sedative drugs and anti-depressants.
Drugs used to treat cancer.
Some anti-ulcer drugs.
Some hormones, particularly anti-androgens and anti-oestrogens used in severe acne or hirsutism.

Be sure to check with your doctor when you are given a new drug as to whether it will impair your sexual ability and desire. There may be a suitable alternative drug which does not do this, as new derivatives of older drugs which have a lesser incidence of side effects are becoming available every day.

Coping with a partner who has sexual problems

Some women find themselves having to cope with a partner who has difficulty in obtaining or maintaining an erection hard enough for penetration of the vagina – this problem is called impotence or erectile dysfunction. Another common problem is that of the man who becomes overexcited and comes to orgasm too quickly – this is called premature ejaculation.

What can you do to help such a man?

The most important thing is not to overreact – treat his sexual problem as a non-event, at least initially. To most men with sexual dysfunction, their problem is of enormous importance and is usually equated with loss of self-esteem and a loss of manliness. The most important thing you can offer to a man with sexual dysfunction is to be a caring and supportive friend, who can openly discuss the problem without giving it heavy emotional connotations. You should work together optimistically and patiently and not judge your love life purely on the basis of its sexual aspect.

There are several facts you need to know before you can help your partner. They are:

1 An erection is not necessary for a man to enjoy sex and experience a satisfying orgasm and ejaculation. You can stimulate an impotent man to the point of orgasm by affectionate fondling, kissing or oral sex. Masturbation and sexual fantasies can also help in this area. All this can happen without an erection ever occurring.

2 If your partner becomes impotent you should not let it prevent regular expression of your sexual desires, as this in itself can be detrimental to normal sexual function. Your partner can still give you sexual pleasure through masturbation and some impotent men become wonderful lovers because their techniques of foreplay and affectionate fondling, tickling and massage become much more developed and sophisticated, especially compared to those of the man who thinks that thrusting the penis in the vagina is all that is needed for a woman's sexual satisfaction. Remember you can still have a wonderful love life while your man is recovering from impotence.

3 You cannot force a man to have an erection, nor can he force it upon himself; rather you can both only allow it to happen. Some

women find that repeated and frantic masturbation of a deflated penis will not coerce it to become erect, and indeed may have the opposite effect.

4 You have equal responsibility in achieving mutual satisfaction, and you cannot always expect the man to take the dominant role. Try to take the initiative and let your man lie back, free from pressure, while you make love to him.

5 The stress of sexual performance is greater for a man than for a woman because he cannot fake a good, lasting erection whereas a woman can fake enjoyment and orgasm. Try not to be demanding in the early stages.

6 It is rare for couples to have a simultaneous orgasm, or 'to come together'. Just because he has an early orgasm, this should not mean that you give up your efforts to have one.

7 As men get older their sexual performance very gradually decreases and the lag time between new erections increases. If this is understood, unrealistic expectations and disappointment can be avoided.

8 The sexual performance of the male is most commonly reduced by stress, so take a good look at your relationship as friends and confidants. You may need to give your man some psychotherapy and relaxation therapy, with the aim of increasing his self-esteem and confidence. For example tell him he is a wonderful sexy man who knows how to please you, while his erections are still recovering.

9 Excessive consumption of alcohol, cigarettes or recreational drugs is a common cause of impotence, and if your partner is seriously trying to overcome sexual dysfunction he should give up or drastically reduce these toxic dependencies.

10 Patience is a virtue, as most impotent men take several months to overcome the problem, and quite a bit longer to regain their confidence. Your unfaltering support will be needed.

Once you have these ten points in mind you can work together, perhaps under the guidance of a sex therapist, to overcome the sexual dysfunction. Get your partner talking so that you know what he likes in bed, and if he needs you to modify your behaviour try to accommodate him, as he may need a certain environment or type of stimulation to achieve an erection.

If impotence continues for more than three months, get him to see a medical doctor with a special interest in sexual dysfunction, as a physical examination will be needed to exclude a physical cause such as diabetes or a disorder of the spinal nerves. If no medical cause for chronic impotence is found, it is best to see a psychiatrist or psychologist with a special interest in sexual dysfunction (a sex therapist). Most sex therapists will get you to follow a programme whereby you learn to make love again, without vaginal penetration being allowed, no matter how big an erection occurs. Only when the therapist feels your partner is cured will he give him permission to attempt vaginal penetration.

During sex therapy a couple often rediscover each other in a new and exciting way and acquire a new dimension to their love life, a dimension they might otherwise have missed in their obsession with an erect penis.

Adolescent sexuality

Nowadays women are becoming sexually active at a younger age and statistics show that nearly 50 per cent of women between the ages of sixteen and nineteen have had sexual intercourse. Under the age of sixteen, around 13 per cent of women have had sexual intercourse and by the age of nineteen, 70 per cent of women have had sexual intercourse. Thus the days when a woman was told to keep herself pure for her future husband on the premise that 'no man wants a secondhand rose' are gone, and women are now as free as men to explore their adolescent sexuality.

The main reasons behind this increase in adolescent sexuality are the social acceptance of de facto couples and the availability of the oral contraceptive pill. However, this increase in adolescent sexuality does not mean that young women are becoming promiscuous. The majority of adolescents prefer to stay in a steady relationship.

Adolescent couples usually indulge in a lot of 'necking' or 'petting' before trying intercourse, and this is an important phase in their physical and sexual development. Many adolescent girls make a game of this petting, and give their partner a little more each time they meet, until eventually mutual masturbation is occurring. This allows the couple to experience full sexual enjoyment and, more importantly, allows the woman to feel in control and maintain her virginity for as long as she wants.

The age at which an adolescent girl becomes a sexual creature varies tremendously and depends upon several factors:

1 The time of awakening of her hormonal glands, namely the hypothalamus, pituitary and ovaries. The production of the female hormones from the awakening ovaries results in rounded breasts and a curvaceous figure, as well as creating sexual desire for the opposite sex. Mother Nature does not always spread her favours equally, and some young adolescent girls seem to blossom into hormonally active women overnight, while others complain bitterly that they cannot shed their childlike tomboy form as they enviously watch their flirtatious girlfriends. Each side has its advantages, however, and the late bloomer will eventually arrive at sexual maturity, often with a taller and more slender figure than her precocious sisters.

2 The psychological attitude of the people around a blossoming adolescent is important. If it is hostile or indifferent to her new beauty and charm, the young woman may feel like hiding or suppressing her sexuality. This may create a guilt complex and retard her sexual development.

3 The psychological attitude of the young woman to her own development is the most important factor. If, for example, she is disgusted by the appearance of menstrual blood, pubic hair or by her sudden surges of sexual desire, she may suppress all her thoughts or feelings on the subject. This strong negative emotion can in turn switch off her hormonal glands and her sexual development may slow down, to return later when she can psychologically cope with it.

Sex and the older woman

Jane Fonda tells us that a woman's sexual desire increases as she ages and that for most women, there is more sexual interest, pleasure and capacity for orgasm with increasing maturity. She says that for many women enjoyment of sex appears to rise continuously into the middle years and remain stable from that time on.

At the time of writing this chapter I am thirty-four years of age and cannot speak personally for this phenomenon, yet I feel there is much truth in these ideas for many women. As a very young doctor I had believed that women generally lost interest in sex as they aged and that by forty-five sexual intercourse would be quite a rare event for most women. How mistaken I was! It is through communicating with thousands of women of different cultures that I have realized that sexual interest remains an eternal thing for the majority of women.

While working in India, I was surprised to see women in their seventh or eighth decade eager to go home to their husbands after having a vaginal repair operation. They would be very pleased that their little operation had restored a normal capacity for sexual intercourse. As they say, life is a great teacher and my naïve concepts soon vanished.

Notwithstanding all this, women passing through the menopause often notice a reduced libido and capacity for an enjoyable sexual response. This is because the deficiency of the female hormones, oestrogen and progesterone, reduces sexual desire and causes shrinkage of the uterus and vagina. The pelvic muscles become weak without their hormonal support and the vaginal mucosa becomes dry and fragile. Little wonder that sex for many menopausal women may become unwelcome and painful. This unfortunate situation can be reversed by the use of hormone replacement therapy and, indeed, a woman's sexual organs can be transformed into their former youthful state. Hormone replacement therapy can also increase the capacity for orgasm.

For menopausal women who do not want to take hormone tablets, the use of a vaginal oestrogen cream can also bring back vaginal lubrication and tone.

Other products can be used to improve vaginal elasticity and lubrication, such as vegetable oils (cold pressed) and vitamin E cream applied to the vaginal walls. For annoying vaginal irritations 'aloe vera' gel or lotion is excellent for the fragile menopausal vagina. All these products can be applied directly to the vulva and also inserted high into the vagina with a vaginal applicator available at chemist shops.

Many menopausal women have problems with urinary frequency or incontinence which means that during coughing, straining or laughing, a small amount of urine uncontrollably leaks out of the bladder and urethra, soiling the underpants.

The previously described exercise for the pelvic floor (see page 41) is excellent for these bladder problems and will also aid your muscular performance during sexual intercourse.

If this exercise is not sufficient to overcome the problem, a vaginal repair operation will be necessary. This is a simple operation and involves removing loose, excessive tissue from the vagina and tightening the muscles around the neck of the bladder. The time spent in hospital is usually around four to five days and the post-operative period is not very painful compared to an operation involving an abdominal wound.

During middle age and beyond, both men and women usually take a longer time to achieve orgasm, and thus love-making tends to become a more emotional, warm, romantic affair compared to the sudden strong urges of younger couples. This is perhaps the reason that more mature sex is said to be very satisfying, with each partner taking their time to please the other. If orgasm does not occur, there is no major trauma, as the act of true love-making can create many beautiful sensations and feelings that are not just physical responses.

Sexual problems between long-term couples

Routine and fatigue are the most common problems to erode an interesting and active sex life between long-term couples. The male who stays late at the office and comes home, drained, to find his partner who is equally drained, having managed to juggle the needs of three children and a job all day, creates the setting for a non-event. The last hour of the day before retiring to bed is usually spent in essential yet mundane chores and the bed itself becomes a place for quickly falling asleep. Indeed, many overworked women come to see sex as the last chore of a busy day. It would be so different if she was going out on a romantic date, expecting to have the undivided attention of her man, and yet it is just the opposite, as she often feels she will be expected to accommodate the sexual needs of a partner who seems to have rather lost his air for romance. She doesn't feel sexy, gorgeous or excited and would probably prefer to make an excuse.

Also, this type of 'time economy rushed sex', although it suits many men who come to orgasm quickly, often leaves women still hanging in the plateau phase of stimulation until around two in the morning when they finally drift off into unconsciousness. No wonder women avoid this sexual frustration and feign fatigue.

Another common reason for sexual discord between long-term couples is a feeling of anger and resentment towards one's partner. This hostility may be conscious or subconscious and can quickly lead to sexual barriers. It may be due to a sudden off-the-cuff argument, or to a longstanding deeply buried conflict, but the result will be the same in that the injured partner wants to create distance. Often the injured partner will deny sexual gratification to the other as a form of punishment for previous hurts. A common cause of anger is when a sexual partner is concerned only with fulfilling his or her own needs and not those of the partner. In these cases, people tend to suppress anger instead of communicating their sexual needs.

If both partners are feeling anxious and resentful, deep down both may really want to be soothed and calmed by an affectionate encounter; and yet the stretched rubber band inside each person will not relax and neither one can become humble enough to make the initial warm overture. Both are left without relief and the hostility continues to increase.

A significant percentage of women find that they are no longer 'turned on' by their partner. Sexual desire rarely disappears totally from a good relationship, rather it comes in waves but only occasionally does it appear simultaneously in both partners. When sexual desire fades totally and for long periods of time, there are usually serious underlying problems. These problems may be such things as serious personality clashes, financial conflict, mistrust and infidelity. An unfaithful man will often subconsciously tell his partner that she is too tired, overworked or a nymphomaniac, so that the blame lies on her shoulders. The woman begins to see herself as sexually unattractive and can develop depression and a rejection and inferiority complex.

Unhygienic habits can also be a real turn-off to a sexual encounter, especially when they are chronic. Such things as lack of washing and shaving, failure to change clothes and heavy smoking are common problems. Some people get cleaned up to go out but not to go to bed and really don't put in any effort. Obesity and unfitness are also common off-putting things for some aesthetically minded persons.

The sexual evolution of a person is a totally individual thing and depends so much on finding a tender loving partner who cares about the other's needs and is flexible enough to grow and change with them; of course, this is a reciprocal thing.

Some women never find Mr Right and they learn to live with Mr Compromise who is better than nobody or a vibrator. Some women are extremely sexual beings and need to experience different lovers in their life to be fulfilled and really to feel that they are beautiful and desirable. Other women are more domesticated and need a faithful husband, good provider and traditional family life.

Whatever you may be, don't take sex too seriously and don't place orgasm and physical satisfaction on a pedestal. Don't force your sexuality when the opportunity is not there; rather, learn to use your basic energies wisely and usefully and let your sexual self mature and mellow, along with your mental and emotional self.

Sex is meant to be simple and good fun, just like eating. It is the exaggerated emotional connotations that we give it that create many of the problems.

Sexual assault

Sexual assault is best described as the sexual use of a female against her desire. It is often the expression of a man's physical power and dominance over a woman, rather than uncontrollable sexual desire, and thus has become a political issue that illustrates the continuing struggle of women for equal human rights.

Not only must the law protect women from sexual abuse, but society as a whole and the family unit must take responsibility to educate women of all ages on how to protect themselves against this ever-present threat. The legal system is still the end point in the process called into play after the abuse has occurred and prevention must lie in educating women and their children about services that help potential victims of sexual abuse before their problem becomes serious.

Sexual abuse often begins in childhood and can be terrifying and confusing for the victim at this age. It can be particularly horrifying for a child who has not been forewarned by the parents to be confronted with a man exposing or playing with himself, especially if the child is constrained by the assaulter. Young boys are just as much at risk and both sexes need to be forewarned during childhood.

Some mothers have told me that they are loath to tell their innocent five-year-old about dirty old men who play with children's genitals or carry out sadistic acts, lest they create premature neurosis in the child. However, we live in an epoch of sensationalism and children should be forewarned that rape, assault and drug addiction are everyday occurrences on the streets, not just on the television.

I well remember my parents telling me, when I was not yet four, that the man who lived across the road was horrible, dirty and not to be trusted. I was warned never to be caught alone in the lane with him as he was likely to chase me with his penis. From that point on, whenever he smiled at me from across the street, I saw devil's horns springing from his head and an evil glint in his eyes – needless to say this kept me well away from him!

Although I did not understand the significance of sexuality or eroticism at this tender age, the warning put into my sub-conscious mind instilled a healthy respect for big male strangers with a penis and this awareness conferred a lasting protection upon me throughout my vulnerable years.

It is often the pretty, extrovert young girl, who is an early bloomer, who is particularly at risk.

The school system, as well as the parents, should take responsibility for telling pre-adolescent children about the risk of sexual abuse. If children are sexually abused without any comprehension on their part, they will be less likely to report it and the potential for ongoing abuse is much higher. This will often leave permanent mental scars and cause chronic psychosexual problems that will prevent happy healthy sexual relationships in adulthood.

The National Society for the Prevention of Cruelty to Children has an 'at-risk' list and estimates that there are 44,000 children in the UK at risk of sexual abuse, most of them girls. An investigation carried out by the National Children's Home of 11,000 children in its homes reported that 15 per cent of the children had been sexually abused in earlier life and this represents one in four of this particular population. Government estimates of abuse are more conservative than the NSPCC's – 39,000 children are at risk of abuse.

There is a special helpline for children who have been abused or at risk which they can ring free themselves – 0800 1111.

Incest

This refers to the sexual abuse of a young child by a member of the family, most commonly the father, stepfather, brother, uncle or cousin. Many cases of incest go unreported and thus an accurate incidence is difficult to estimate. However, we do know that it is not uncommon and it is thought that around one in twenty girls may have been sexually violated during childhood. The age of the victim varies from less than five to, more commonly, the years of puberty from ten to thirteen.

The child who is a victim of incest is often in a more difficult situation than the child who is sexually abused by a stranger. Such a child is often threatened not to talk to the only person who could help them and made to feel that the sexual activity is their fault and will be punished if discovered. Even if the child talks, it is not uncommon for parental reaction to be unfriendly, if not hostile, which may be even more psychologically damaging to the child. The mother may be fearful of breaking up the family, creating a public scandal, losing her husband or sending him to jail, and may rationalize that the child is exaggerating or fantasizing. This hush-hush attitude may be practised in front of professionals called in 'to help' and it is easy to see how such a situation can become buried or allowed to smoulder on.

This failure to take the child affected by incest seriously was reinforced by the exaggerated ideas of the famous psychiatrist, Sigmund Freud, who did not accept that incest could be so common, and rationalized away his disbelief by propagating the idea that all little girls fantasize about their fathers making sexual advances towards them and are jealous of their mothers, who receive his favours instead. Another reason why incest is commonly swept under the carpet, is that people find it more comfortable to believe that they have a sexually precocious and provocative child, rather than a deranged male in the family. Unfortunately, the truth of the matter is that these children are usually bribed into sex by means of lollies, picnics, toys and other childlike things and are totally innocent victims.

One can create all sorts of rational excuses for the occurrence of sexual abuse of children, but they are only academic, and our energies should be spent in preventing it, right from the moment the nappies change to knickers.

Rape

This term refers to a forcible and often violent sexual attack against the victim's will. It is not uncommonly associated with battering or torture of the victim and some rapists have a predilection for maiming their victims or cutting them up into little pieces. One third to one half of all rapes are done by the victim's husband or regular partner, but as the law stands now, a husband cannot be charged with raping his wife, unless they are not living together, when he can be charged. However, in 1989 the Scottish High Court ruled that a husband could be charged with raping his wife, and this was upheld on appeal at the Scottish Court of Criminal Appeal. It remains to be seen whether this historic decision will percolate through to English courts.

If children are raped, it is not always by a stranger and relatives are not uncommonly implicated.

It is sad to know that three out of four rapes go unreported because women are inhibited by the attitude held by many males that it is impossible to rape a woman without some participation on her side. Many women also dread the need to relive the experience while recounting the minute details to the police and examining medical doctor, who may not be overly sympathetic or ready to believe.

The law used to be weighted in favour of the accused, and the victim had to rely on her own strength to prove that she was raped without provocation, that penile entry occurred, and that she resisted the assault. It is not surprising that previously the conviction rate of reported rapists was improbably low. Sentencing in the United Kingdom has often been controversial in rape, with individual judges causing outrage with lenient sentences. Sometimes it would appear that rape is sentenced more lightly than for damage to property (as in the Ealing Vicarage rape case). Whereas rape is a specific charge in Britain, more advanced thinking on rape legislation such as, for example, that enacted in 1981 in New South Wales, Australia, allows for a wider definition of rape to be applied and divides rape into varying levels of severity, each with a corresponding level of punishment. The aim of this is to bring more sexual offenders to trial, to facilitate court procedures for sexual assault victims, and make it easier to report a rape.

What sources of help exist for rape victims?

For counselling after rape, GPs and police surgeons should automatically refer the victim to a Rape Crisis Centre. You can also refer yourself simply by ringing the helpline (24 hours) on 071-837 1600. There is another line, operating between 10am and 6pm Monday–Friday, on 071-278 3956. Rape Crisis Centres exist throughout the country and can be found in local telephone directories. The Centres do offer legal advice, but this can also be offered by the Rights of Women group on 071-251 6577.

Workers at these centres can explain the normal procedure for undertaking legal action, as well as discussing with you the normal stages of court procedure, before you actually need to participate in the courtroom. Support from these workers is highly desirable as there may be several months between the rape and the hearing in court.

What medical care should a rape victim receive?

All rape victims should seek medical attention, whether they wish to proceed with legal charges or not, and workers at the sexual assault centres or rape crisis centres can refer you to sympathetic doctors.

If you have been raped, do not wash or change your clothes before seeing the doctor as you may be removing legal evidence of sexual assault and venereal disease. If you have been lucky enough to escape without physical injury, it may be impossible for a doctor to prove forcible penile entry into the vagina, and thus bloodstains, damaged clothes or dirty finger marks may be the only valid signs of assault that could support legal charges. The doctor will do a careful physical examination, looking for general bodily injury as well as injury to the genital organs. After this the following procedures should take place.

Certain laboratory tests should be done:

1 Swabs of the vagina and vulva should be taken to examine secretions for the presence of the enzyme 'acid phosphatase' which is found in semen.

2 If semen is found it can be tested to identify the blood group of the rapist.

3 Swabs of the upper vagina and vulva should be taken to examine for the presence of mobile sperm.

4 Swabs from the vagina, cervix and anus should be taken to test for venereal infections, such as gonorrhoea.

5 A blood test to screen for syphilis, herpes and AIDS should be done. These are called baseline tests and are to confirm that you were not already a carrier of these diseases before the rape attack.

Certain medical treatment should be given:

1 Every sexually assaulted woman should be given antibiotics to prevent venereal disease. An injection of benzathine penicillin G, 2.4 million units, should be given intramuscularly with the aim of preventing gonorrhoea and, hopefully, syphilis. If allergy to penicillin is a problem, other antibiotics can be substituted.

2 Unwanted pregnancy can be prevented if the victim goes to the doctor within 72 hours of the rape and gets a 'morning after pill', or other high dose oestrogen preparation. The rape victim should be advised against unprotected sexual intercourse during the remainder of the menstrual cycle. If the menstrual period following the rape is delayed, a pregnancy test should be done on the blood and, if positive, most doctors advise a therapeutic termination of pregnancy.

3 The victim will need advice as to when she can resume normal sexual intercourse, especially if genital injury has occurred.

Certain follow-up procedures should take place:

1 If the initial swabs show that the woman caught a venereal infection, further swabs and treatment will be needed to eradicate the infection completely.

2 Even if the initial blood test for syphilis was negative, it should be repeated at six weeks and three months after the rape. If the three month blood test is negative, the victim can be certain she has not caught syphilis.

3 AIDS and herpes – if the initial blood tests for AIDS and herpes were negative, they should be repeated at six weeks and three months after the rape. If they are still negative at this time it is extremely unlikely that these diseases have been contracted. They need only be repeated if symptoms develop in the future.

4 The woman should receive counselling from a sympathetic doctor or a worker from one of the sexual assault or rape crisis centres to reduce the chances of long-term psychological damage.

4 Pandora's Box
– the premenstrual syndrome revealed

For centuries the premenstrual syndrome (PMS) has been treated as a 'Pandora's Box' and the lid pushed down tightly to keep the inexplicable demons out of the way. This is because of a fear born out of ignorance, scepticism and condescension. Until the lid is removed and the demons of PMS are exposed for therapeutic and rational exorcism, we shall remain in the dark ages. Just because the cause of PMS is a complicated matter this does not mean that its numerous symptoms cannot be dealt with in a practical way.

The female is physiologically a very different creature from her male counterpart, and in particular she is subject to changes in metabolism produced by a cyclical ebb and flow of ovarian hormones. In contrast, the production of male hormone from the testicle is constant and not cyclical. The ebb and flow of a female's hormones produces a corresponding change in her physical and mental state and normally this is within tolerable and even pleasant limits. There is a richness and a completion in the moods and sensations produced by a normal physiological change in hormones. Under such circumstances a female can rejoice and enjoy her cyclic physical and mental changes and indeed take great interest in the symptoms and signs which reflect them.

Man has taken great pains to discover the cycles of our solar system's planets and yet, often in his eyes, the biological cycles of a woman have been seen to be the stamp of an inferior species, inevitably unpredictable and not worthy of serious study. It is interesting to surmise from where this stigma originates. Perhaps in the old-fashioned religious ethic of Eve bearing the curse in the garden of Eden; and yet even this explanation does not suffice as the stigma has existed for centuries in diverse cultures and religions.

I have done much research into the causes of PMS and I have concluded, along with many other researchers in this area, that it is the result of an imbalance in the normal monthly hormonal cycle. There are three definite phases in the monthly hormonal cycle of a normal woman and these can be compared to the cycles of Mother Nature, such as the phases of the moon, the tides and the passing of the seasons. For example, if perchance spring and summer were too short, the earth did not receive her maximum sunlight and the winter lasted too long, then the produce of the earth's soil would suffer. Similarly, if the natural flow of female hormones from the ovary is insufficient or ends too soon, the metabolism of many tissues and organs of the female body is disrupted.

The obvious role of the medical profession, and the female herself, is to learn how to promote and sustain the best natural cyclic production of hormones from the ovaries. This will ensure a normal and tolerable state of physical and mental well-being during the monthly cycle.

How common is PMS?

It is surprisingly common and one could say that approximately 50 per cent of all women in the reproductive age group suffer from some degree of PMS, and of these some 5 per cent suffer from severe and devastating symptoms.

The PMS is no respecter of socio-economic status, race, colour or intelligence and is seen in all countries of the world.

Why is PMS so common?

1 Modern-day women have far fewer pregnancies than women of sixty years ago, a fact which is largely due to the existence of the oral contraceptive pill and legalized abortion. In round figures, the average modern-day woman has four hundred menstrual cycles to experience and therefore four hundred possible episodes of premenstrual difficulty, unless she decides to remain pregnant for many years of her life.

2 Modern-day women are better educated and more liberated in their attitudes to their bodily changes, and thus PMS has finally been recognized as a real and common entity. Before this time it

was mislabelled as a neurotic and inexplicable illness and its incidence was therefore grossly underestimated.

3 Modern-day women are exposed to the stressful and often toxic life-style of the twentieth century involving addiction to alcohol, junk foods, heavy smoking and pollution, processed devitalized diets and demands for multiple role-playing. For the busy working mother, or indeed for any mother, there is little time left for herself, for contemplation, recuperation and unwinding. All these factors aggravate and many precipitate PMS.

What is the social and legal importance of PMS?

In the past, many doctors 'pooh-poohed' the whole concept of PMS and relegated it to the 'too hard basket', or just simply ignored it as a silly female peculiarity. However, those days have gone and statistics have undoubtedly shown that the incidence of crime, accidents, emergency admissions to hospital, and child battering are much more common in the one to two weeks before the period. When non-accidental injury of a child with an apparently loving mother is suspected, one of the most important questions the doctor should ask is the date of the last menstrual period.

A female expert on PMS, Dr Katharina Dalton, has spent thirty years of her life investigating the symptoms of PMS and she has discovered the staggering statistic that the incidence of suicide is seven times higher in the premenstrual phase.

These are some of the really tragic aspects of PMS and they highlight the fact that it should no longer be considered an insignificant, silly female disorder, but rather a poignant issue in women's health, demanding urgent research.

Two unprecedented legal decisions in the United Kingdom have forced the medical profession, and society in general, to look at PMS with new spectacles. In one of these legal cases a barmaid was charged with the attempted stabbing of a policeman and was put on probation by the judge with the understanding that she continue regular medical treatment for PMS. In this case the judge accepted her PMS as a mitigating circumstance. Perhaps the reason for the judge's lenient verdict was the statement by the defence witness, Dr Katharina Dalton, that this woman was a true PMS sufferer and that she had greatly reduced her dosage of progesterone at this time.

In the other case a divorcee ran her car into her lover, crushing him against a telegraph pole which resulted in his death. She was conditionally discharged for twelve months after pleading guilty to manslaughter by reason of diminished responsibility due to PMS. Again, Dr Dalton was witness for the defence. Dr Dalton told the story that this woman was pliant and law abiding for most of the month but that once every twenty-nine days she would attempt arson, violent suicide or smash windows. She had been in prison on and off for ten years and accurate records showed twenty-six episodes of violence occurring every twenty-nine days. She was judged to be in the grip of a biological force beyond her control – PMS – which transformed her cyclically into a violent creature – and she was acquitted.

PMS also went on trial in the United States of America in 1982. A female legal aid lawyer argued before a criminal court judge in Brooklyn, New York, that the case of her client who was accused of child battering should be thrown out of court because the accused was a sufferer of severe PMS. The lawyer argued that her client needed treatment not punishment, and the criminal charges against her were dropped in exchange for her pleading guilty to violation and harassment which are lesser charges. This was the first American legal acknowledgement of PMS. Conversely, in France, PMS has long been recognized as a legal cause of temporary insanity.

Many people are worried that the use of PMS as a mitigating circumstance in criminal acts will open the door for abuse of PMS by dishonest lawyers desperate for a reason to prove the innocence of their client. However, this has not proven to be true, and it is interesting to note that similar fears were expressed after the 1845 trial of Martha Brixey who was acquitted for the murder of her employer's child, on the grounds of insanity due to 'obstructed menstruation'. You see we are not dealing with anything new, it is just the media who like to sensationalize events.

The use of PMS as a defence is indeed a hot subject and the rationale behind it could be brought into the defence of all crimes committed by people with psychiatric disorders; in other words, these people need treatment not punishment. However, unlike PMS, not all psychiatric disorders have a biochemical or hormonal cause and are therefore not all amenable to drug treatment. The only solution for psychiatric crimes which have no physical cause is confinement and forced rehabilitation.

The new legal angle carries with it the good news that many women who have endured PMS distress in confusion and guilt are now being listened to at last. Their suffering is gaining credence in social, medical and legal dimensions and, in the long run, this will bring greater compassion and understanding for women. This can only be encouraged.

These major social-legal implications will never need to be considered for the majority of PMS sufferers. But for the minor group who suffer from severe and devastating PMS and lose control, their behaviour will now be given special compassion and credence in criminal matters.

These major legal decisions have worried some feminists because they feel that all women will be labelled as hysterical and unpredictable as a consequence, and that this may impair women's status. However, cases of PMS which are severe enough to incur legal repercussions will always be a small minority. Furthermore, with better education and understanding such cases would never have reached this desperate point. PMS *is* treatable.

Most women who suffer from PMS are never so affected that they express violent and criminal behaviour. Rather, their suffering is usually lonely and internalized and manifested mainly as a loss of self-esteem and well-being.

Women have no need to feel guilty about PMS; it is simply a treatable physical disorder, not an emotive political drama.

What causes PMS?

Although we have come a long way since the time of Hippocrates, there are still many strange ideas put forth to try to explain this troublesome group of symptoms. Hippocrates thought that PMS was caused by a 'wandering uterus' which travelled around the body and somehow upset the brain. His treatment was quite incredible and consisted of burning aromatic incense at the vaginal opening to entice the uterus back home to its rightful position in the pelvis.

It was Dr Franks, in 1931, who first used the term 'premenstrual syndrome' and he thought it was due to excess oestrogen. He decided to try to flush this excess oestrogen out of the body with large doses of laxatives and he claimed great success. Little wonder, as the poor PMS sufferers were probably so distracted by their frequent loose bowel actions that they had little time to remember the symptoms of their PMS!

In retrospect these ideas are laughable and today are of historical and curiosity interest only. If one makes a thorough research of the current literature existing on PMS, one finds several different theories as to its cause. Let us take a look at some of these:

1 Allergy of the woman to her own sex hormones – hard to believe!

2 Salt and water retention – this is a result of PMS and not the cause.

3 Low blood sugar – this is a result of PMS and not the cause.

4 Imbalances in the chemicals of the body known as prostaglandins (see page 375) – this may increase various types of physical pain, but does not explain the mental symptoms of PMS.

5 Disturbance in the balance of brain chemicals – once again a result of PMS not the cause.

6 Overactive nervous system resulting in an overproduction of stress hormones – this factor can operate in all stressful conditions, not just PMS.

7 Excessive levels of the hormone prolactin which comes from the pituitary gland. This may be a factor in PMS sufferers with very painful breasts and infrequent periods and this hormone should be checked in these cases. It is not, however, a universal finding.

8 Psychological defect or personality disorder – undoubtedly the underlying personality and environment can influence the

development of PMS. However, more commonly, mental problems arise secondary to the biochemical and hormonal imbalances of PMS. Personality factors may intensify PMS symptoms but they cannot be held responsible for causing them.

There are many more such theories but none give a satisfactory answer and, after ten years of treating thousands of women with PMS, my clinical research has made me certain that the fundamental cause of PMS is a hormonal imbalance. This may be only of a subtle degree, but it is enough to produce PMS.

If you look at Figure 14, you will see that there are three phases in the normal monthly cycle:

1 A slow peak in the hormone oestrogen.

2 A peak in both female hormones, oestrogen and progesterone.

3 A gradual smooth reduction in both female hormones premenstrually.

In contrast, Figure 15 illustrates the monthly cycle in a typical PMS sufferer. You can see that phase 1 is normal but that in phases 2 and 3 there is a premature and excessive reduction in the female hormones. It is this relative deficiency in both female hormones that is the basic cause of all the physical and mental PMS symptoms.

My ideas concur very closely with those of one of the international experts on PMS, Dr Katharina Dalton, who has treated over 30,000 PMS sufferers. Dr Dalton believes that a deficiency of progesterone is more important than a deficiency of both female hormones and that is why she treats PMS exclusively with natural progesterone injections or pessaries. Furthermore, Dalton believes that women who take some brands of the oral contraceptive pill have a high incidence of PMS because the synthetic progesterones in the oral contraceptive pill falsely indicate to the body that there is enough progesterone, so the ovaries stop making the real thing. The result is relatively too much oestrogen, not enough natural progesterone and heaps of PMS. I believe there is much truth in her theories.

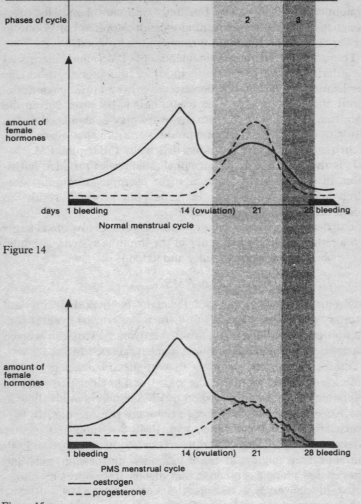

Figure 14

Figure 15

This explanation of hormonal deficiency is corroborated by the high incidence of post-natal depression which occurs in the month subsequent to the birth of a child – a condition which is directly due to the sudden drop in female hormones that occurs straight after the birth. Furthermore, the depression and anxieties common in menopausal women are often partly due to the very low levels of female hormones in their blood.

There is an increased incidence of PMS and menstrual irregularities after division (ligation) of the uterine tubes for sterilization, especially if procedures involving burning (cauterization) of the tubes have been used. This is because, during the operation, the blood supply to the ovary may be damaged with a resultant decrease in hormone production from that ovary. This in turn causes a relative hormonal deficiency and regular PMS.

It is thought that these hormonal deficiencies produce imbalances in several brain chemicals (for example, serotonin, noradrenaline, dopamine and the endorphins), which results in emotional and psychological disorders.

The deficiency of female hormones also causes low blood sugar and a reduction in the efficiency of the immune system, although the reason for this is not yet fully understood.

Can stress and a poor diet worsen PMS?

Environmental stress can act through the hypothalamus and pituitary gland (see page 20) to disturb the normal cyclical production of female hormones from the ovaries. This can worsen the deficiency of female hormones and exaggerate PMS.

Another important factor is that of dietary deficiencies. An American gynaecologist by the name of Dr Goei performed a computerized study into the diets of PMS sufferers in his clinic in Los Angeles and obtained some very interesting results. In particular, he found that women with PMS consumed far greater amounts of refined carbohydrates, dairy products, sugar and salt and consumed far less of the B vitamins, magnesium, zinc and manganese. Thus it is obvious that dietary imbalances may worsen or, in some cases, even cause the symptoms of PMS.

Another study was done by Dr Guy Abrahams in England and he found that PMS sufferers have low levels of magnesium in their blood. It is well known that stress, processed diets, excess coffee, alcohol and diuretic drugs will all cause a loss of magnesium. Dairy products may interfere with magnesium absorption and thereby increase the need for this mineral. And stress stimulates the adrenal glands which results in a loss of magnesium from the body.

Over a period of time, a diet high in refined and processed carbohydrates may deplete the body of its reserves of chromium, manganese, zinc, magnesium and most of the vitamins, and this will aggravate many symptoms of PMS. We shall discuss a suitable diet for PMS sufferers a little further on.

What is the definition of PMS?

PMS is a cyclical recurrent deterioration in the physical and/or mental well-being of a woman in the reproductive age group. It can only occur *after* ovulation and may begin as early as sixteen days before menstrual bleeding, if ovulation occurs early, or as late as a few days (one or two) before menstrual bleeding begins.

It is often relieved by the onset of menstrual bleeding, but in some women it may persist until menstrual bleeding finishes.

If symptoms occur before ovulation they are not part of the PMS and indeed during this time the PMS sufferer usually feels at her best.

A common misunderstanding is that the term PMS is exactly the same as PMT, and that the two terms can be used interchangeably. This is quite wrong as PMT stands only for premenstrual tension, which means anxiety and irritability, whereas PMS stands for premenstrual syndrome, which encompasses a group of emotional symptoms, including tension, and also a group of physical symptoms.

What are the many possible symptoms of PMS?

Psychological
Depression, guilt, negativity, loss of self-esteem, insomnia, changeable moods, anxiety, irritability, sudden angry outbursts, regret, muddled thinking and changes in sexuality.

Physical
1 Painful breasts.

2 Fluid retention, weight gain and swelling of the body.

3 Headache.

4 Skin problems – flare-up of acne, herpes, eczema and so on.

5 Low blood sugar with fatigue, light-headedness, drowsiness and a craving for sweets, junk foods and coffee.

6 Backache and increase in muscular or arthritic pains.

7 Other possible symptoms are a mixed bag – constipation, dizziness, hay fever, a runny nose.

A very interesting association has been noted between some unrelated chronic diseases and the premenstrual phase, in that these diseases may flare up during this time. For example, sufferers of arthritis, collagen diseases, asthma, hay fever, epilepsy, schizophrenia and bowel diseases may notice a deterioration premenstrually. This is probably because the female hormones have an anti-inflammatory effect and increase general resistance and immune function. That is also why these chronic diseases often improve during pregnancy.

By noting these cyclical premenstrual flare-ups in unassociated chronic diseases, a patient can be reassured that a continual deterioration in her disease is not occurring.

As you can see, there are many possible symptoms for the PMS sufferer and it is little wonder that doctors often find it difficult to treat the syndrome holistically by going to the root cause.

How do you know if you have the dreaded PMS?

Timing of symptoms is the key to diagnosis. There are no blood tests that can tell you, yes or no, nor is there any particular type of symptom necessary to prove the diagnosis. The clue to diagnosis is to key the time relationship of your symptoms to your menstrual bleeding. As stated before, if you truly are a PMS sufferer your symptoms will be worse after ovulation and up to menstruation, with an improvement occurring at the beginning of menstrual bleeding, or at least by the end of menstrual bleeding.

The best way to discover this is to record the dates of symptoms and menstrual bleeding on the same calendar.

Let us take a look at the charts of three hypothetical PMS sufferers, using the following codes:

M = menstrual bleeding
H = headache
D = depression
F = fluid retention
A = anxiety
S = skin problems
B = breast pain
P = menstrual pain

You can make up others for your own particular symptoms.

You can see by looking at the charts of Mary, Teresa and Christine that they are typical PMS sufferers in that their various physical symptoms recur each month during the premenstrual time and are relieved during the first few days of the menstrual flow.

Should you visit a doctor if you think you have PMS?

Very definitely yes, and you can help the doctor enormously by keeping an accurate symptom–menstrual calendar. Because PMS has many possible symptoms, other more serious diseases can masquerade as PMS. For example, diseases of the thyroid gland, a pituitary tumour or disorders of the adrenal gland may all produce depression, fatigue, anxiety and menstrual irregularity and your doctor will need to check for such diseases.

Also, some women with personality disorders or severe depression may wrongly attribute their symptoms to PMS and fail to seek correct treatment from a psychiatrist or hypnotherapist. In all these other diseases, symptoms will be present constantly, whereas the PMS sufferer is only unwell premenstrually as shown on the menstrual charts of Mary, Teresa and Christine.

The treatment of PMS – the natural approach

There are two essential prerequisites in the treatment of PMS:
1 Because PMS is a recurrent disorder, it is essential that any treatment be safe and free from side effects that could accumulate on a long-term basis.

	January	February	March	April
1		H B D	M	
2	B	M P	M	
3	B	M P	M	
4	B	M		
5	H B D	M		
6	H B D	M		
7	H B D			
8	M P			
9	M P			
10	M			
11	M			
12	M			D
13				B D
14				B D
15				B D
16				B D
17				H B D
18				M P
19			D	M
20			B D	M
21			B D	M
22		D	H B D	M
23		B D	H B D	
24		H B D	M P	
25		H B D	M P	
26		H B D	M	
27	B	M P	M	
28	B	M	M	
29	B D			
30	H B D			
31	H B D			

Mary's Chart

Mary has a 5 day bleeding cycle every 25 days.

	May	June	July	August
1				
2				
3				
4				
5				
6		F D		
7		F D		F
8		F D	F	F
9		F D H	F	F
10		M P	F	F
11	F	M P H	F	F
12	F D	M	F D	F D
13	F D	M	F D	F D
14	F D H	M	F D H	F D
15	M P H		M P	M P H
16	M P H		M P H	M P
17	M		M	M H
18	M		M	M
19	M		M	M
20	M		M	
21	M			
22				
23				
24				
25				
26				
27				
28				
29				
30				
31				

Teresa's Chart

Teresa has a 5 to 7 day bleeding cycle every 26 to 35 days. In other words she has a variable menstrual cycle.

	September	October	November	December
1				
2				
3				
4				
5				
6				
7				
8				
9				
10	A			
11	D A			
12	D A	A		
13	D A	A	D A	
14	D A H	D A	D A	
15	M D A H	D H	D A	
16	M D	D H	D A	A
17	M D H	M D H	D A H	D A
18	M	M D	M D H	D A
19	M	M	M D	D A H
20		M	M H	M D A H
21		M	M	M D
22			M	M H
23				M
24				M
25				
26				
27				
28				
29				
30				
31				

Christine's Chart
Christine has a 5 day bleeding cycle every 32 days.

2 Because PMS has many possible symptoms, any effective treatment must be broad based and capable of treating all those symptoms.

There are two main aims in the natural treatment of PMS:

1 To improve the woman's own ovarian function
Each ovary has an amazing potential, provided it is free from serious disease, and every one of the hundreds of thousands of ovarian eggs is capable of producing female hormones.

The ovaries require the nutrients vitamin E, B6 and zinc to manufacture hormones, and if taken in supplemental dosage these nutrients will help to optimize natural ovarian function. The ovaries also require adequate stimulation from the pituitary gland. Supplemental vitamin B6 and the avoidance of stress, along with a healthy life-style, will help to regulate the pituitary gland and therefore the ovaries.

Your ovaries will not be efficient hormone factories if you do not supply them with sufficient oxygen-rich blood – yes, a reasonable blood circulation is very important. To improve circulation of blood to the ovaries, simple measures such as avoidance of heavy smoking, regular aerobic exercise and yoga, along with extra vitamin C, E and garlic can really help. Many women find that with these simple yet powerful measures, they can prime and 'feed' their ovaries to a better performance and do not need to resort to taking hormone treatments. Your own sex hormones are the most natural and best for you.

2 To alleviate each individual symptom of PMS using physiological and harmless substances
In my experience this translates into using vitamin-mineral and herbal medicines which will not disturb the normal metabolic systems of the body. These naturopathic medicines can also be used to treat PMS in women on the oral contraceptive pill and they can safely be used in combination with hormones and drugs that may be necessary for other medical diseases.

Let us take a look at the most notorious symptoms of PMS and attack each one systematically.

(a) Psychological and emotional symptoms

Vitamin B6 (pyridoxine) has been shown in clinical trials to relieve headaches, depression, anxiety, irritability and fatigue in over 50 per cent of PMS sufferers. This is partly because B6 is essential for the production of the mood-regulating brain chemicals, serotonin and noradrenaline (see page 121).

Some women are worried by sensational media reports of B6 toxicity or poisoning and it is necessary to clarify these reports.

Over the last ten years B6 has been widely prescribed for such diverse conditions as schizophrenia, autism, hyperactivity in children, morning sickness in pregnancy and PMS, and in general one can say that it has been very safe in correct dosage.

The daily requirement of B6 for normal adults is two milligrams and this can usually be obtained from a well-balanced diet. In some conditions this daily requirement is increased, for example pregnancy complicated by anorexia and nausea, alcoholism, some cases of infantile convulsions and rare anaemias. Many oral contraceptive pill users and patients on drugs for tuberculosis may also need more.

In some conditions, for example, PMS, carpal tunnel syndrome and certain types of arthritis, B6 has been proved to exert a beneficial therapeutic effect in reasonably high doses. In other words, in these cases the vitamin is acting as more than just a vitamin (essential factor) – it is acting as a pharmacological agent, in the way that a drug would act. However, we all know that any drug in high doses (overdose) can have toxic side effects, for example, aspirin, antibiotics or anti-arthritic drugs and thus the dosages of these drugs are controlled by instructions written on the packet or by a doctor's script.

Unfortunately this has not been the case with vitamins used in a pharmacological way, and thus patients have sometimes decided to control their own dosage, usually with the logic that the more the better, and this has resulted in some cases of extremely high overdosage and toxic effects.

Published reports show that the daily dosage of B6 required to produce toxic effects is 2000 milligrams or 1000 times the daily requirement! This means that if you buy standard tablets containing fifty milligrams each you must swallow forty tablets a day to cause problems; however, people will do anything to feel well again. In the *New England Journal of Medicine*, 1983, there was a report of seven women who suffered from clumsiness and numbness of the hands and feet after taking between 2000 and 6000 milligrams of B6 daily for several months without supervision; all improved greatly after vitamin B6 was stopped.

It can be categorically stated that the average therapeutic dose of B6 which ranges from *50 to 200 milligrams daily*, depending on the condition and the response, is very safe; this dosage range should not be exceeded, as if improvement is not noted at 200 milligrams daily, then increasing this dosage will not give any more improvement.

Overall, it is safer to take B6 in recommended dosage than it is to take aspirin, oral contraceptive pills or tablets against arthritis, and a useful therapeutic substance should not be abandoned because of exaggerated and poorly explained media reports.

If trying to overcome premenstrual depression and anxiety with vitamin B6, it will be necessary to take it with two other B vitamins for optimal results. They are vitamin B1 (thiamine), 50 to 100 milligrams daily, and niacinamide, 100 to 200 milligrams daily.

Essential metabolic minerals for the brain and nerves should be taken in supplemental dosages. These are magnesium, potassium and calcium, as if they are severely deficient, symptoms of anxiety, irritability, palpitations and in extreme cases convulsions may occur. Good sources of these minerals are raw vegetables and fruit juices, but we shall delve more deeply into a special diet for PMS later on.

With the above mentioned vitamins and minerals a natural tranquillizing effect is produced and the PMS sufferer will find that if she takes these substances regularly, a gradual reduction in her psychological problems will occur. Furthermore, these substances may be taken on a long-term basis with absolutely no side effects and will eliminate or drastically reduce the requirements for sedative drugs. The brain may be seen as a 'soggy computer' that requires these metabolic nutrients to function correctly. If a deficiency of these vital nutrients exists, the chemical and electrical messages passed between the cells of the soggy computer become deranged, and this may result in mental and emotional symptoms.

(b) Fluid retention and weight gain

For centuries European doctors have prescribed herbal diuretics to stimulate the kidneys to excrete excess fluid and salt (sodium) which is retained by many women premenstrually. In contrast to synthetic diuretic drugs, these herbal diuretics do not produce a loss of the vital minerals, potassium and magnesium.

Some severe PMS sufferers may need to take synthetic diuretic drugs from time to time; however, they should try to use the smallest dose possible and should always ask for 'potassium sparing diuretic drugs' as opposed to ordinary diuretics. You need a prescription for these. It is best to take a diuretic drug every second or third day, rather than every day, and to combine it with a magnesium supplement.

For those women who wish to try diuretic herbs, I recommend the following ones: uva ursi, parsley piert and juniper. These will reduce abdominal swelling, pelvic congestion and weight gain due to fluid retention.

If swelling and aching of the legs is a problem, particularly if associated with easy bruising and varicose veins, the following herbs are excellent: aesculus, hamamelis, ruscus aculeatus and beta rutosides. Don't forget the precious vitamin C in all cases of fluid retention – you can take it in the form of pure calcium ascorbate powder, a quarter of a teaspoon four times daily in raw fruit and vegetable juices.

Many PMS sufferers find that fluid accumulates in their breasts premenstrually, contributing to the painful lumpy breast syndrome known as 'benign breast disease'. These women should follow the treatment programme detailed on page 193.

(c) Headaches

Some women are plagued by predictable premenstrual headaches which typically start a few days before menstrual bleeding is due and are relieved by the onset of the menstrual flow. These are called 'hormonal headaches' (see page 378). They can be very debilitating with a severe throbbing pain localized to one side of the head, or a constant dull ache all over the head. There may be nausea and vomiting and visual changes such as black spots and flashing lights before the eyes. It is very difficult to cope with housework and small children at these times and little wonder that these women often become depressed and irritable.

Women who suffer from these types of headache will benefit from the regular ingestion of the minerals calcium and magnesium. They should also avoid excessive consumption of coffee and avoid missing meals. Because congestion of the brain is often incriminated as a cause of many headaches, it will be found that the diuretic action of juniper, uva ursi and parsley will have a beneficial effect on premenstrual headaches.

These hormonal headaches are due to the low levels of female hormones premenstrually and, if all else fails, a low dose contraceptive pill or the prescription of a small dose of oestrogen, for example, ethinyl oestradiol, ten micrograms daily, during the headache periods can be very effective.

The amino acid 'phenylalanine' is a useful preventative against headaches and can be taken in a dosage of 400 milligrams two or three times daily, to give a natural painkilling and mood-elevating effect. It is available without a prescription but should not be taken during pregnancy nor by people suffering from the rare metabolic disease, phenylketonuria.

(d) Pelvic congestion and premenstrual pains in the lower abdomen

These symptoms can often be reduced by the herb 'crampbark' which has been used by the American Red Indians for centuries to bring relief of period pain. Crampbark contains an alkaloid substance which has an anti-spasm effect on the uterine muscle and therefore reduces the pain of the muscular contractions of the period. The botanical named for crampbark is viburnum opulus. The minerals calcium and magnesium also have an anti-spasm effect on the uterus, thereby reducing premenstrual period pains.

Sexual frustration and failure of orgasm can lead to congestion of the blood vessels around the uterus and ovaries, resulting in dull dragging pains in the lower abdomen and upper thighs. A healthy sex life, masturbation, aerobics and yoga can all bring relief.

(e) Low blood sugar (hypoglycaemia)

As the oestrogen and progesterone levels drop premenstrually the blood sugar levels (BSL) may become a little unstable, with a roller coaster effect being produced. When the blood sugar level reaches a low point, a craving for food, particularly sweets, becomes very strong and, in many cases, irresistible. A woman with premenstrual hypoglycaemia may be able to control her diet and weight at most times, but premenstrually she often loses control and will regain the weight she has fought so strenuously to lose during the first part of the cycle. She will crave for chocolate, sweets, soft drinks and coffee and find these things give her a temporary high of energy, only to leave her feeling flat and tired two hours later, and the cravings return.

Thankfully this vicious cycle is preventable by taking supplemental doses of the minerals chromium and zinc along with B vitamins 1 and 6. The dosage of chromium required is 500 micrograms daily, and zinc, fifty milligrams daily. Chromium and zinc help to stabilize blood sugar levels because they aid the insulin hormone to regulate the entry of sugar into the body cells. The B vitamins help the cells to break down the sugar for energy and therefore the metabolism of the sugar becomes more efficient.

Chromium and zinc are available in several different forms: some comprehensive multivitamin tablets or in trace mineral yeast powder.

Other measures that women who suffer from low blood sugar should take are the ingestion of small frequent meals containing protein, and the avoidance of refined carbohydrates, sugar, excessive alcohol and coffee.

(f) Skin problems
The immune system seems to be adversely affected by the low levels of female hormones premenstrually and this is why an outbreak of acne, herpes or eczema is more likely at this time.

To aid the immune system, zinc and manganese should be taken along with the vitamins B1, B6 and vitamin E. Oil of evening primrose and high dose garlic capsules will also boost the immune system to help overcome these premenstrual skin disorders.

Now we have dealt a deathly blow to the most notorious symptoms of PMS, you may be left feeling that it is just all too complicated to remember or attempt. I will admit that even for the most 'together' lady it is hard to recall, so for a woman in the throes of PMS it is surely impossible to remember all the above indicated substances.

However, take heart, for you can obtain the vast majority of these vitamins, minerals and herbs described as being of benefit during PMS in one tablet. Many good multivitamin preparations are available, but make sure you find one that has the essential factors I have mentioned. You can also be guided by your doctor's opinion.

To make it easier for you I have designed a practical reference table (Table A) which will enable you to choose the best natural treatments for your individual PMS symptoms.

Handy diet tips to overcome PMS

Many dietary recommendations have been made in Table A and need not be repeated here. There is no need to be fanatical regarding your diet as I have seen health food fanatics almost collapse from a nervous breakdown in trying to avoid the least trace of chemicals and preservatives in their meals – relaxed moderation is the key.

1 Basic diet proportions should be approximately:
Protein 20 to 30 per cent
Complex carbohydrates 45 to 60 per cent
Fats 15 to 20 per cent

2 Eat a wide variety of natural and raw foods as these are living foods which can regenerate a stagnant metabolism.

3 Grow some fresh fruit, vegetables and herbs in your garden. If you live in a flat you can still do this using pots.

4 Eat regularly:
(a) high calcium foods – figs, dates, almonds, fish, low fat milk and yoghurt.
(b) high potassium foods – olives (unsalted), beans, peas, lentils, raisins, bananas, raw fruit juices.
(c) high magnesium foods – almonds, barley, figs, dates, walnuts, oats.
(d) high iron and sulphur foods – spinach, lentils, strawberries, beetroot, liver, lettuce, figs, carrots, cabbage, dates.

5 Include fibre in your diet in the form of unprocessed bran, wheatgerm and raw fruit and vegetable salads – celery, apples and fenugreek are especially high in fibre.

6 If you have a tendency to low blood sugar you should have small frequent protein meals (for example every three to four hours), as opposed to three large meals per day. Some of this protein can be obtained from low fat meats and dairy products but a significant proportion should come from vegetarian sources. Excellent first class protein can be obtained by combining any three of the following – nuts, seeds, legumes and grains *at the same meal*.

In summary, if you follow the recommendations in the naturopathic table, along with the suggested dietary changes, you will have a 70 to 80 per cent chance of relieving your PMS. It may take three to four months before full relief comes, and there will be the occasional blue day despite your efforts. But take heart, for the benefits will be sure and lasting and there are thousands of your sisters out there with exactly the same challenge to overcome.

However if you find that after three to four months on this programme you are still suffering from PMS, particularly if you are approaching the menopause, hormonal therapy may be just the thing to tip the scales in your favour. Let us now take a look at the fascinating subject of hormonal treatment for the premenstrual syndrome.

Table A

Premenstrual symptom	Vitamin required	Mineral required	Herbs and oils required	Life-style and dietary modifcations
Fluid retention with swollen limbs, bloated abdomen, pelvic congestion, congestive headaches, weight gain due to fluid	B6 (pyridoxine) C – best form is pure calcium ascorbate powder	potassium, magnesium	diuretic herbs: juniper, parsley, uva ursi, buchu, crampbark, ruscus aculeatus, beta rutosides, hamamelis, aesculus	**Avoid:** 1 excessive fluid – restrict fluids to 1½ litres daily premenstrually 2 salt and processed packaged foods **Increase:** fresh fruit and vegetables
Breast tenderness and lumpiness	B1 + B6, E + C	potassium chloride, iron phosphate, selenium	garlic capsules, primrose oil	**Avoid:** 1 excessive saturated animal fats 2 salt 3 coffee and alcohol **Increase:** 1 fish 2 cold pressed vegetable oils and raw seeds 3 fresh fruit, vegetables and garlic 4 wheatgerm and soya beans

Skin problems – acne, herpes, eczema	B1 + B6, C, A	zinc	garlic capsules, primrose oil	**Avoid:** 1 smoking cigarettes 2 alcohol and drugs **Increase:** 1 cold pressed vegetable oils and raw seeds 2 sardines, seafoods and fish liver oils 3 raw vegetable and fruit juices, especially carrot and citrus 4 dandelion, alfalfa, capsicums, watercress and parsley
Emotional and psychological symptoms	B1 + B3, B6	zinc, magnesium, calcium	passiflora, camomile, valerian, scullcap, hops	**Avoid:** 1 excess alcohol 2 heavy smoking **Increase:** 1 high calcium foods, for example, fish, low fat dairy products and raw seeds 2 high magnesium foods, for example, green leafy vegetables, raw nuts and seeds, low fat cheese, eggs, brown rice, bananas and avocado 3 foods high in vitamin B6: wheatgerm, yeast, cabbage, oranges, lemons, wholegrain cereals, vegetables, malt, bananas and molasses

Premenstrual symptom	Vitamin required	Mineral required	Herbs and oils required	Life-style and dietary modifications
Low blood sugar (hypoglycaemia)	B1 + B6, C	chromium, zinc, manganese	liquorice root, oats, ginseng	**Avoid:** refined carbohydrates, lollies, chocolate, sweets, white flour, caffeine beverages and soft drinks **Increase:** foods with a high chromium and zinc content, for example, chicken, liver, shrimps, cabbage, carrots, green beans, peppers, lettuce, potatoes, apples, bananas, oranges, wholegrains and trace mineral yeast

Hormonal treatment of PMS – progesterone therapy

This is a rather controversial subject as some researchers believe staunchly in its effectiveness while others feel it is unproven and a last resort. I feel it has a role in severe PMS that interferes with normal working capacity and life-style and, particularly, where there is a risk of premenstrual suicide, child battering or alcoholism.

Dr Katharina Dalton has been the greatest advocate of natural progesterone therapy and she has achieved great success with it in her thousands of PMS patients. She believes that natural progesterone is superior to the synthetic progesterones. Some of the synthetic progesterones have masculine properties and tend to cause a worsening of PMS.

How is natural progesterone administered?

Unfortunately it cannot be taken by mouth as it is rapidly broken down by the liver and inactivated. It can only be given by deep oily intramuscular injections, vaginal and rectal suppositories, or by surgical implantation into the fat of the abdominal wall.

Dosages:

1 *Injections*: 25 to 100 milligrams daily.

2 *Vaginal pessaries or rectal suppositories*: 200 to 400 milligrams three to four times daily.

3 *Implant*: five to twelve pellets of 25 or 100 milligrams are implanted surgically into the abdominal wall.

Very severe PMS sufferers may find that the effect from suppositories is too shortlived and will require daily injections. The injections or suppositories are begun five days *before* symptoms of PMS are expected to occur and given daily, up until menstruation. Every woman is different, as can be seen by her menstrual symptom calendar, but the usual initial course of natural progesterone injections or suppositories is from day 14 up until the onset of menstrual bleeding. If PMS persists during menstrual bleeding, progesterone may be continued during the first few days of bleeding. The dosages and duration of treatment can easily be juggled by your doctor and yourself, to suit your individual pattern of PMS. Once a woman is established on natural progesterone therapy she may be given permission to use an extra suppository if she feels an increase in very distressing symptoms during the day.

For how long does a progesterone implant provide relief?

This may vary from three to twelve months and the effect will gradually wear off with a recurrence of mild PMS symptoms which will tell the woman it is time for another implant. Interestingly it is often her family who first notice that the implant is wearing off.

For how long is natural progesterone given?

Natural progesterone suppositories, called Cyclogest, are available on prescription. A three month course is usually necessary, after which time the course can gradually be reduced and finally stopped. If PMS recurs when the progesterone is stopped, it may be necessary to continue it for a much longer time and in some severe cases up to the menopause. There does not appear to be any risk of addiction to progesterone and resistance to its beneficial effects does not develop.

Are there any side effects from natural progesterone?

1 If the dosage chosen is excessive there may be euphoria, restless energy, insomnia, faintness and menstrual cramps. If these are present the dosage needs to be reduced.

2 The menstrual cycle may be altered in length with either a reduction or increase being noted, and there may be some premenstrual spotting of blood.

3 Occasionally mild breakthrough bleeding may occur, but the actual menstrual bleed will usually be lighter than normal.

4 Weight gain is usually not a problem.

5 Change in libido may be noted, either increase or decrease.

6 The oily injections may create painful areas in the buttocks and occasionally oil may collect there which can result in an abscess.

7 In a small number of women progesterone may raise blood sugar levels and thus is best avoided in diabetic women.

8 The vaginal pessaries contain wax which melts and may cause an unpleasant vaginal discharge. The rectal suppositories may result in soreness of the anus, diarrhoea and excessive wind from the bowels.

Can you fall pregnant while taking natural progesterone for PMS?

Yes, as it will not act as a contraceptive when taken in the routine fashion for PMS and thus other methods of contraception will be required. If, however, a small dose of progesterone is begun early in the cycle, that is at day 8 and continued until day 13, when the high doses required for PMS can be started, a reasonable contraceptive effect can be obtained. Even so, it should not be fully relied upon.

Are there any synthetic progesterones
which have efficiency in relieving PMS?

Fortunately, for those women who do not like the idea of daily injections or suppositories, there is one 'synthetic' progesterone which has proven value in relieving PMS. This particular progesterone is called 'dydrogesterone' and is the most 'natural' progesterone available that can be taken by mouth and still be active in its effect. It is available on prescription.

Dydrogesterone is almost identical in chemical structure to the natural progesterone produced by our own ovaries and that is why it is so effective and safe.

In Europe, there has been widespread use of dydrogesterone in PMS and it has been found to be more than 70 per cent effective in relieving fluid retention, fatigue, low blood sugar, depression and menstrual cramps. Furthermore, dydrogesterone has been found to be remarkably free from side effects and does not cause changes in the blood, liver or weight and, very importantly, does not induce masculine side effects.

Dosage of dydrogesterone tablets is 10 milligrams twice daily from day 12 to day 26 of the cycle. In very severe cases, and especially if heavy painful menstrual bleeding follows PMS, then dosages can be safely doubled and the tablets started much earlier in the cycle.

My personal view is that dydrogesterone tablets should be tried before resorting to injections or suppositories of progesterone. I have found that dydrogesterone tablets are just as effective as progesterone injections and suppositories and they are much easier to administer.

Other synthetic progesterones, such as medroxyprogesterone, norgestrel and norethisterone are not very effective in relieving PMS.

In general, when treating a PMS sufferer with any type of progesterone, the long-term goal should be gradually to wean the woman on to the smallest possible dosage which relieves symptoms. I feel progesterone is very safe provided the woman remains under continual supervision to safeguard against any long-term side effects.

In the United States, natural progesterone injections and suppositories have not been approved by the US Food and Drug Administration for treating PMS although a few clinics have been given permission to use small doses of up to 200 milligrams daily for research purposes. This will not be enough for some severe sufferers; however, doctors may prescribe larger doses as long as they tell the patient that the drug has not been approved.

Other methods of treating PMS

Does the oral contraceptive pill have a role in relieving PMS?

This is a very individual matter and clinical trials have not provided a definite yes or no answer. I have found that in some PMS sufferers the symptoms are greatly worsened by the combined oral contraceptive, whereas others gain great benefit. It is a matter of trial and error. The oral contraceptive pill helps some women because it prevents the natural hormonal fluctuations and produces a constant level of synthetic hormones throughout the monthly cycle.

I have found that oral contraceptive pills containing the very masculine progesterones, norgestrel or levonorgestrel, often worsen PMS and are best avoided. In preference, use oral contraceptive pills containing the progesterone, norethisterone.

In women approaching the menopause I think a standard oral contraceptive pill is too strong and potentially dangerous as a treatment for PMS. However, a tailor-made pill of natural oestrogen and a progesterone such as dydrogesterone or medroxyprogesterone, administered in twenty-one-day cycles, can often be of great benefit to premenopausal women. This type of hormone replacement therapy can be started before the menstrual periods have stopped completely and will be effective in overcoming symptoms of both PMS and the menopause. It is often not realized that premenopausal women have a high incidence of PMS and need treatment for both imbalances.

What other special drugs may be tried in overcoming PMS?

1 Bromocriptine
This drug blocks the production of the hormone, prolactin, in the pituitary gland. Excessive production of prolactin has been associated with depression and breast pain. However, although bromocriptine has been shown to be effective in reducing breast pain, it is not helpful in overcoming the mental and emotional symptoms of PMS. Although the dosage is small, it often produces nausea, vomiting and fainting and I would not recommend it as a standard treatment for PMS.

2 Anti-depressant drugs
These drugs are sometimes prescribed in the hope of overcoming premenstrual depression. However, in practice, they tend to cause drowsiness and fatigue and do not help the physical symptoms. They can also cause a rise in prolactin which may exaggerate breast pain and cause weight gain. They need to be taken every day as they require two weeks to exert the full effect. I cannot recommend anti-depressant drugs as a standard treatment for PMS.

Answers to some common questions on PMS

1 Is PMS more common in women with a family history of PMS?
Yes, there is a definite hereditary influence and the type of PMS symptoms are often similar in mother and daughter.

2 Can women suffer from PMS after a hysterectomy?
Yes, if the ovaries are left behind they will still have fluctuations in hormone production which may produce PMS even though menstrual bleeding does not occur.

3 Is PMS more common in women with a past history of toxaemia of pregnancy or post-natal depression?
Yes, definitely so.

4 Can a woman passing through the menopause with irregular and infrequent periods suffer from PMS?
Yes, she may notice cyclical PMS symptoms for as long as two years after her menstruation ceases, and the severity of PMS can be great at this time.

5 Does PMS become more common with advancing age?
Yes, PMS is usually not severe in women under twenty years of age, and becomes more noticeable after the age of thirty, and for this reason it has been called the 'mid-thirties syndrome'.

6 Does the incidence of PMS increase with increasing numbers of children?
Yes, it appears to do so, and particularly if a woman has suffered from significant post-natal depression.

Post-natal depression

The problem of depression after childbirth is a common one, although it may seem surprising that after nine months of waiting the baby does not bring infinite joy. Long-term post-natal depression occurs in 5 to 10 per cent of women and about 2 in every 1000 suffer so severely that hospital admission is required. Mild post-natal depression (third-day blues) occurs in up to 50 per cent of women.

What are the symptoms of post-natal depression?

1 Depression with unhappiness, crying, loss of interest and motivation, loss of self-esteem and feelings of guilt.

2 Loss of sex drive.

3 Fatigue and irritability.

Typically the symptoms last only a few days but some women take many months before they feel like their old selves again.

What causes post-natal depression?

After childbirth the levels of oestrogen and progesterone come rocketing down and, by the third day after birth, have reached very low levels. This causes the miserable and irritable feelings, especially as the woman has been accustomed to a sense of well-being due to the very high levels of hormones during pregnancy, levels which can make some women quite euphoric.

Another factor which may aggravate this depression is a feeling of isolation. The new mother is often confined to the house with the baby. This feeling of isolation can be particularly difficult for single mothers. The demanding and exhausting routine of caring for a new-born, excessive weight gain during pregnancy and a painful vaginal wound or cracked nipples can all add up to create a negative experience.

How can you cope with post-natal depression?

In exactly the same manner as you cope with PMS, as their causes are similar – a lack of the precious female hormones. I advise women with post-natal depression to take a naturopathic preparation made up of the amino acid supplements, tryptophan 1000mg, tyrosine 1000mg and phenylalanine 500mg daily, on an empty stomach with a sweetened beverage. These are approximate dosages and you should be guided by your own doctor or naturopath.

You should also take:

1 AB complex vitamin, one tablet with every meal.

2 A suitable iron supplement, 200mg daily.

3 A calcium supplement, providing 1000mg of elemental calcium daily.

The diet should consist of large amounts of raw fruits and vegetables and small frequent protein meals.

Fluid intake should be high and raw vegetable and fruit juices are an excellent source of the much needed mineral potassium.

If hormonal therapy is required, dydrogesterone is the most suitable preparation and is safe to take while breastfeeding. Natural progesterone injections, suppositories or implants may also be used.

Some women find breastfeeding aggravates post-natal depression, possibly because it stimulates increased levels of prolactin, so it may not be advisable to continue breastfeeding for longer than three months in cases of severe post-natal depression.

If you have a painful vaginal wound (episiotomy), please take:
Vitamin E, 200 milligrams daily,
Zinc chelate, 50 milligrams daily,
Vitamin C, 1000 milligrams three times daily.

Is life-style important?

Very. Excercise regularly and do not smoke heavily. Every woman is an individual and some women love to stay at home with the baby, while others need to get back into their individual hobbies and professions. They should plan to have a nanny or arrange daycare as soon as possible and in no way feel guilty about their choice. It is *most* important not to feel guilty as post-natal depression has a physical cause and is not a personality inadequacy on your part. With effective treatment you will soon get over this difficult milestone of motherhood.

Can you prevent post-natal depression?

Yes, simply by starting treatment immediately after delivery of the child. This is really good news as some women are literally terrified to have another baby, not because of labour pains or episiotomies, but simply because they vividly remember their last bitter episode of post-natal depression.

In summary

Some women who suffer from PMS may not want to stop taking sedatives or hormones and that is their prerogative. But at least women should have the bare facts upon which to make a rational decision for themselves and not be victims of a politicized health-care service in which different approaches to treatment are not mixed.

PMS is a disease that is shrouded in old-fashioned theories and prejudices, and a naïve sufferer can fall prey to treatments that are inappropriate and harmful on a long-term basis. Hopefully the veil of mystery has been lifted and the lid of Pandora's Box flung off. Now you can make your own well-informed choice in a market-place that is overbrimming with alternatives.

The minority of women who suffer from severe PMS may need to seek help from the best of both worlds, but the vast majority who have moderate to mild PMS will get complete relief from entirely natural substances that do not interfere with body metabolism. Remember, PMS is not a valium deficiency, a defect of personality or a synthetic hormone deficiency. PMS is a deficiency of your own ovaries which is aggravated by nutritional deficiencies. In the vast majority of cases the ovaries can be stimulated and sustained to be productive of an optimum amount of natural hormones without recourse to synthetic drugs.

5 Dysmenorrhoea (period pains) – we have come a long way!

As far as dysmenorrhoea or period pains are concerned, there is much water under the bridge and its currents sing a woeful and sad song.

Thanks to modern pharmacology, women can nowadays find humane and scientific relief, but our sisters of ancient and not so ancient times paved this road of progress with their suffering and shame. Let's listen to a few of their salutary stories.

Amongst Kolosh Indians of Alaska, when a girl showed signs of womanhood, she was shut in a little hut or cave which was completely blocked up with the exception of a small airhole. In this dark and filthy abode she had to remain for a year, without fire, exercise or associates. As for the Indians of Rio de la Plata, they used to sew a menstruating woman up in a hammock, as if she were dead, leaving only a small hole for her mouth to allow her to breathe. In this state she continued as long as the symptoms lasted. The Australian Aborigine, during the menstrual period, may not walk on any path frequented by men, nor touch anything used by men; she may not eat fish, nor go near the water, much less cross it. For, if she did, it is believed that fishermen would have no luck.

Dysmenorrhoea was first described as a medical disorder by the father of medicine himself, Hippocrates, who ascribed it to obstruction of the cervix. His treatment was unusual, to say the least, namely fumigation of the vulva with vapours of a decoction of sweet wine, fennel seeds, fennel root and rose oil! This idea reached its surgical conclusion in the early 1800s when successful treatment of dysmenorrhoea by dilatation of the cervix was first documented to have taken place.

Unfortunately, the story goes downhill from there. In Victorian

England, women had leeches applied, whilst across the Atlantic, women were fitted with a galvanic belt – galvanism (the use of electrical current) being in fashion at the time to cure all manner of ills. One doctor claimed great success from applying suction cups to the breasts of the sufferer!

These medical curiosities may seem amusing today, but they are insignificant compared to the confusion which led doctors to treat dysmenorrhoea by surgically removing the ovaries. This drastic treatment became so popular that, by the end of the last century, dysmenorrhoea was recorded as the major reason for the surgical castration of premenopausal women and, by 1906, 150,000 castrations had been carried out for this condition. Very severe sufferers were advised to have a hysterectomy. Naturally, many women became too frightened to complain lest they received such treatment.

After all these methods had failed, the frustrated medical profession next turned to the theory of 'psychological disturbance' as being the reason behind dysmenorrhoea, and women were subjected to half a century of psychological counselling for presumed mental disease. The belief that women with dysmenorrhoea were neurotic and ambivalent regarding their sexuality was very popular among doctors. One doctor even went so far as to warn his colleagues that 'interference with a woman's defences, such as period pains, might lead to outright psychosis'.

Thankfully, such confusion has gradually been cleared away by scientific medicine. The first big breakthrough in the treatment of dysmenorrhoea was the discovery in the 1930s that dysmenorrhoea was associated with ovulatory cycles and therefore could be prevented if ovulation was suppressed. The use of the oral contraceptive pill to suppress ovulation provided the first *real* pain relief for dysmenorrhoea and is still a valid and effective treatment today.

An even greater breakthrough came in 1957, when a certain Dr Pickles suggested that excessive prostaglandins in the menstrual blood could cause strong spasms of the muscular uterus, resulting in period cramps.

In the 1970s, it was realized that prostaglandins are found in nearly every cell of the body and therefore, must have a crucial role to play in human physiology. They were discovered to regulate the tone of the smooth muscles in the blood vessels, the uterus and intestines. If there are excessive prostaglandins in the menstrual fluid, there will be strong contractions of the uterine smooth muscles with resultant period pains. The smooth muscles are not under our voluntary control, in contrast to our skeletal limb muscles, and that is why we cannot reduce period pains by will-power alone. At last, a physical cause for period pains, not a psychosomatic one, had been discovered and woman's mind and soul were freed from guilt and shame.

What causes dysmenorrhoea or period pains?

At the end of each menstrual cycle, the fall in oestrogen and progesterone secretion by the ovaries precipitates the shedding of the layer of cells lining the uterine cavity (endometrium), in the form of blood. This shedding is accompanied by the release of prostaglandins into the uterus and menstrual blood. In some women there is an excess of prostaglandins in the menstrual blood and especially in the concentration of one particular prostaglandin known as 'prostaglandin F2 alpha' or PG2. In the search for the culprit responsible for producing painful contractions of the uterine muscle, this prostaglandin is the prime candidate. This can be easily proved, as if PG2 is injected intravenously into women it causes uterine cramps, bleeding, nausea, vomiting, diarrhoea and headaches.

Uterine contractions are painful when they are strong because they compress the blood vessels to the uterus and so cut off its blood supply. This lack of blood supply to an organ is called 'ischaemia' and it is the same phenomenon that occurs in a heart attack – perhaps dysmenorrhoea should be called a 'uterine attack'.

Not all menstruating women have this high level of PG2 in their uterus and not all women have equal sensitivity to its contracting action. This is why not all women suffer from period pains and yet, when they do, prostaglandins are always the main culprit.

How common is dysmenorrhoea?

Dysmenorrhoea affects over 50 per cent of menstruating women and there is no particular 'personality type' predisposed to suffer –

all menstruating women are susceptible. Even though suffering may be severe, women are reluctant to seek medical advice and fewer than a quarter visit their doctor about it.

How severe is dysmenorrhoea?

Perhaps the best way to judging the severity of dysmenorrhoea is to look at how much it interferes with a woman's normal daily activities. It is the most common cause of women being unable to attend school or work. In one study, 38 per cent of young adult women needed to take time off from their work or studies every so often, and a lower percentage regularly stayed at home. For a small but significant percentage of women with severe dysmenorrhoea, the pain can result in a total inability to participate in any normal activities and extreme debilitation.

It is not always realized that dysmenorrhoea sufferers may experience various other symptoms as well as period pains. Indeed it may be difficult to separate some of these from the premenstrual syndrome – for example fatigue, mood changes, headaches, as well as diarrhoea, nausea and vomiting.

Who gets dysmenorrhoea?

There are many unproved theories as to what sort of woman gets dysmenorrhoea. The fact is, virtually any menstruating woman can be a victim. However, it is uncommon in the first year after commencing menstrual bleeding and becomes more common in the early twenties. It probably gets less common in later adult years but this is not a straightforward trend because it may be more that the character of the pain changes. There have been suggestions that it is more frequent in women who smoke or are overweight but, again, the evidence is not categorical.

Before we delve into the relief of dysmenorrhoea, it is important for you to understand that there are two kinds of dysmenorrhoea, as the treatment required is different in each case.

1 Primary dysmenorrhoea

This type of pain is entirely due to the muscular contractions of the uterus as it expels its contained blood. These pains begin with, or just before, the onset of the blood flow, reaching a climax and gradually going away after twenty-four to forty-eight hours.

They are caused by prostaglandins inducing strong uterine contractions.

2 Secondary dysmenorrhoea

This type of pain is the result of some underlying cause other than strong muscular contractions of the uterus. The underlying cause will usually be some disease of the female organs in the pelvic cavity. The diseases most commonly implicated are infection of the tubes, ovarian cysts, uterine fibroids and endometriosis and these diseases require specific treatment by a gynaecologist.

Some other causes of secondary dysmenorrhoea are congenital abnormalities of the uterus and cervix which prevent a free flow of blood from the uterus. These can result in so-called 'obstructive dysmenorrhoea', with distension of the uterus by blood. Women with such a congenitally abnormal uterus will experience severe pain from the very first period.

The intra-uterine contraceptive device is a common cause of secondary dysmenorrhoea and heavy bleeding.

In some women with a hormonal imbalance, the uterus may become enlarged and congested, resulting in secondary dysmenorrhoea and heavy bleeding; this is quite common in pre-menopausal women and is called congestive dysmenorrhoea.

A very heavy and painful menstrual flow, especially if somewhat delayed, may be due to a miscarriage, so if you have not been using contraception it is important to see your doctor to exclude this possibility, as well as to determine whether you need a curettage to clean out the uterine cavity.

How can you tell if you have primary or secondary dysmenorrhoea?

Table B gives helpful distinguishing features between the two types of dysmenorrhoea.

What investigations will your doctor do if you are suffering from dysmenorrhoea?

Your doctor will do a vaginal pelvic examination during which the uterus, tubes and ovaries will be palpated. In a woman with primary dysmenorrhoea this examination will be normal.

Conversely, in a woman with secondary dysmenorrhoea, the

doctor will feel evidence of underlying disease in the pelvis, such as a uterus fixed in a retroverted (backwards pointing) position, tender lumps in the ovaries or tubes, an enlarged boggy tender uterus, and so on. If these signs of disease are found, usually a laparoscopy and ultrasound scan of the pelvis will be done. Using laparoscopy, the doctor will be able to visualize directly, by means of a telescope passed through the abdominal wall, diseases such as endometriosis or tubal infection, while the ultrasound scan will show up lumps and cysts in the tubes and ovaries.

Table B

Feature	Primary	Secondary
1 Timing in cycle	Pain only occurs around the time of bleeding	Pain often occurs at other times in cycle, apart from bleeding, and may be present continually
2 Relationship of pain to blood flow	Pain begins just before or with onset of bleeding and goes away once the flow is minimal	Pain often begins before bleeding starts and gets worse during the later days of bleeding
3 Consistency of pain	Pain remains the same with each period	Gradually worsens over time
4 Age at onset of pain	Young, usually within one or two years of first period	Older (20 to 30 for endometriosis, 30 to 40 for fibroids), but pain may begin with the very first period
5 Associated symptoms	Nausea, vomiting, diarrhoea, headache, depression	Painful sexual intercourse, bowel disturbance, fever, fatigue, infertility, breakthrough bleeding, urinary symptoms

If disease is found in the pelvis, a diagnosis of secondary dysmenorrhoea will be made and treatment will need to focus on eradicating the underlying disease, rather than suppressing the pain of dysmenorrhoea. In severe cases, such as large fibroids, tubal abscess or widespread endometriosis, surgery will be necessary, along with the use of antibiotics or strong hormonal therapy. In severe cases of secondary dysmenorrhoea, occurring in women who have finished childbearing, a hysterectomy may be the best solution.

In the majority of women, dysmenorrhoea is not caused by severe underlying disease and is just simple primary dysmenorrhoea.

Treatments for primary dysmenorrhoea

Anti-prostaglandin drugs

The obvious treatment is to give drugs which directly block the production and action of prostaglandins in the uterus. This will prevent painful uterine contractions which are the cause of primary dysmenorrhoea. These drugs are known as anti-prostaglandin drugs and include aspirin, naproxen, mefenamic acid, indomethacin and ibuprofen. Clinical trials with anti-prostaglandin drugs in over 400 women, treated during nearly a thousand painful menstruations, showed them to be extremely effective, so that when used by themselves no other type of analgesic was required. Patients were advised to take medication at the first hint of pain and repeat it four hourly – this gave an almost ninety per cent success rate in achieving total relief.

We know that anti-prostaglandin drugs will be effective if taken at the *first sign* of the period, whether this be pain or bleeding, but if you delay taking them, the results will be disappointing. Usually quite high doses are needed on the first day and these may be repeated every three to four hours. It may be necessary, however, for each individual woman to juggle the dosage and timing of her medication under her doctor's supervision to suit her particular needs. If treatment is started early enough, there may be no need to continue it into the second day.

What are the side effects of anti-prostaglandin drugs?

When they are used to treat dysmenorrhoea, they are usually only taken in high dosage for one to four days and when taken like this, they are very safe, as opposed to when taken daily over a long period of time.

Nevertheless, anti-prostaglandin drugs may occasionally cause some temporary damage to the kidneys and stomach, and women with underlying kidney disease or stomach ulcers should avoid them. Special care also needs to be taken by asthmatics, as these drugs can induce an acute asthma attack.

Women should also be aware that if they have an intra-uterine contraceptive device, anti-prostaglandin drugs may cause a reduction in the contraceptive efficiency of the device.

Hormonal therapy

1 The oral contraceptive pill

The combined oral contraceptive pill will stop ovulation and, in most cases of primary dysmenorrhoea, is a very effective preventative against pain and heavy menstrual bleeding. For women also desirous of effective contraception, it is the perfect solution; however for those not needing this, some might argue that it is a bit excessive to take the oral contraceptive pill for twenty-one days in every twenty-eight, just to prevent forty-eight hours of pain. It is a very personal choice and some will prefer to take anti-prostaglandin drugs for one to four days each month instead.

2 Progesterone

If dysmenorrhoea is associated with heavy bleeding, the prescription of a progesterone tablet may be reasonably effective in preventing these problems, if taken from day 5 to day 26 of every twenty-eight-day cycle. I personally recommend 'dydrogesterone', as it is the closest oral progesterone that we have to our body's natural progesterone.

Another suitable oral progesterone is medroxyprogesterone acetate, although it may stimulate appetite in some women.

Remember, progesterones alone do not provide contraception and you will need to use other means.

3 Beta-sympathomimetic drugs

These drugs resemble adrenalin and act on the uterine muscle to produce relaxation; that is why they are often used to stop the contractions of premature labour. Unfortunately, when given in doses effective against dysmenorrhoea, there are usually adrenalin type side effects, such as fast heart beat, palpitations and anxiety, and thus this treatment is restricted to women who have very severe dysmenorrhoea resistant to the previously mentioned treatments.

A versatile approach

We are living in an interesting epoch in medical history – with the bringing together of the modern and the old, the allopathic and the naturopathic or, in other words, the synthetic and the natural. For many years there has been animosity and scepticism separating these two fields of medicine, but fortunately many medicos are realizing that by combining the two it is possible to achieve a better result. In other words, drugs and naturopathic medicines can work well together and enable smaller and less toxic doses of drugs to be used.

Being a twentieth-century woman is not always easy as women nowadays have far fewer pregnancies than their predecessors, which, although it has certain advantages, means that they must experience the discomfort of many more menstrual cycles. Why not take advantage of the best of both worlds to ease the dilemma of being a modern woman?

Suitable analgesics to take at the first sign of period pain are aloxiprin 600mg and codeine phosphate 15 to 30mg. They can be repeated every four hours. They can be combined with the herbs crampbark 100mg and cimicifuga 75mg, and the anti-spasmodic minerals calcium phosphate 500mg and magnesium phosphate 500mg. These naturopathic remedies can be taken along with the above mentioned analgesics every four hours.

Miscellaneous questions concerning dysmenorrhoea

Will having a dilatation and curettage relieve dysmenorrhoea?

No, not for more than two or three menstrual cycles and indeed, if it is overdone, the circular fibres of the cervix will be disrupted, resulting in a weak and lax cervix that can later cause premature labour in pregnancy.

Does the old notion that having a baby cures dysmenorrhoea hold any truth?

Perhaps a grain of truth because after a first pregnancy the density of nerve fibres within a given area of uterine muscle is reduced. However, in practice, it is not always the case and seems to be a little mythical.

Now we know that dysmenorrhoea has a physical cause, is it possible that psychological factors still play a role?

Not usually, although in a woman who is dominated by her mother's attitudes and experiences, there may be a transference of the mother's suffering to that of the daughter. If a woman is really under a lot of pressure, this can act to produce a hormone imbalance which may worsen dysmenorrhoea and increase the amount of menstrual bleeding.

Can women with lower back pain suffer from a greater degree of dysmenorrhoea?

This seems to be a common association, and not always a fortuitous one. It appears that lower spinal problems may cause imbalances in the nerve and blood supply to the pelvis and this may worsen pelvic congestion and pain. Thus, yoga and a visit to a reputable chiropractor who can give spinal exercises and gentle spinal manipulation may bring significant relief. Some women find that acupuncture to points in the inner legs and lower abdomen and back, combined with massage of tender body points, is worthwhile.

Can a change in life-style aid women with dysmenorrhoea?

An abundant oxygen supply to the pelvic organs is necessary for optimum health and thus heavy smoking should be curtailed and replaced with deep breathing and regular exercise. The diet should include high magnesium and calcium foods, such as raw vegetable and fruit juices, figs, low fat dairy products, nuts and raw seeds. Furthermore, it may be possible to alleviate dysmenorrhoea by improving the balance of prostaglandins in the body. To do this you should reduce saturated animal fats and increase polyunsaturated fats such as fish, raw seeds, cold pressed vegetable oils, vegetables, grains and fish liver oils. See Table 2 on page 376 which outlines this in more detail.

Pain at the time of ovulation

A significant percentage of women experience pain at the time of ovulation, as the egg bursts through the capsule of the ovary into the abdominal cavity. Ovulation occurs twelve to sixteen days before the onset of the next menstrual bleeding and its associated pain may last from a few minutes up to twelve hours. Ovulation pain rarely lasts longer than this and is usually a sharp pain felt low down in the abdomen on one side. If ovulation occurs from the right ovary, the pain will be right-sided and vice versa. There may be a slight vaginal blood loss at the time of the ovulation pain.

German doctors have named ovulation pain *Mittelschmerz*, which means literally 'middle pain', as it occurs around the middle of the menstrual cycle.

What treatment is available for ovulation pain?
1 The combined oral contraceptive pill will stop ovulation and is entirely effective.

2 Analgesics such as aspirin or codeine combinations can be taken to relieve acute pain.

Some women notice that from the time of ovulation up to the onset of the next period, they feel a dull ache or heaviness and bloating in their lower abdomen.

In the majority of cases, this ache is due to congestion of the blood vessels in the pelvis and can often be relieved naturally without drugs by taking:

1 Odourless garlic capsules, two capsules three times daily with food.

2 Vitamin E, 100 milligrams daily.

3 Calcium ascorbate (vitamin C) powder, a quarter of a teaspoon, four times daily in juices.

4 A naturopathic preparation containing beta-hydroxy-rutosides 100mg, nicotinic acid 10mg, bioflavonoids 100mg, calcium ascorbate 150mg and the herbs ruscus aculeatus 50mg, aesculus 20mg, hamamelis 20mg, ranunculaceae 10mg. Dosage: two tablets three times daily.

In summary

This chapter has given practical suggestions and, if applied, you should gain significant relief. Life is not always easy for the female species, particularly when the passing of PMS is only followed by more pain and suffering as the blood flow commences. Many women feel trapped by recurrent cycles that are fraught with pain and tension which seem to serve no purpose. They often ask, 'Does my life revolve around my role of procreation and why can't males go through this?' These questions are valid enough but unfortunately they don't change the irrevocable facts. However, rather than grin and bear it, or worse, feel guilty, be prepared to beat it.

6 Contraception – the bare facts

The oral contraceptive pill (OCP)

The oral contraceptive pill contains various amounts of the two synthetic female hormones, oestrogen and progesterone. Most women take a combined OCP, which is a standard type of pill containing both oestrogen and progesterone. A minority of women use the 'mini pill' which contains only the hormone progesterone – this pill is also known as the 'progesterone only pill'.

The combined OCP is the most effective contraceptive available because it prevents ovulation and is 99.9 per cent effective, if taken correctly. The mini pill is less effective as a contraceptive with a failure rate of four per cent. This means that if a hundred women take the mini pill for one year, four of them will become pregnant.

The combined OCP

1 A fixed dosage OCP
A fixed dose of oestrogen and progesterone is taken for twenty-one days every twenty-eight days and gives a regular twenty-eight-day cycle, with menstrual bleeding occurring during the seven-day break. Some women prefer to take lolly pills during the seven-day break which contain only sugar, as this way they don't have to rely on their memory to know when to stop and start again.

2 Variable dosage OCP
In these pills the amount of oestrogen and progesterone is gradu-ally increased over twenty-one days. The seven-day break is still taken and the cycle will still be a regular twenty-eight-day one.

The variable dosage OCPs are known as biphasic or triphasic and their great advantage is that over the whole twenty-eight-day cycle a lower *total dose* of oestrogen and progesterone is taken.

3 Sequential OCP

In the sequential OCP, oestrogen only is given for the first part of the cycle, and then progesterone is added for the last ten to twelve days. See Figure 16.

The length of the cycle can be twenty-eight days if desired, or longer, with a regular menstrual bleed occurring during the seven-day break. The sequential pill is also called the 'tailor-made pill' as it is necessary that your doctor write a special prescription for a pill combining the types of oestrogen and progesterone that suit your particular requirements. It is very good for women who are sensitive to progesterone and get such side effects as increased appetite, acne and depression when using a fixed or variable dosage OCP. The sequential OCP is not as effective a contraceptive as the fixed and variable dose OCPs and has a two per cent failure rate.

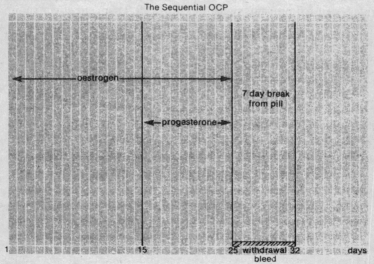

Figure 16

A great advantage of the various kinds of combined OCP is that a woman can control her cycle and if she does not want a menstrual bleed, because of a honeymoon or sporting event, for example, she can simply keep on taking the active pills for as long as two to three months without the usual seven-day break. When she is ready for a menstrual bleed, she then takes the seven-day break from the pills.

Which type of combined OCP should you choose?

In general, stick to the lower dose pills as they are safer as regards possible side effects. Table C shows the best type of OCP to take if you have a tendency to any of the listed problems.

Apart from contraception, for what other reasons is the combined OCP prescribed?

1 Heavy painful periods – the OCP will usually make your periods lighter and less painful.

2 Irregular periods – the OCP will make your periods regular and you can control their timing.

3 In some cases of PMS, certain types of OCP will reduce many of the symptoms. It is wise to avoid pills containing the progesterones norgestrel or levonorgestrel as they can deepen depression. In PMS cases, Anovlar 21 is often a suitable OCP. A tailor-made sequential OCP is another appropriate choice.

4 Improvement in acne and oily hair. Once again Anovlar 21 is a good OCP for this, or a suitable alternative is to have a special sequential tailor-made OCP made up by an endocrinologist. The tailor-made OCP should contain a high dose of oestrogen and a feminine progesterone.

5 Ovulation pain – the OCP will prevent this completely.

6 In some cases of endometriosis the OCP can reduce symptoms and in early cases may actually result in a cure.

7 Some women with recurrent ovarian cysts find that the OCP reduces this problem, but this is not universal.

8 In women with some auto-immune diseases such as rheumatoid arthritis and collagen diseases, the OCP can have a beneficial anti-inflammatory effect.

9 In women who are worried by the small size of their breasts, the OCP, particularly the brands with a higher oestrogen content, may produce a desirable increase in breast size.

Table C

Problem	Avoid	Use
Acne, oily skin and hair, excess facial hair, depression, aggression and increased appetite	Masculine progesterones such as levonorgestrel and norgestrel	More feminine progesterones such as norethynodrel, and medroxyprogesterone acetate. In severe cases, a tailor-made sequential OCP may be best
Breakthrough bleeding	Very low dose OCP	OCP containing a higher dosage of oestrogen or OCP containing a stronger more masculine progesterone or triphasic OCP
Painful breasts	High oestrogenic OCP	Use OCP containing a masculine progesterone or a low dose OCP
Poor circulation	Masculine progesterones and high dose OCP	Low dose OCP containing the more feminine progesterones or triphasic OCP
Fluid retention	OCP containing a high oestrogen dose	Low dose OCP

Is the OCP safe?

Although deaths as a result of side effects of the OCP affecting the circulation occur, they are no more common than deaths due to the complications of other types of contraception, and are far fewer than the deaths that occur during pregnancy and childbirth.

There are certain medical conditions which make it dangerous for a woman to take the OCP and in these cases it should be completely avoided. These conditions are:

1 Pregnancy.

2 Cancer of the breast or female reproductive organs such as the ovaries, uterus, cervix and vagina.

3 Blood clots in the circulation.

4 Some heart diseases.

5 Liver tumours or active severe hepatitis.

6 Bleeding from the vagina of unknown cause.

7 Severe migraine headaches.

8 Some diseases of the circulation.

There are certain medical conditions which make it necessary that special precautions and supervision be exercised if the OCP is to be taken. Often it is safer to use another form of contraception. These conditions are:

1 Diabetes.

2 High blood pressure.

3 Obesity (weight over 30 per cent of ideal).

4 Gall bladder disease and gallstones.

5 Disorders that were caused or worsened by pregnancy such as jaundice, herpes, some ear diseases and skin pigmentation.

6 Smoking more than ten cigarettes a day.

7 Recent hepatitis or liver disease.

8 Fibroids of the uterus.

9 Breastfeeding.

10 Migraine headaches of the ordinary variety.

11 Age over thirty-five years, especially if a smoker or if suffering from poor circulation. If over forty-five years of age it is unwise for a woman to take the combined OCP.

12 High blood fats, for example, elevated cholesterol and triglycerides.

13 Very irregular menstrual cycles or a late onset of menstruation.

14 Multiple sclerosis.

15 Epilepsy.

16 Depression.

17 Large or tender swollen varicose veins.

What are the possible risks of taking the OCP?

When the OCP was first introduced, its oestrogen and progesterone dosage was too high and side effects such as nausea, vomiting, acne and weight gain were common. Over the last decade the dosage of hormones in the OCP has gradually been reduced, which has resulted in a dramatic reduction in these annoying side effects. Still, certain side effects do occur and these will be looked at individually.

1 Breakthrough bleeding
Breakthrough bleeding is bleeding occurring at other times in the cycle apart from the regular monthly menstrual bleed. It is a frequent complication with low dose OCPs and will often settle down after several months. If it does not, a higher dose OCP will be required. If breakthrough bleeding occurs on the same day in each cycle it is likely to be due to the OCP; however, if the bleeding is very irregular or heavy a vaginal examination, Pap smear and curettage of the uterus should be done.

2 Weight gain
This can be a real problem for some women and it is the OCPs containing a high dose of progesterone, particularly the strong

masculine (androgenic) progesterones, which cause an increase in appetite and facilitate fat deposition. It is necessary to change to a low dose OCP containing a more feminine progesterone and also to reduce intake of fats and sugars.

3 Pigmentation of the skin

In some OCP users the skin develops darker areas of brown pigmentation. This is called chloasma and is due to the oestrogen and progesterone hormone content in the OCP. To prevent chloasma use a sunscreen lotion and wear a broad-brimmed hat. Other skin and mucous membrane disorders that may be increased in OCP users are acne and vaginal thrush.

4 Circulatory disorders

There is an increased risk of high blood pressure, clots forming in the deep veins, heart attacks and strokes in OCP users. These problems are now rare with the modern low dose OCP, but they are far more likely in women over thirty-five years who smoke. In women at risk from these disorders, OCPs containing the masculine progesterones should not be used as they may increase the risk of blockage and hardening of the arteries.

The symptoms of these disorders may be severe chest pain, severe leg pain or swelling, sudden severe headaches, blurred vision or loss of sight. If any of these things occur, they should be reported immediately to a medical doctor and the OCP should be *stopped at once*.

5 Gall bladder disease

The risk of stones forming in the gall bladder is increased in OCP users.

6 Failure of menstruation (amenorrhoea)

For up to twelve months after stopping the OCP one per cent of women will not have their menstrual periods return. This results in temporary infertility until menstruation recommences, either naturally or with the help of ovarian stimulating drugs. Women who are more likely to suffer with amenorrhoea after taking the OCP are those who began menstruation late in life (after the age of fifteen), or whose periods were infrequent or very irregular before beginning the OCP.

7 Risk of cancer

If oestrogen is taken by itself there will be an increased risk of cancer of the uterus. However, the good news is that if progesterone is given along with oestrogen, as in the OCP, there is a *reduced* chance of cancer of the uterus and ovaries.

At the present time we are not sure if the OCP increases the chances of cancer of the breast and cervix, but it seems not to and, if any risk does exist, it is extremely small.

The risk of liver tumours is slightly increased in women who take high dose OCPs for a prolonged period.

8 Congenital abnormalities of the unborn child (foetus)

There is no evidence to show a higher incidence of abnormalities in the foetus of women who conceive *immediately after* stopping the OCP.

If a woman inadvertently continues to use the OCP for several months *during* early pregnancy there is a possible increase in limb shortening, heart defects and a variety of other congenital defects.

9 The control of epileptic fits

Control may be made more difficult by the OCP as oestrogen increases the electrical excitability of the brain, and may increase the number of fits.

The mini pill

The mini pill contains only one hormone, progesterone, in a small dosage and is totally free of oestrogen.

How does the mini pill work?

When taking the progesterone only pill, ovulation still occurs in 60 per cent of women, and thus the mini pill does not work in the same way as the combined OCP. The mini pill prevents pregnancy mainly by thickening the mucus in the cervix and thus making it difficult for the sperm to pass through and reach the egg. Thus, although an egg may be available to be fertilized the sperm cannot reach it in time.

What are the disadvantages of taking the mini pill?

1 An increased contraceptive failure rate of four per cent. This compares favourably with the intra-uterine contraceptive device.

2 Menstrual bleeding may be unpredictable and you will not be able to control its timing as you can with the combined OCP.

3 Increased risk of breakthrough bleeding.

4 A small percentage of mini-pill users complain of an increase in acne and weight gain.

5 The risk of a tubal pregnancy (ectopic pregnancy) is slightly greater in women taking the mini pill and thus it should be avoided in women with a previous history of ectopic pregnancy.

How do you take the mini pill?

It is necessary to take the mini pill *every day at the same time*, until the pack is finished, then another pack is started straight away. You do not take a seven-day break from the mini pill. The maximal contraceptive effect occurs three hours after taking the mini pill and thus if intercourse occurs at night, it is best to take the mini pill with the evening meal rather than just before retiring.

For whom is the mini pill suitable?

1 Women who are breastfeeding, as it does not affect the amount or composition of breast milk. Only small traces of the mini pill reach the breast milk and these are so low that they are of no importance to the baby.

2 Women for whom oestrogen is dangerous, for example, because they form blood clots or have liver disease.

3 Women who are overly sensitive to oestrogen and find that the combined OCP causes breast pain, nausea, fluid retention, migraine, high blood pressure and so on.

4 Women over thirty-five years of age who smoke heavily.

5 Women over forty-five years of age.

6 Women who have poor circulation.

7 Women who are diabetics and require long-term contraception.

In general, side effects of the mini pill are rare, since it does not cause such a large metabolic change in the body as does the combined OCP, and it can be an excellent method of contraception for many women.

The morning after pill (MAP)

It is possible to prevent a pregnancy if a very high dose of oestrogen and progesterone is taken *within seventy-two hours* of unprotected sexual intercourse.

In a woman not using contraception the risk of pregnancy varies greatly depending on the time of the cycle when intercourse occurred. It is greatest just before and after ovulation, around mid-cycle (i.e. in a twenty-eight-day cycle the days of risk are from days 7 to 17 inclusive) and some sources have estimated the risk in these days to be between 10 and 30 per cent. This risk goes up if there are multiple episodes of unprotected intercourse.

If intercourse has occurred a number of times and provided not more than seventy-two hours have passed since the first occasion, the MAP may still be used.

In what situations is the MAP useful?

1 Rape.

2 Unprotected mid-cycle intercourse.

3 For the woman who has intercourse rarely and does not wish to stay on the pill continually, or use barrier methods.

How effective is the MAP in preventing pregnancy?

The failure rate is fairly low and various reports put it between 0.16 per cent and 5 per cent, meaning that the MAP will prevent pregnancy in 95 per cent of cases and usually more. However, if the MAP fails and pregnancy still occurs, there is an increased risk that the pregnancy will occur in the Fallopian tubes (ectopic pregnancy).

Not all doctors believe in using the MAP and some are even unaware of its effectiveness; indeed it is often the informed woman who demands it. The MAP is very safe and may be used by any woman and, in many cases, it can provide a speedy relief from anxiety and guilt.

How is the MAP given?

A high dose OCP containing 50 micrograms of oestrogen (ethinyloestradiol) and 250 micrograms of progesterone (levonorgestrel) is required. Two of these tablets should be taken immediately and then another two twelve hours later.

This high hormone dosage may cause nausea and vomiting in a minority of women and it is wise to ask your doctor for an anti-nausea tablet or suppository to take in conjunction with the pills. If you vomit up the pills they must be taken again.

What do you do after you have taken the MAP?

Do not have unprotected intercourse for the rest of your cycle and see your doctor one week after the expected date of your next menstrual bleed. If your menstrual bleed does not arrive or is very light, a pregnancy test should be done as the MAP may have failed.

If pregnancy does occur, the hormones in the MAP will not damage or deform the growing baby if you do decide to keep it.

Handy hints for taking the OCP

1 If you are given a course of antibiotics by your doctor for an infection the OCP may not give adequate contraceptive protection during that time and you should use another method of contraception, such as condoms, during that particular cycle.

2 If you are taking long-term medication for epilepsy, tuberculosis or severe tinea infection of the skin you will need one of the high dose OCPs.

3 Remember, if you are starting the OCP for the first time, or after a break which is longer than the regular seven-day break, it will not be effective until you have taken it for fourteen days.

4 If you have a bout of vomiting or diarrhoea the OCP may not be effective, so avoid intercourse or use another method of contraception until your next period arrives.

5 If changing from a high dose OCP to a low dose OCP you will not be protected until you have taken the low dose OCP for fourteen days.

6 Check the date of your pill pack at the same time every day, to make sure you have not forgotten a pill. Take your pill at the same time every day.

7 Keep at least one month's supply of the OCP at home, so you don't run out, and always take it with you on holiday.

8 If you miss a menstrual period, don't panic, as this is not rare in OCP users. However, it is wise to have a pregnancy test done (on a blood sample) once your period is two weeks overdue, especially if you have been forgetful.

9 If you are booked to have a major surgical operation under a general anaesthetic, it is safer to stop the OCP six weeks before the operation date.

10 If you are less than sixteen years of age and in need of contraception the OCP is usually the safest choice. It is advisable to tell at least one of your parents and, although there may be initial objection, parents are usually relieved that you will not be at risk of an unwanted pregnancy. However, teenagers under sixteen are legally entitled to contraception without parental consent and help can be obtained from your GP or a family planning clinic.

11 While on the OCP visit your doctor every six months for a check-up of your weight, urine, blood pressure and breasts. Ideally, before beginning the OCP, a pelvic and vaginal examination should be done. A Pap smear of the cervix should be taken every one to three years, and every six months if you are a carrier of herpes or have genital warts.

12 If you have risk factors which increase the danger of taking the OCP such as age over thirty-five, smoking, obesity, high

blood pressure, a family history of diabetes or circulatory disease, it is wise to have some blood tests done before beginning the OCP and also every twelve months while taking the OCP.

The recommended blood tests are:
− blood sugar level
− blood fat level

13 If you forget to take a pill at the usual time, take it as soon as you remember, even if this means taking two pills in the same day. If you are more than a day late with the combined OCP or more than three hours late with the mini pill you can no longer count on the pill to protect you from pregnancy. If this happens continue your pack as normal but use additional methods of contraception for at least two weeks or until you start your next pill pack.

14 There are no medical reasons for taking a break from the OCP. The only reason to stop is the desire to fall pregnant or a lack of need for contraception.

Metabolic secrets of the OCP

Sometimes the OCP can be a mysterious drug in that it affects women quite differently according to their 'metabolic type', and yet the metabolic changes it induces in the body are constant and easy to categorize. Some women doggedly avoid the OCP because they find it brings depression, fatigue, weight gain and loss of sex drive, while others become more or less addicted to the happy equanimity and sense of physical well-being that the OCP gives them. Let us examine the various nutritional imbalances and symptoms that may be produced by oestrogen and progesterone in the OCP and how they may be relieved with various nutritional and naturopathic medicines. The OCP is an excellent method of contraception and it is a pity that many women discard it prematurely because of a few annoying side effects which could have been overcome by changing the type of OCP, as well as by using specific vitamins, minerals and herbal diuretics.

1 Depression
Depression is a common complaint of women on the OCP and

typically they complain of unpleasant moods, pessimism, dissatis-
faction, tension, crying and loss of libido. In OCP-induced
depression, sleep and appetite are relatively normal and this
differentiates it from constitutional depression which is a more
profound biochemical disturbance and does interfere with sleep
and appetite.

How can the OCP cause depression?

The OCP can cause an imbalance in the production of some
important brain chemicals, especially one named serotonin. Serotonin is a brain protein that exerts a controlling influence on
moods, psychological drive and sexual desire. Serotonin is made
in the brain from the amino acid (small protein), tryptophan.

To make serotonin, tryptophan needs adequate supplies of
vitamin B6 (pyridoxine), an essential enzyme for the conversion.
The OCP, however, can cause tryptophan to be shunted away
from its usual job of making serotonin, and this results in two
things:

(a) Increased requirement for B6.
(b) Less serotonin production.

These abnormal biochemical changes are induced in 80 per
cent of women on the OCP and this is why they are more likely to
suffer from depression, loss of libido and a relative deficiency of
vitamin B6. I hope you can now see that a little bit of boring old
biochemistry can be good for your mind and spirit!

OCP users with this type of depression will usually respond to
supplemental vitamin B6 and tryptophan which overcome the
metabolic imbalance in the brain and return production of serotonin to normal. In most cases, depression and fatigue will be
gradually eliminated and libido improved.

Doses of vitamin B6 should be between 50 and 200 milligrams
daily and B6 should always be taken along with its helper factors,
namely vitamins B1 and B3, manganese and zinc. A word of
warning here – dosage of vitamin B6 should never exceed 200
milligrams daily as overdosage is not only expensive, but also
detrimental to the nerves.

Tryptophan can be taken in a dosage of 400 milligrams three
times daily, and is far more effective on an empty stomach,

meaning two hours before or after meals. Good food sources of vitamin B6 and tryptophan are milk, eggs, whole grains and green leafy vegetables.

The depression may take four to six weeks to lift, so a little patience will be required to avoid throwing away an excellent form of contraception. If the depression is severe, it is often useful to change from the conventional OCP to a tailor-made sequential OCP which is less likely to cause depression.

2 Sugar metabolism

The OCP has a slight tendency to increase the blood sugar level (BSL) and this may be beneficial in women who suffer from a low blood sugar level (hypoglycaemia). Hypoglycaemic women find they are intermittently tired and hungry when the blood sugar level drops below 2.6 millimoles/litre and the OCP tends to even out this 'roller coaster' pattern of their blood sugar level. This can enable them to keep going for longer periods after eating, reducing cravings for carbohydrates and sugars and, thereby, aiding weight reduction. Conversely, in women with a predisposition to diabetes, the OCP may actually cause them to get it, and it must be withdrawn.

Blood sugar level control is aided by small regular meals (four to five meals daily) containing first class protein such as fish, eggs, dairy foods or low fat meat. Everyone these days knows that too much saturated fat is bad news and an excellent alternative source of first class protein is to combine any three of the following four food groups – nuts, seeds, legumes and grains – at the same meal.

3 Metabolic changes in the blood

Overall the OCP tends to increase the blood fats, cholesterol and triglyceride, although the increase is usually not drastic and not outside normal limits. In some women, cholesterol may actually decrease, presumably because of reduced appetite.

If a woman on the OCP has a family history of circulatory diseases, especially hardening of the arteries, she should have her blood fats measured after being on the OCP for six months to detect any adverse changes.

It is important for women with a tendency to high blood fats to avoid the masculine (androgenic) progesterones, such as levonorgestrel, norgestrel, norethisterone and lynoestrol. In preference, they should use the feminine (non-androgenic) progesterones such as medroxyprogesterone and norethynodrel. This is because the masculine progesterones tend to increase the undesirable low density fats, and reduce the desirable protective high density fats.

There are several naturopathic supplements which can help to reduce and maintain a desirable balance of blood fats to protect against possible changes induced by the OCP. They are:

(a) Calcium ascorbate powder, one quarter of a teaspoon in fruit or vegetable juices, four times daily.
(b) Garlic and lecithin capsules – these should be of the cold processed, high allicin variety, and an odourless form of these is available. To be effective, dosage must be high and please ensure that each capsule contains at least 270 to 300 milligrams of garlic, otherwise results will be disappointing. Dosage is two capsules, three times daily with food.
(c) Vitamin E with pectin, 250 milligrams daily, except in people with high blood pressure, who must not take vitamin E supplements.

Diet will also influence the blood fats and it is necessary to increase polyunsaturated fats to twice the amount of saturated animal fats before a reduction in cholesterol will be achieved. Good sources of polyunsaturated fats are fish (unfried), cold pressed vegetable oils, raw seeds, walnuts, primrose and blackcurrant oils and vegetables.

4 Metabolic changes in the liver

Oestrogen stimulates the liver to increase the production of many different proteins. This can result in confusion for doctors when interpreting some laboratory tests, as women on the OCP have a false appearance in their blood tests of excess thyroid hormone, cortisone, iron and copper, but this is of no metabolic consequence.

However, some important liver proteins are increased by the OCP, and among these are the clotting factor proteins which circulate in the bloodstream as raw materials for formation of a blood clot, in case you cut a blood vessel.

Thus women on the OCP form blood clots more easily, and sometimes unnecessarily in the blood vessels, causing blockages and deep venous thrombosis.

If you have been on the OCP for many years, or are over the age of thirty-five and have a suspect family history, you should get your doctor to measure the levels of clotting factor proteins in your blood – if they are very high it would be safer for you to go on a progesterone only pill.

The useful naturopathic supplements to reduce risk of clots are:

(a) Vitamin E with pectin, 250 milligrams daily.
(b) Garlic and lecithin capsules in the same form and dosage as detailed under 'Metabolic Changes in the Blood'.
(c) Cod liver oil, primrose oil, blackcurrant oil and deep ocean fish.

Another liver protein which is increased by oestrogen is renin, and this can result in an increase in blood pressure and fluid retention in susceptible women. These women should try to avoid conventional diuretic drugs on a regular basis as they can result in mineral deficiencies and fatigue. The most suitable diuretic drug is 'Aldactone' as it does not produce mineral deficiencies.

For women who find that the OCP induces fluid retention, swollen aching legs, or a worsening of varicose veins, I recommend a herbal diuretic tablet containing beta-hydroxy-rutosides 100mg, nicotinic acid 10mg, bioflavonoids 100mg, calcium ascorbate 150mg, and the herbs ruscus aculeatus 50mg, aesculus 20mg, hamamelis 20mg, ranunculaceae 10mg. Dosage is two tablets three times daily. This is extremely effective in reducing fluid retention without causing any side effects.

5 Skin metabolism

There is no doubt that OCP produces changes in our cellular immune system which can make some women more susceptible to fungal infections. These infections may not be dangerous, but they can still produce annoying symptoms. Various skin infections which may be worsened by the OCP are:

(a) Acne.
(b) Fungal skin infections: an infection with a fungus called pityriasis may really take off, causing pink, brown and white scaly skin patches of unpleasant appearance.
(c) Tinea.
(d) Warts: there is a suggestion that the growth of venereal warts due to the wart virus is encouraged by the OCP; however, the risk of catching this infection is not increased.

6 Vaginal metabolism

The growth of the fungus, candida albicans, is increased by oestrogen and vaginal thrush may be more difficult to eradicate in OCP users. A useful measure to increase vaginal resistance to thrush is to douche once or twice weekly with a culture of lactobacilli. This helps to maintain a healthy vaginal acidity. (See page 230 for more information on douching.) The OCP does not increase the risk of recurrences of herpes.

In all the above skin and vaginal infections, specific supplements to boost cellular immunity should be taken. They are:

(a) Zinc supplement 50mg, twice daily with food.
(b) Pure calcium ascorbate powder, one quarter of a teaspoon four times daily in raw juices. This is very useful as some studies have suggested that the OCP reduces blood levels of vitamin C and also reduces the effectiveness of vitamin C supplements.
(c) Garlic capsules are a useful antibiotic against a broad range of fungi and bacteria. The dosage for these is two capsules three times daily with food.
(d) Extra folic acid should be obtained from a high consumption of raw fruits and vegetables as well as their juices.
(e) Vitamin B12 injections or tablets should be taken by vegetarians on the OCP.

Tea tree oil cream is helpful if applied directly to patches of skin affected by fungal infections such as candide.

In summary

It can be seen that the OCP induces widespread metabolic changes, just like all drugs. In most women these changes remain within normal limits and do not produce distressing symptoms. However, when they do, these symptoms can be reduced and moderated by correct diet and specific naturopathic supplements. If you visit your doctor regularly the OCP is very safe, as obvious signs of metabolic derangements, such as high blood pressure or blood fats and high sugar levels and depression, will be detected before any permanent damage results.

Even if you are currently taking the OCP without any obvious side effects, you may be surprised at the benefit obtained by taking some of the nutritional supplements mentioned in this chapter. These may induce a worthwhile increase in your energy reserves and improvement in your mood and libido, as well as skin appearance.

Mechanical methods of contraception

The intra-uterine device (IUD)

The IUD is a small metal and/or plastic object that is placed inside the cavity of the uterus, where it acts as a contraceptive because it prevents implantation of the fertilized egg. See Figure 17.

There are various shapes and sizes of IUDs (see Figure 18) and the copper ones have a copper wire coiled round their plastic stems. There is a fine string attached to the end of the IUD which passes down through the cervix into the upper vagina. This string is not noticeable during sex, and is useful as a woman can check its length. If it remains the same, she will know that the IUD is in the correct intra-uterine position.

The use of the IUD goes way back in history. Arabian camel riders used to place a stone in the uterus of their female camels to prevent conception during their long treks in the desert.

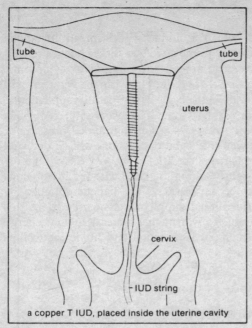

a copper T IUD, placed inside the uterine cavity

Figure 17

How does the doctor insert an IUD?

Firstly, the doctor will do a vaginal and pelvic examination to check the size and position of your uterus. A long thin graduated metal rod will be passed through the cervix into the uterus to measure the length of its inside cavity.

The IUD is compressed into a thin plastic introducer tube which can easily be slipped through the cervix into the uterine cavity, after which the introducer is removed, leaving behind the IUD.

The procedure can usually be done with a local anaesthetic in the cervix or with some intravenous analgesia if necessary. However, in younger women, who have never been pregnant and have a small uterus, a general anaesthetic may be more desirable.

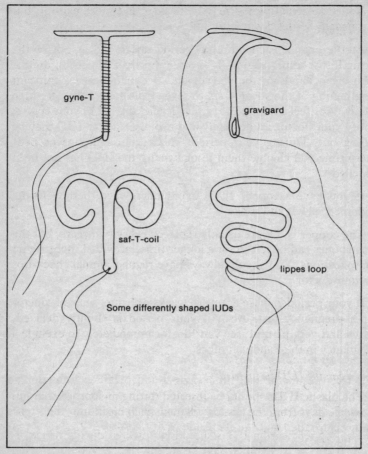

Figure 18

What happens after the IUD has been inserted?

1 You should avoid sex or the use of vaginal tampons for forty-eight hours.

2 You may notice some cramps in the lower abdomen along with some light spotting of blood. This should settle down after three months.

3 Your menstrual period may be heavier and more painful, but this usually settles down with time.

4 At the end of each monthly period check the length of the string in the upper vagina. It is often most convenient to do this with clean hands in the shower and if you notice a significant lengthening of the string – six to seven centimetres (two to three inches) – or feel a hard piece of plastic sticking out of your cervix, notify your doctor immediately and avoid sex as the IUD may be falling out. During your period, check your tampons or pads every time you change them to make sure the IUD has not been expelled.

5 If you have a copper IUD, avoid microwave therapy to the abdomen, pelvis and back.

6 The copper IUDs are usually replaced every two years, but the plastic ones can be left in for a longer time, provided there are no complications. You should always have regular annual check-ups by your doctor.

7 If your period is more than two weeks overdue, see your doctor for a pregnancy test. Also, if your period is slightly delayed, heavy and very painful, see your doctor immediately to exclude a pregnancy in the Fallopian tubes.

When can the IUD be inserted?

1 The plastic IUDs should be inserted during menstruation or up to twelve days from the first day of menstrual bleeding.

2 The copper bearing IUDs should be inserted during menstruation or up to seventeen days from the first day of menstrual bleeding in a twenty-eight-day or longer cycle. If an IUD is inserted after these days it can be very dangerous as a newly fertilized egg may have deeply implanted into the uterus and this pregnancy will then continue with the IUD present.

3 At the same time as a termination of pregnancy.

4 Six weeks or longer after childbirth.

5 The IUD can be used like the morning after pill in a woman

who has had unprotected sexual intercourse during mid-cycle. If a copper IUD is inserted by day seventeen of a twenty-eight-day or longer cycle, this should prevent the fertilised egg from implanting in the uterus.

What are the risks in having an IUD?

1 Pelvic infection

The risk of all degrees of pelvic infection involving the tubes, ovaries, uterus and vagina is increased in IUD wearers. If this is not diagnosed or if it is treated incorrectly, scarring and blockage of the tubes may occur with resultant infertility. The symptoms of pelvic infection include lower abdominal cramps, fatigue, fever, painful sex, offensive vaginal discharge, heavy breakthrough bleeding and extremely painful periods. If you have any of these symptoms see your doctor immediately to check the IUD.

2 Expulsion of the IUD

The IUD may be rejected by muscle spasm of the uterus, or if the uterus and cervix allow it, it may simply slip out! The IUD can only go down into the vagina, it will not travel back up through the tubes into the abdomen. Thus it is very important that you check your upper vagina with your fingers after every menstrual bleed to see if the string has lengthened or if you can feel a hard plastic object. Of course, if the IUD is not in the correct position you will not be protected against pregnancy.

3 Perforation of the uterus

If the IUD is inserted with a rough technique or if the uterus is very soft, as in just after childbirth, the IUD may be forced through the uterus into the abdomen during insertion. If this occurs an abdominal operation will be necessary to retrieve the IUD. This occurs rarely (less than 1 in 1000 insertions) but it is important to have your IUD inserted by a doctor with special expertise in this area.

4 Ectopic pregnancy

It is known that pregnancies occurring in women using IUDs are more likely to be in an abnormal or ectopic position, than in women without IUDs. This is particularly so if pelvic infection is present. The pregnancy usually grows in the Fallopian tubes but may also, very occasionally, grow in the ovary.

Recently the copper 7 IUD has been withdrawn from use in the United States because the manufacturing company has been faced with hundreds of lawsuits. This is not because IUDs are extremely dangerous, but rather because Americans love to sue each other in a legal system which encourages the overuse of lawyers. The plaintiffs were litigating against some of the common complications of IUDs that I have just mentioned, and yet, any woman who has an IUD these days should be aware that she is taking a calculated risk, and must be willing to accept this. The manufacturing companies disclose all these facts and are not at fault. A woman contemplating an IUD should make sure she knows all the facts, including the risks, before making a final decision. These risks are not small and if they are unacceptable an IUD should be avoided.

What medical conditions can make it dangerous for a woman to use an IUD?

1 Pregnancy already existing.

2 Pelvic infection.

3 Abnormal shape of the uterus, for example, congenital abnormality or large fibroids.

4 Abnormal shape of the cervix.

5 Cancer of the uterus or cervix.

6 History of previous ectopic pregnancy.

In women who already have heavy painful periods, especially if associated with anaemia, the IUD should generally be avoided as it is likely to worsen this complaint.

In women with a small uterine cavity, the IUD is likely to be expelled or cause painful cramps and, for this reason, it may not be acceptable to young women who have never had children.

Women with certain diseases of the heart, especially of the

heart valves, would be safer to avoid the use of the IUD as it may act as a source of infection to these valves.

Should women who have never had children use an IUD?

If a woman wants to have children in the future she should think very carefully before having an IUD fitted. She must accept that an IUD brings an increased risk of pelvic infection and thus infertility, and if she cannot accept this risk she should use an alternative method of contraception. If a woman has several sexual partners she would be well advised to avoid the use of the IUD until she has had her family.

Is an IUD a reliable contraceptive?

IUDs are second to the OCP as a reliable method of contraception. The failure rate is estimated at three to four per cent.

What do you do if you become pregnant while an IUD is in place?

If your period is overdue, first have a pregnancy test done. If you are pregnant, this test usually shows positive ten days after conception. If the pregnancy test is positive you may request a termination or continue with the pregnancy.

If you decide to continue with the pregnancy it is desirable to get your doctor to remove the IUD gently. You should not try to attempt the removal of the IUD yourself. If it is not possible for your doctor to remove the IUD by pulling on its string, it should be left in place and unfortunately there will be a 25 per cent chance that the IUD will cause a miscarriage. Also, the continuation of the pregnancy with the IUD in place increases the risk of infection finding its way into the uterus and causing premature labour. The risk of a deformed baby is not increased if you become pregnant while an IUD is in place.

Diaphragms and spermicides

The vaginal diaphragm is another popular method of mechanical contraception and some women use it happily for many years, preferring to avoid chemical hormones and the risks associated with the IUD. Others find it intolerable to have a mechanical object in their vagina during love-making, although it is really only a mental block, as if the correct size of diaphragm is used, both sexual partners should be completely unaware of its presence. It is most important to be measured by your doctor to determine the correct size of diaphragm for you.

What is a vaginal diaphragm?

A diaphragm is a shallow rubber cup with a flexible metal rim. When it is properly fitted and inserted it covers the cervix and is 'locked' in place behind the pubic bone and the rear wall of your vagina – see Figure 19. The diaphragm is designed to serve two purposes:

1 It stops sperm from entering your cervical canal.

2 It holds a jelly or cream which kills sperm that may manage to swim around the rim of the diaphragm.

The diaphragm should *always* be used in combination with a spermicidal jelly or cream.

How do you insert the diaphragm?

Before inserting a diaphragm for the first time, it is important that you understand how to place it properly. Put your index finger, or your index finger and your third finger, in your vagina. Keeping your fingers straight move them inwards (up to the last knuckle) and back (towards the rectum) along the rear wall of the vagina. As you can see in Figure 20 your vagina does not go straight up but angles backwards.

Moving your fingers slightly forward, you will be able to feel a knob that is slightly harder than the walls of the vagina and shaped a bit like the end of a dented nose. That is your cervix, the opening to your uterus, and that is what your diaphragm must cover during intercourse. To the front of your cervix, you will feel your pubic bone. The front rim of the diaphragm must go above the pubic bone while the opposite rim goes against the rear wall of the vagina.

When the diaphragm is in place, the rubber will be wrinkled rather than lying flat. You should be able to feel the cervix through the rubber.

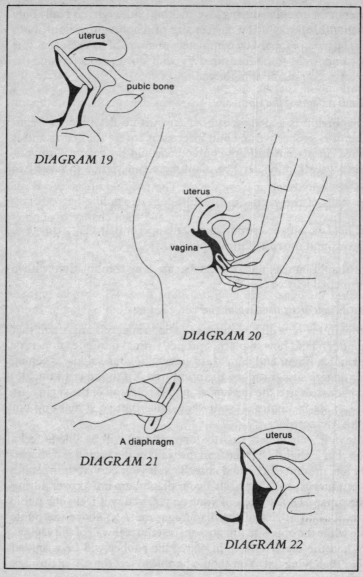

DIAGRAM 19

DIAGRAM 20

A diaphragm

DIAGRAM 21

DIAGRAM 22

Figures 19, 20, 21, 22

Preparing for insertion

1 Urinate and wash your hands.

2 Place one to two teaspoons of spermicidal jelly or cream into the dome of the diaphragm. Spread the spermicide around the inner surface of the dome and also a small amount around the rim. The spermicide on the rim makes the diaphragm easier to insert and helps seal the diaphragm in place. Too much jelly or cream can make the diaphragm too slippery to handle during insertion.

3 You can insert the diaphragm while you are standing with one leg up, squatting, or lying down. The position of the cervix and the walls of the vagina will be different depending on your position. If you are used to one position and then change to another, take extra care in positioning the diaphragm to be sure the cervix is covered.

Inserting the diaphragm

1 Hold the diaphragm with the dome down (spermicide up) and press the opposite sides of the rim together between your thumb and third finger – see Figure 21. The diaphragm can be held from above or below.

2 Spread the lips of your vagina with your free hand. Hold the compressed diaphragm dome down (spermicide up) and push it gently inwards along the rear wall of the vagina as far as it can go. Your index finger, kept on the outer rim of the diaphragm, will help you guide the diaphragm into place – see Figure 20.

3 With your index finger, push the front rim of the diaphragm up until it is locked in place just above the pubic bone – see Figure 19.

4 Using your index finger, check that the diaphragm is in place and is holding the contraceptive jelly or cream over the cervix. It is important that the cervix be covered by the diaphragm and spermicide and that the diaphragm be locked in place between the upper edge of the pubic bone and the rear wall of the vagina. You should be able to feel the cervix through the rubber shield. You

can feel the front rim of the diaphragm above the pubic bone, but you may not be able to follow the rim all the way around as your fingers may not be long enough – see Figure 22.

5 If, after some practice, you still find insertion awkward or difficult, vary your body and hand position slightly until you can insert the diaphragm comfortably, and get your doctor to check your insertion technique.

When should you have your diaphragm checked?

1 If you change your weight up or down by more than three kilograms (half a stone) you may need a new size.

2 If you or your partner are aware of the diaphragm during sex or if it slips down when you cough or strain.

3 After a pregnancy or termination of pregnancy you may need a new size.

4 After one year of use as it can develop holes.

When should you insert the diaphragm?

You may insert it any time in the six hours before sex commences, which is very comforting as you don't have to race off to the bathroom just when your partner gets in an amorous mood. A further application of spermicidal jelly or cream must always be inserted, without removing the diaphragm, before each recurrent episode of intercourse.

When and how should you remove the diaphragm?

It should not be removed for six to eight hours after intercourse. It can remain in position for twenty-four hours.

To remove the diaphragm put your index finger behind the front rim and pull the diaphragm down and out.

Is the diaphragm a reliable contraceptive?

Failure rates are quoted at the 10 to 15 per cent level, which is rather high, but I am sure this is often due to incorrect insertion or forgetfulness on the part of the user. It is a very safe method of contraception, the only possible side effect being allergy to rubber or spermicide. In these cases a plastic diaphragm may be preferable.

Condoms and spermicides

A woman may go through phases in her life when she is tired of shouldering all the burden of contraception and in this situation it may be an opportune time to remind a man that he is equally responsible; condoms are a good answer.

Condoms and spermicides *when used together* provide an excellent form of contraception, with a failure rate of only three to four per cent. They also protect women against the very real threat of sexually transmitted diseases, such as gonorrhoea, herpes, warts and possibly AIDS.

How do you use a spermicide?

The spermicide may be in the form of foam, cream, a pessary or jelly. Whichever it is, it is necessary to insert it no more than twenty minutes before intercourse. (Please see Figure 23 for method of using an applicator.) You must also insert a new application before each recurrent episode of intercourse.

Some women are worried that spermicides will increase the risk of congenital abnormalities in their babies if they conceive while using a spermicide, but there is no proof of this.

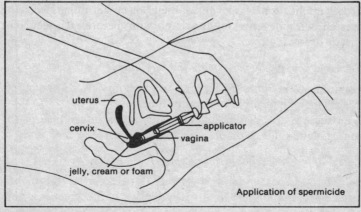

Application of spermicide

Figure 23

Surgical contraception

This is commonly known as sterilization; when it is performed in a woman it is called tubal ligation and when it is performed in a man, vasectomy.

In tubal ligation a small length of each Fallopian tube is either cut and tied, burnt, or crushed with plastic rings or clips – see Figure 24.

In vasectomy the tube which carries sperm from the testicle to the penis is cut and tied – see Figure 25.

Tubal ligation may be done through a small four to ten centimetre (two to four inch) surgical incision in the lower abdomen just above the pubic bone and this will not even leave a noticeable bikini scar.

Alternatively, tubal ligation can be done using the special surgical telescope known as a laparoscope, through two very small punctures in the abdominal wall.

Nowadays, burning of the tubes using a localized electrical current is usually avoided because it may cause burning of other

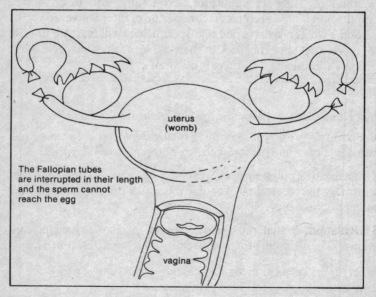

uterus
(womb)

The Fallopian tubes
are interrupted in their length
and the sperm cannot
reach the egg

vagina

Figure 24

adjacent structures, increase the risk of ectopic pregnancy and, if excessive tissue is burnt, result in premature menopause. Burning of the tubes is also avoided because it has a higher failure rate than other methods, and if a woman changes her mind, it is more difficult to reverse.

How effective is ligation of the tubes?

Overall, taking all the different methods into account, the procedure fails and results in pregnancy in three out of one thousand women. This is a very low failure rate.

If you later regret the decision can tubal ligation be surgically reversed?

If microsurgical techniques are used to repair the tied and cut tubes, subsequent pregnancy rates can be as high as 70 per cent, but a 100 per cent guarantee can never be given; thus, from the outset, the woman who chooses sterilization should regard it as an irrevocable act. Also the microsurgery needed to repair the tubes and reverse the ligation involves a difficult and tedious operation taking three hours.

Reversal is most likely to be successful if clips have been used on the tubes. If there has been significant destruction of the tubes as in the burning technique, or if the featherlike ends of the tubes have been removed, surgical reversal has a very poor chance of resulting in pregnancy.

What are some of the common myths concerning sterilization?

1 Fertility = virility is a common male misconception, and sexual potency, desire and performance are not changed by sterilization.

2 Sterilization will help sexual problems or marital conflicts – this is entirely untrue, unless of course the sexual problems are related to fear of pregnancy.

3 Ovulation, sexual satisfaction, sperm production and ejaculation will be different after sterilization – this is entirely untrue.

What factors should be taken into account when deciding whether to undergo sterilization?

Statistics have shown that the decision should be entirely voluntary

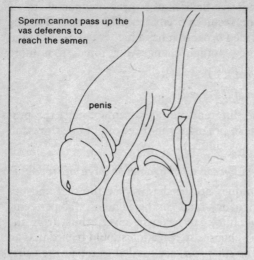

Figure 25

and not done because of spouse pressure. If a spouse is against the decision for sterilization of the partner, and it goes ahead, marital conflict and relationship breakdown often result.

It is very important to consider your future and look at how you would cope if your spouse died, your marriage broke up or some of your existing children died, before closing your options. It is especially important not to make the decision for sterilization during a crisis in your life, and also in general it is best to avoid making the decision immediately after the termination of a pregnancy or after childbirth, or during pregnancy. Indeed, it is best to wait at least six months after childbirth, in case the new-born child is not normal or dies.

Does tubal ligation have any physical side effects?

Some women find that their menstrual bleeding is heavier and more painful after sterilization, especially if they were on the OCP beforehand, and this has dissuaded a significant number of women from having the procedure done.

In very rare instances, a premature menopause may result if

there has been excessive destruction of the blood vessels to the ovary during the operation. This is particularly likely with the burning technique, if care is not taken.

Contraception after childbirth

When can normal sexual activity be resumed?

There is no special rule about this and whenever you feel like it, then that is the right time. There are no medical dangers in having sexual intercourse within the first few weeks of a normal childbirth. If you have had an episiotomy, however, you should check with your doctor first.

In a woman who has had a complicated labour involving forceps, drips, wires, an episiotomy and so on, it is understandable that sexual libido may take longer to return than in a woman who has had a totally natural birth with her husband closely involved.

After childbirth and during lactation the blood levels of the female hormones, oestrogen and progesterone, will be low and, for this reason, your sexual appetite and vaginal lubrication may very well be reduced, at least temporarily – don't feel guilty about this as it will pass and you will eventually regain your previous sexual abilities and desires.

Breastfeeding, will it prevent you from falling pregnant?

Breastfeeding has a potent anti-fertility effect, but only if suckling is very frequent, and it can never be relied upon completely. During breastfeeding there are high levels of the hormone prolactin which reduces ovulation and thus fertility, and it is very rare for ovulation to occur in the first three months after childbirth in a woman who is fully breastfeeding. If the baby is receiving supplementary bottle feeds or solids and suckling is less frequent, ovulation can return earlier than three months after birth.

An interesting study in India amongst women not using modern contraceptives reveals to us the long-term contraceptive efficiency of breastfeeding. If women lived in the country and suckled frequently, the pregnancy rates were only 50 per cent, twenty-three months after childbirth. If, however, women moved to the city where they suckled less, pregnancy rates reached 50 per cent after only nine months.

For the Western woman we can say that additional contraception during breastfeeding becomes necessary if:

1 The baby takes supplementary milk feeds or solid feeds.

2 The baby sleeps through the night.

3 The mother goes out to work all day leaving a long gap between morning and evening feeds.

Remember, you may fall pregnant *before* your menstrual periods resume, so if you are not taking precautions, monthly pregnancy tests may be a good idea. Once regular menstruation has resumed, your chances of falling pregnant are considerably increased, even if you are breastfeeding.

What contraception can be safely used after childbirth?

1   *The combined OCP*
(a) *If breastfeeding:* this should generally be avoided because a reduction in milk production may occur, and also some of the hormones contained in the combined OCP may pass through the milk to the suckling infant.
(b) *If not breastfeeding:* the combined OCP can be started two weeks or more after childbirth, but not before, as if given too early it may increase the risk of blood clot formation in the veins.

2   *The mini pill (progesterone only pill)*
This is an excellent method of contraception for women who are fully breastfeeding and if suckling is frequent it need not be started until eight weeks after childbirth. If breastfeeding is less frequent, it is better to start earlier, at about five to six weeks after childbirth.

The amount of the hormone progesterone contained in the mini pill is very small and only tiny amounts reach the breast milk – indeed it has been calculated that a breastfed child whose mother takes the mini pill would receive only one mini pill every two and a half years!

3 The IUD

This is a reliable method whether breastfeeding or not. Insertion is generally not done until six to eight weeks after childbirth, otherwise the device may be expelled from the enlarged uterus which is still in the process of shrinking. If insertion is delayed more than eight weeks after childbirth a pregnancy test should be done before insertion.

In a breastfeeding woman who is not menstruating, it is best not to use a copper IUD because of the theoretical risk of copper poisoning. A plastic IUD should be used instead.

4 Barrier methods

Condoms and spermicides are effective if used consistently. The vaginal diaphragm is also a suitable alternative, although it should be refitted six weeks after childbirth as a larger size may be needed. In women with a slight degree of prolapse of the vagina or uterus, a special cervical cap can be tried – these are fitted at family planning clinics.

Natural family planning (NFP) and the rhythm method

This method of contraception involves the avoidance of sexual intercourse *during the fertile days of the menstrual cycle*, although other forms of sexual enjoyment may be practised, provided there is no entry of the penis into the vagina or sperm contact with the vaginal opening during the fertile days. NFP has been approved by the Second Vatican Council and this allows Catholic couples one form of contraception.

To become proficient at NFP, it is necessary to educate yourself to recognize the signs of ovulation and fertility in your own body. This is most accurately done by:

1 Using a menstrual calendar.

2 Measuring body temperature changes.

3 Observing the type of cervical mucus.

Some women also find that they can recognize ovulation time

because they feel a sharp lower abdominal pain (ovulation pain) and experience abdominal bloating and increased sexual desire.

Keeping a menstrual calendar

It is necessary to keep a calendar for *six menstrual cycles* to get an overall picture of your pattern. Even after this difficulties can arise and there will be around a 20 per cent chance that a subsequent cycle will not fall into your previous pattern. So you can see that the calendar method, if used by itself, has a significant risk of failure, particularly if you tend to have irregular cycles – and these are common in the adolescent and menopausal years.

Some important facts to know when using a menstrual calendar:

1 The first day of menstrual bleeding is day one.

2 Ovulation is judged to take place twelve to sixteen days before menstrual bleeding begins.

3 Sperm can survive for up to four days in the reproductive tract of the woman before fertilization occurs.

4 The egg can survive for up to two days before fertilization by the sperm.

Let us take a look at the menstrual calendar of a hypothetical woman called Jenny which shows her safe and unsafe (fertile) days.

Jenny has kept a record of the required six menstrual cycles. She has found her cycle lengths, calculated from the first day of bleeding to the next first day of bleeding, to be as follows:

August 29 days
September 32 days
October 31 days
November 31 days
December 34 days
January 30 days

Jenny will use the longest cycle (34 days) to calculate the 'late safe days' in her cycle and the shortest cycle (29 days) to calculate the 'early safe days'. See Figure 26.

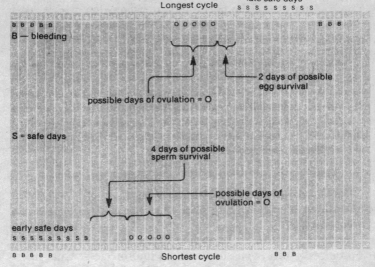

Figure 26

Now that Jenny has this record, she can assume that in subsequent cycles she will be safe from day 1 to day 9 and from day 26 onwards. As you can see she is unsafe or fertile from day 10 up to and including day 25 of each cycle. This means a whole sixteen days during which unprotected sexual intercourse can result in fertilization and pregnancy. It is easy to understand why many women find it unacceptable to have to abstain for sixteen days, especially when these fertile times are associated with an increase in well-being and sexual desire.

Matters can be helped quite a bit if body temperature and vaginal mucus observation are used to try and pinpoint more precisely the time of ovulation.

Body temperature measurement

This is also discussed on page 289 of the chapter on infertility and you should refer to this section for more precise information. Basically, the body temperature will rise by 0.3 to 0.5°C during the one to two days *after ovulation*, and will remain elevated until the next menstrual bleed occurs twelve to sixteen days later.

You can use one of the new digital thermometers which takes approximately one minute to give an accurate reading. Otherwise you should use a basal body temperature thermometer and it should be left in the vagina for five minutes.

Note that a falsely high reading can be obtained by sleeping in late, alcohol the night before, an infection such as the flu, a high protein meal late at night, a tooth extraction or having the electric blanket on.

It is important to take the vaginal temperature every day for the whole cycle, so that you can be aware of subtle changes. You should keep a regular record on a temperature chart. See Figure 35 on page 290.

As soon as three consecutive daily temperatures have been recorded, all of which are above the level of the previous six consecutive daily temperatures, you can assume that ovulation has occurred.

To be really safe, you should avoid unprotected sexual intercourse until the temperature has been elevated for at least three days.

The observation of cervical mucus

There are three types of cervical mucus, which correspond to the three phases of the menstrual cycle.

1 Dry
This is observed during the first few days after menstrual bleeding ends; during this time there is very little oestrogen being produced by the ovaries and, as a result, the cervix does not secrete very much mucus and the woman will feel dry at the opening of the vagina (vulva). The majority of women can sense this *dry time* and they may find they do not lubricate adequately for sex.

2 The fertile phase
As ovulation gets nearer, more oestrogen is produced. This causes the cervix to secrete more mucus and there is a sensation of wetness at the vulva. The mucus continues to increase and becomes watery, clear and elastic up until ovulation occurs. The

last day of this type of mucus corresponds to ovulation in most women, and is the day of peak fertility. Unprotected sexual intercourse should be avoided for three days after this day of peak mucus as the sperm can easily penetrate it.

3 The infertile or 'after ovulation' phase

After ovulation has occurred, progesterone changes the nature of the cervical mucus and it becomes less in amount, thicker, opaque and sticky and a dry feeling at the vulva gradually returns. The sperm cannot traverse this type of mucus.

Try to sample mucus from your cervix rather than the vulva. You should get your doctor to show you how to do this.

Getting it all together – calendar, temperature and mucus

Let us take a look at the hypothetical example of Christine who is using all these three pointers of ovulation to avoid the fertile days in her average 28-day cycle. See Figure 27.

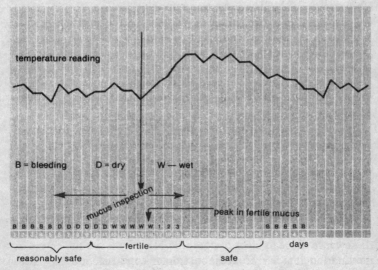

Figure 27

1 Sexual intercourse is reasonably safe during her menstrual bleeding.

2 She starts to examine her cervical mucus from day 6, after menstrual bleeding has finished. She finds six dry days followed by five wet days. Sexual intercourse is reasonably safe on alternate dry days, after the mucus has been checked.

3 Once the cervical mucus starts to increase, or no later than the tenth day of the cycle in any case, she begins to measure her temperature and continues this until the third day of sustained temperature rise. Ideally it is best to measure the temperature every day.

4 Christine notices a temperature rise on day 16, associated with a peak in clear slippery cervical mucus, ovulation pain and increase in libido. This gives her a high degree of confidence that ovulation occurred on day 16. Three days after ovulation, that is on day 20, she can resume unprotected sexual intercourse until menstrual bleeding finishes.

How effective is NFP as a contraceptive?

The failure rate is quite high, mainly because of a high dropout rate and an inability to follow carefully the signs of ovulation and fertility. Also, some women do not realize that sperm contact with the vaginal opening can result in pregnancy even though the penis has not entered the vagina.

The effectiveness of NFP can, however, be quite high, as long as avoidance of sexual intercourse during fertile days is strict. If intercourse is only allowed after ovulation has occurred and not during the 'reasonably safe' days of bleeding and between the end of bleeding and up to ovulation, it can be a very safe method indeed. In these cases failure rates are as low as three to four per cent.

For a significant percentage of women, the long periods of abstinence from sex during the fertile days are very stressful. In these cases one can elect to combine NFP with the use of barrier methods such as a vaginal diaphragm or condoms, until ovulation has occurred. Unfortunately, the use of spermicides, which increase the safety of barrier methods, may change the cervical mucus, making it difficult to interpret.

Contraception in the future

The unisex pill

Within the next decade, we will see the evolution of contraceptive pills that are equally effective in men and women. However, now that women have effectively won control over their own bodies and destinies, they may find it hard to sacrifice autonomy and trust men to be reliable in taking a contraceptive pill.

The unisex contraceptive pill will be the result of genetic engineering. Strategic chromosomes grown in the laboratory will manufacture the hormone 'inhibin'. Inhibin acts on the pituitary gland to regulate production of follicle stimulating hormone (FSH), which in turn controls ovulation and sperm production. A unisex contraceptive pill containing inhibin could block sperm and egg production without interfering with sex hormone production or libido.

The race for a unisex pill is on, and a handful of countries are already involved in what is becoming a cut-throat business to exploit inhibin commercially.

The vaginal pill

Clinical trials using vaginal pills containing an anti-oestrogenic 'progesterone' have revealed that these pills are a safe and effective alternative to the oral contraceptive pill. Side effects at this stage appear to be minimal, and a big advantage of the vaginal pill over the oral contraceptive pill is that it does not result in high levels of hormones in the blood.

Anti-sperm vaccines

This could easily become a realizable form of fertility control. Both men and women could be vaccinated with a fragment of the sperm structure and this would result in the production of antibodies which would attack and immobilize sperm, thus preventing fertilization of the ovum. This vaccine could be designed to produce immunity to sperm for a limited time or an anti-anti-sperm vaccine could be given to reverse the contraceptive effect. One great advantage of an anti-sperm vaccine would be that hormonal function and ovulation would be left undisturbed and the undesirable side effects of the oral contraceptive pill and the IUD would be avoided.

The contraceptive implant

The contraceptive implant consists of small pellets of the hormone levonorgestrel, which are inserted surgically into the fat layer of the skin. More than 30,000 women in thirty different countries are using these new contraceptive implants. The pellets have a contraceptive effectiveness that lies in between the regular oral contraceptive pill and the mini pill. Tests have shown a pregnancy rate of between 0.8 and 2 per cent in women with the implant. The only side effect of the implant is that it tends to make the menstrual cycle a little erratic by producing irregular vaginal bleeding or spotting.

The implant will definitely be a useful form of contraceptive in the near future, especially for women who sometimes forget to take their pill and for women who are hypersensitive to oestrogen.

The new French pill

A new birth control pill, soon to be released in France, is still undergoing trials in the United Kingdom. The new pill is known officially as RU-486 and need only be taken once a month within a day or two of missing a period, or two to three days before a period is due. At this early stage a woman would be unaware if she had fallen pregnant, unless she had blood tests.

How does RU-486 work?

RU-486 is a drug which washes away newly fertilized eggs, thus preventing them from implanting into the uterus and bringing on a late period.

It has been tested on thousands of women in fifteen countries with much success, and no serious side effects have been reported. RU-486 is said to be 93 per cent effective provided it is taken within one week of a missed period. Thus it is only effective in interrupting very early pregnancies.

It is still a very new drug and there are many unanswered

questions. For example, if a woman used RU-486 and it did not prevent pregnancy continuing, we have no information, except for animal studies, about its effect upon the developing foetus if the woman decided to continue with the pregnancy.

In some women, RU-486 may result in heavy bleeding, especially if it is taken too late. In the future we may find that RU-486 has other side effects of which we are currently unaware.

There is still much controversy amongst doctors regarding its proper use and, at the present time, its role seems to be as a back-up to prevent pregnancy continuing when conventional contraceptive methods have failed. It will also be very useful for victims of sexual assault.

Other doctors are more enthusiastic about its use and feel it will be a good alternative to the oral contraceptive pill and the IUD which have their dangers, and also to barrier methods which have a significant failure rate.

More conservative doctors feel RU-486 should be restricted to use in women who have a definite diagnosis of pregnancy and want an abortion. This would avoid a surgical termination of pregnancy and would undoubtedly be a less traumatic way, both emotionally and physically, of terminating a pregnancy.

Whatever the final use of RU-486, it should always be given under medical supervision and should not be freely available over the counter.

The anti-abortion lobby is outraged by RU-486 and has labelled it the 'death pill' because it interrupts a pregnancy after fertilization has occurred. They are alarmed that women will be able to wash away a tiny embryo in the comfort and privacy of their own homes, without any personal suffering.

However, the issue of whether RU-486 actually causes abortion depends upon whether you believe human life begins with fertilization of the egg by the sperm, or after the fertilized egg has implanted and begun to grow in the uterus. If you believe in the latter, you would see the action of RU-486 as being to prevent human life rather than to destroy it as in an abortion.

Despite debates of morality and the sentiments of politically and socially powerful individuals, women will eventually demand RU-486 as, since time immemorial, they have searched for an agent that will bring on a missed period. This demand is understandable as RU-486 will enable them to terminate an unwanted pregnancy without pain, fear or guilt. The World Health Organization has hailed RU-486 as the drug of the year for family planning and some are proclaiming it as the biggest development in birth control since the oral contraceptive pill.

Termination of pregnancy

Unfortunately, there will always be unwanted pregnancies and since ancient times women have looked for ways to induce termination of such pregnancies. Before termination of pregnancy (TOP) was legalized women often resorted to desperate and dangerous methods, such as oral mixtures of quinine, iron and toxic herbs. Other antiquated methods consisted of filling the uterine cavity with solutions of soap or caustic materials and the introduction of sharp instruments such as knitting needles through the cervix into the uterus. The death rates from these do-it-yourself or backyard abortions were terribly high, not to mention the denigration and suffering undergone by the women who often had to beg for an abortion.

The availability of safe and early TOP is a basic human right belonging to all women, and nowadays 60 per cent of women live in countries where abortion is legal and easy to obtain. This availability should be 100 per cent and women need to continue the struggle for control of their fertility.

The conservative anti-abortion lobby will always try to obstruct the availability of TOP and use exaggerated statistics and moralistic propaganda to make women feel guilty and humiliated. These opponents of abortion really have no right to interfere in the private life of a woman, nor in the relationship between a woman and her doctor. The doctor is the only professional legally qualified to judge the necessity of TOP, and the mental health of the woman is just as important as her physical health when making this decision. For this reason TOP can justifiably be performed if the continuation of the pregnancy is deemed detrimental to a woman psychologically or emotionally.

It is all very well for conservative right-wing committees to pontificate academically over an individual's destiny. However, it is the individual woman who has to go through the nine months of pregnancy, labour and perhaps years of unwanted commitment. Surely the decision should be made by the individual responsible for the pregnancy and birth.

If you think you may be pregnant and do not want to continue with the pregnancy, it is best to have a pregnancy test as soon as possible. By measuring the level of the hormone beta-human chorionic gonadotrophin (B-HCG) in the blood or urine, a pregnancy can be detected ten to fourteen days after conception, meaning before or at the time of the next usual menstrual period. You can have a pregnancy test from your GP, a family planning clinic, or you can buy a home pregnancy test over the counter from a chemist. If the test is positive and you feel that a TOP is absolutely necessary for your mental and/or physical well-being, make an early decision and stick to it. Do not torture yourself with guilt or excessive introspection and try to think about it clinically, in much the same way as you would think about having a regular medical procedure, such as a tooth extraction, done.

Some women who really want a TOP procrastinate for too long with guilt feelings and end up having a TOP when their pregnancy is beyond twelve weeks, which is far more dangerous than an early TOP. The decision to have a TOP is your own, and do not let others make you feel guilty or force you into something you are not sure of.

If you decide to have a TOP, your GP or family planning doctor can refer you to the NHS for a free hospital abortion. For this you will need two doctors to agree that your family or mental health will suffer if your pregnancy continues. Your own GP can be one of the signatories for the purposes of the 1967 Abortion Act. When first seen you will be asked to give an explanation for your request. At this stage you will receive counselling and also afterwards in the hospital. Theoretically it should work smoothly like this, within a twelve-week span, but there are sometimes delays. When this happens, some women may opt for private clinic abortions. Abortion is illegal in the Isle of Man and in Northern Ireland and Eire.

Currently used methods of inducing a termination of pregnancy – therapeutic abortion

1 Menstrual extraction

Since 1970 the technique of menstrual extraction has been widely used to induce an abortion. It must be done within forty-two days after the first day of the last menstrual period or within seven to fourteen days of the missed period.

Menstrual extraction is also known as menstrual regulation or the 'instant period technique' and involves passing a very thin tube through the cervix into the cavity of the uterus to suck out the tiny embryo and placenta from its attachment to the uterine lining.

Menstrual extraction has a failure rate of one per cent and, if any suspicion arises that the pregnancy has not been effectively terminated, follow-up pregnancy tests should be done so that the menstrual extraction can be repeated if a test proves positive.

Menstrual extraction is much safer and easier than the methods used to terminate a pregnancy at a later date, and indeed, because the embryo has not really taken shape at this early stage, many women feel that with menstrual extraction they are not having an abortion, but rather just a procedure to bring on a late period. Many women find that menstrual extraction is ethically easier to accept than a 'real abortion'.

Other advantages of menstrual extraction over a late surgical TOP are that it is pain free, cheaper and can be done without a need to dilate the cervix. A general anaesthetic is not necessary and the procedure can be easily tolerated with a local anaesthetic or even just reassurance.

2 Vacuum aspiration

This method of TOP is suitable for pregnancies under twelve weeks in duration. A thin plastic flexible tube is passed through the cervix into the uterus and is connected to a vacuum pump. The embryo and placenta are sucked out of the uterus through the plastic tube.

A vacuum aspiration can be done under a local or general anaesthetic. Some women find a general anaesthetic 'kinder' than a local, mentally and physically.

Vacuum aspiration is fast, easy to perform and very safe if done by an experienced operator. Blood loss is usually small and the dilatation of the cervix required to clean out the uterus is less than that with a conventional dilatation and curettage.

Vacuum aspiration is also convenient, as it can be done in the morning and the patient can return home in the evening.

3 Dilatation and curettage

Once a pregnancy has progressed beyond fourteen weeks in duration, a vacuum aspiration is no longer the method of choice for termination of the pregnancy. The embryo and placenta grow rapidly after the fourteenth week of pregnancy and, to remove the large mass, it is necessary to dilate the cervix and scrape out the uterus, often in a piecemeal fashion with forceps and a blunt curette.

4 Prostaglandins

Once a pregnancy has progressed beyond twelve weeks, the technique of injecting prostaglandins into the fluid surrounding the baby (amniotic fluid) is often used. This stimulates the uterus to contract and results in a miniature labour. Injections of prostaglandins can be used to abort pregnancies of up to twenty-eight weeks' duration. After injection of the prostaglandins into the amniotic fluid, the average time required for completion of the abortion is sixteen hours.

Prostaglandins have also been used in the form of intravenous infusion or vaginal suppositories, or in combination with an intravenous infusion of oxytocin.

Prostaglandins can have unpleasant side effects such as nausea, fever and abdominal pain.

The prostaglandin technique has a particular role in inducing abortion in women with such foetal abnormalities as Down's syndrome, spina bifida and genetic diseases when these have been revealed by screening tests such as amniocentesis or chorionic villus biopsy after the twelfth week of pregnancy.

Follow-up after abortion

You should visit your doctor one week after a TOP for a full physical and vaginal examination. You will also need to obtain a reliable contraceptive at this time as ovulation can occur as early as ten days after a TOP.

You should see your doctor immediately after a TOP if you experience lower abdominal pain, fever or heavy vaginal bleeding. It is necessary that intercourse, vaginal tampons and douching be avoided for ten days after a TOP.

If you become depressed after your TOP go and talk to your doctor or a counsellor in one of the family planning clinics to work out any unresolved conflicts and fears you may be harbouring.

Complications of abortion

Now that early and properly performed TOP has been legalized, death rates and other serious complications in women after a TOP have been vastly diminished.

Possible complications include:

1 Heavy bleeding requiring a blood transfusion.

2 Perforation of the uterus during a curettage. This usually heals by itself but if internal bleeding occurs, an emergency abdominal operation will be required.

3 Pelvic and abdominal infection which may result in subsequent infertility.

If TOP is done when the pregnancy is less than ten weeks, it is a very safe operation and the risk of maternal death is ten to twenty times less than that associated with childbirth. The earlier an abortion is done the better, as after twelve weeks the risk of haemorrhage and infection becomes much higher. Also, with a more advanced pregnancy there is the need to dilate the cervix more to clean out the uterus and this dilatation can damage the circular fibres of the cervix resulting in cervical incompetence in later pregnancies. Therefore, make your decision early and do not let other people delay you.

Future termination of early pregnancy – the combination of the French pill with a prostaglandin

Researchers have found that if the French pill, RU-486, is combined with an intramuscular injection of the prostaglandin, PGE2, a 94 per cent success rate is achieved in terminating a pregnancy of eight weeks or less duration. The RU-486 tablet is given for four to six days and, on the last day, an intramuscular injection of the synthetic prostaglandin is added.

By using such a combination, the dose of prostaglandins required is less than the doses previously required for the termination of pregnancy and so unpleasant side effects, such as pain and vomiting, are reduced.

The abortion usually occurs within three days of beginning the above treatment and the bleeding lasts for around ten days.

This combination of RU-486 with PGE2 will be used for termination of pregnancies of eight weeks' or less duration. This technique will greatly reduce the need for surgical termination of pregnancy and will very much increase the safety of termination of pregnancy.

7 Diseases of the female organs

Diseases of the cervix

Cervical erosion

Some women become alarmed when the doctor tells them that they have a 'cervical erosion'. The term is somewhat a misnomer as, in reality, there is usually no ulceration or erosion of the cervix in these women but, rather, simply a pouting outwards of the mucous cells lining the cervical canal. Because these mucous cells are normally red and granular, when they pout outwards they make the inner part of the cervix look red and irritated and create a false impression of an ulcerated area or 'erosion'. This condition is not associated with abnormal Pap smears or cervical cancer.

Usually a cervical erosion does not produce any symptoms, unless it becomes infected, in which case a heavy thick vaginal discharge may occur. This is easily cured by burning or freezing the erosion.

Cancer of the cervix

Of all the pelvic organs, the cervix is the most vulnerable to developing cancer and 2 to 3 per cent of all women will be afflicted with cancer of the cervix. Most cervical cancers are diagnosed between the ages of twenty-five and fifty-five years and, if detected in the early pre-invasive stages, a cure is possible in the vast majority; however, for more advanced cases, the chances of cure drop to less than 50 per cent. In the pre-invasive stage the cancer cells are confined to a small superficial area of the cervix and this stage is called 'carcinoma in situ'.

What are the risk factors for cervical cancer?

Cervical cancer is more common in women who begin an active sex life at a young age and have multiple sex partners. Thus, it is very common in prostitutes but is hardly ever seen in nuns, celibate or homosexual women.

Other risk factors are giving birth before the age of twenty and avoiding regular pelvic examinations and Pap smears.

Women who suffer from genital herpes caused by infection with the herpes simplex virus type II and/or wart virus infection have a higher incidence of cervical cancer and this lends weight to the possibility that this cancer may be stimulated by infections with viruses.

What are the signs of cervical cancer?

Early stages of cancer that have not yet started to invade the cervix do not give any warning signs and detection depends upon the Pap smear. As the cancer grows, it may produce irregular vaginal bleeding and spotting after intercourse. There may be an offensive bloodstained vaginal discharge. If the cancer remains undetected, it will eventually invade the vagina, uterus, bladder and even the bowel, and in these advanced stages the chances of cure become remote with a mortality rate of greater than 50 per cent.

How does one check for diseases of the cervix?

Almost fifty years ago, Dr George Papanicolaou showed that cancer cells shed from the uterine cavity and cervix could be detected in vaginal secretions. His name was given to the test known as the 'Pap smear', in which a small wooden spatula is gently scraped around the cervical opening to collect cells that have been shed from the uterus and cervix. These cells are placed on a glass slide and examined under a microscope to detect abnormal changes that may be pre-cancerous or typical of a fully developed cancer.

The Pap smear has a high degree of reliability and can pick up early cancers of the cervix in over 95 per cent of cases. In the 1 to 5 per cent of cancers that are missed, the next annual Pap smear usually reveals the abnormal cells and, thus, it is most important to have regular annual Pap smears.

The Pap smear in itself cannot prove the existence of cancer and if it is abnormal, it must be followed by more definite tests such as colposcopy in which the doctor stains the cervix with a dye and examines it with a telescope (colposcope). Cancer cells do not take up the dye and often appear white in colour.

The pathologist who reads the Pap smear will report it as fitting into one of five classes:

Class I – Normal cells (negative result).

Class II – Minimal abnormal changes in some of the cells; these slight changes are usually the result of infection in the vagina and cervix and are rarely due to cancer. After treatment of the infection, the class II Pap smear will usually revert to a normal class I smear. A class II Pap smear should be repeated three months after treatment of the infection to ensure it has returned to normal.

Class III – Suspicion of a cancer. The appearance of the cells in a class III smear is called 'cervical dysplasia'. If untreated, the abnormal cells can progress to cancer cells.

Class IV – Abnormal cells (positive result) meaning there is a possibility of cancer.

Class V – Abnormal cells (positive result). In these cases the cells are more abnormal than in class IV and the chances of cancer are much greater.

If your Pap smear is consistently abnormal, the final proof of cancer will rest on the results of a 'punch biopsy' of the cervix, in which suspicious areas are punched out with special forceps and examined under the microscope. If pre-invasive cancer (carcinoma in situ) is found, a 'cone biopsy' of the cervix may be required, and this involves the surgical removal of a cone-shaped section of the cervix, taking tissues from the surface of the cervix and from the inside of the inner canal of the cervix. If the cone biopsy removes all the cancer cells and there are no signs of invasion of the cancer beyond the edges of the biopsy specimen, no further treatment may be necessary.

If the cancer is more advanced but still confined to the surface of the cervix, the preferred treatment is a total hysterectomy, meaning removal of the cervix, uterus and tubes. The ovaries need not be removed in the early stages of cancer and so a premature menopause can be avoided. When a hysterectomy is performed for early stage cervical cancer, the cure rate is almost 100 per cent.

In some lucky women, the cancer may be limited to the exterior surface of the cervix leaving the inner cervical canal non-cancerous, and in these cases the treatment of cryosurgery may be used, thus avoiding the larger biopsy procedure or hysterectomy. In cryosurgery, a special metal probe containing cooling gases (carbon dioxide or nitrous oxide) is directly applied to the cancer cells, freezing them to death. Satisfactory alternatives to cryosurgery are destruction of the cancer cells by the application of heat (cautery) or laser. Laser appears to be becoming the most popular and effective treatment for pre-invasive cervical cancer.

What is the treatment for more advanced cancers of the cervix?

If the cancer has invaded the deep part of the cervix (stage I cancer) there is always some chance that the cancer cells may have invaded some of the lymph glands in the pelvis. In these cases, radiation of the pelvis may be combined with hysterectomy and, in some cases, surgical removal of the pelvic lymph glands. After these types of treatment, cure rates are around 75 to 85 per cent. For advanced stages of cervical cancer in which the cancer cells have invaded adjacent structures such as the bladder and bowel, surgery may be quite difficult and the main emphasis of treatment would be on radiation of the pelvis.

Diseases of the uterus

Cancer of the uterus (endometrial cancer)

Cancer of the uterus usually arises in the cells lining the uterine cavity which are known as the endometrial cells. Thus, uterine cancer is usually synonymous with endometrial cancer. The typical symptoms of this cancer are irregular vaginal bleeding and discharge in a woman approaching menopause or beyond the menopause. The woman most likely to develop an endometrial cancer is one who has previously had irregular heavy periods, irregular ovulation, trouble in falling pregnant or infertility, high blood pressure, obesity, a tendency to diabetes or a late menopause.

The use of unbalanced hormone replacement therapy for the menopause in which oestrogen is given without the controlling effect of progesterone also results in a significantly higher risk of endometrial cancer. It appears that, in some women, the endometrium is overly sensitive to the stimulating effect of oestrogen, which results in the development of a condition of overgrowth of the endometrium known as 'endometrial hyperplasia'. If the endometrial hyperplasia is very advanced, abnormal changes may develop in the endometrial cells and this is considered a forerunner to endometrial cancer. Endometrial hyperplasia will often result in heavy, irregular vaginal bleeding as the thick endometrial lining is shed. In these cases, a dilatation and curettage should be done and the endometrial cells thus scraped away can be checked for cancer changes under the microscope. If no cancer cells are found, the endometrial hyperplasia can be treated with a synthetic progesterone for six months, as this will reduce the thick overgrown endometrial lining to a normal size. In women with endometrial hyperplasia, regular curettages should be done and if there is any suspicion that the endometrial cells are becoming abnormal, a hysterectomy is a prudent choice.

How is uterine or endometrial cancer diagnosed?

There is only one sure way and that is a complete dilatation and curettage of the uterine cavity. A Pap smear is not a reliable test for endometrial cancer and is only used for screening for cervical cancer. It is important to perform a curettage in *all* women who have vaginal bleeding or spotting *after the menopause*, no matter how small or infrequent the bleeding may be, as a significant percentage of these women will be harbouring an endometrial cancer. In younger women the symptoms of extremely irregular periods, vaginal bleeding or spotting between periods or excessively long and heavy periods should be investigated by a curettage as 25 per cent of endometrial cancers occur in pre-menopausal women. Thus, one must not assume that all menstrual irregularities in young women are the result of hormonal imbalance.

How is uterine or endometrial cancer treated?

The standard treatment is a complete hysterectomy and removal of both ovaries which may be combined with radiation to the pelvis before or after surgery, depending on how advanced the cancer is. Unfortunately, removal of the ovaries is necessary as the female hormones that they produce can stimulate the growth of any endometrial cancer cells that may be hidden and resting dormant in the body. For similar reasons, it is not advisable that hormone replacement therapy be given to women who have previously had endometrial cancer, and thus menopausal symptoms may be difficult to relieve.

If adequate treatment is given for an early stage endometrial cancer, the chances of success are good, with 75 to 85 per cent of women surviving five years or more. In advanced cases, when the cancer has invaded structures adjacent to the uterus, the chances of survival are dismal.

The message is that you should *never* assume a vaginal discharge or irregular vaginal bleeding is due to innocent causes – go and find out, as early diagnosis is the key to survival.

Polyps

These are fleshy smooth non-cancerous growths that are attached by a stalk of varying length to the uterine cavity or cervix. If the stalk of a uterine polyp is very long, the fleshy head of the polyp may hang right down through the cervix into the vagina. Polyps may become eroded and infected, which causes them to bleed, so that the woman notices irregular vaginal bleeding and discharge. Polyps attached to the cervix are almost always non-cancerous (benign). However, they should nonetheless be removed and scrutinized under the microscope.

By contrast, women who develop polyps growing from the

endometrium, especially if there are many of them, run a higher risk of developing endometrial cancer and thus they should have a thorough dilatation and curettage of the uterine lining to remove all the polyps. These uterine polyps are then checked under the microscope for any possible cancerous changes. The vast majority are usually benign.

Fibroids of the uterus

Fibroids, also known as 'myomas', are non-cancerous tumours of the uterus, made up of muscle and fibrous tissue. They begin as tiny seeds, scattered throughout the thick uterine muscle and slowly grow to assume many different shapes and sizes. See Figure 28.

Some fibroids grow outwards beyond the uterus, some grow inwards distorting the uterine cavity and some develop a stalk and are known as 'pedunculated fibroids' and hang off the end of their stalk. Although they are non-cancerous, and therefore do not invade other organs, they can assume huge sizes and some have weighed as much as 9 kilograms (20 pounds). Only very rarely will a fibroid tumour become cancerous, the statistics being less than 0.4 per cent.

Fibroids are very common after the age of twenty-five, such that around 20 to 25 per cent of all women over thirty years of age have fibroids. In women who have developed fibroids, there is probably an oversensitivity of the uterus to oestrogen and thus, while regular menstruation is occurring, the tumours slowly grow. Once the menopause arrives and oestrogen production ceases, the fibroids normally shrink in size.

What problems can fibroids cause?

Fibroid tumours can very occasionally block the opening of both Fallopian tubes which will interfere with conception, thus causing infertility.

During pregnancy, fibroid tumours are stimulated to grow by the high levels of oestrogen and occasionally this will reduce the room available for the baby's growth with a resultant premature labour and birth. If a large fibroid is growing near the cervix, a

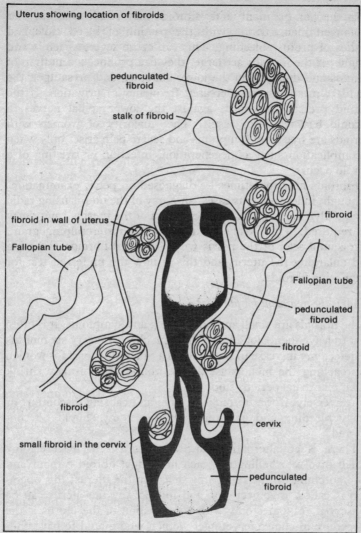

Uterus showing location of fibroids

pedunculated fibroid

stalk of fibroid

fibroid in wall of uterus

Fallopian tube

fibroid

Fallopian tube

pedunculated fibroid

fibroid

fibroid

cervix

small fibroid in the cervix

pedunculated fibroid

Figure 28

normal vaginal delivery may not be possible as labour may be obstructed, necessitating a caesarean section.

In the non-pregnant state, fibroids may result in heavy and prolonged menstruation with the passing of blood clots and gushes of profuse bleeding. This can cause severe anaemia and fatigue. If the fibroids are large, they can produce a sensation of fullness and dragging in the lower abdomen and press upon the bladder, producing an increased frequency of urination. If the fibroid presses backwards against the lower spinal nerves, a chronic backache can result. The majority of women with fibroids are free from symptoms and severe pain arises only when a complication such as degeneration, infection or twisting of a fibroid occurs.

Fibroids may sometimes be diagnosed on pelvic examination, although, in less obvious cases, an X-ray of the uterus using radio opaque dye to show the inner contours of the uterine cavity may be required. This X-ray is known as a hysterosalpingogram. Ultrasound scan of the pelvis will also reveal fibroids distorting and enlarging the uterus and this is now the preferred test for diagnosing fibroids.

What is the treatment for fibroids?

If the fibroids are small and not causing any symptoms, it is often best to leave them alone but have them checked every six months to detect any increase in size. This is a practical choice for women approaching the menopause as the fibroids will usually shrink when menstrual periods stop.

Conversely, if the fibroids are large and causing discomfort or heavy bleeding and anaemia, a hysterectomy should be considered.

There is an alternative surgical treatment to hysterectomy which involves shelling out each individual fibroid tumour and then stitching up the remaining defect in the uterus; this operation is called 'myomectomy' and in this way the uterus can be conserved. Myomectomy with conservation of the uterus is the procedure of choice in younger women who intend to have children and it should also be considered for any woman in whom there is a fear that hysterectomy might produce depression and sexual problems.

After having a myomectomy, some women may find that

several years later a new bunch of fibroids grows in the uterus, and thus it is not always the perfect solution. Also, myomectomy can be a tedious operation for the surgeon as there is frequently a greater amount of blood loss than in hysterectomy. For these reasons, most women with very troublesome fibroids opt for a hysterectomy to rid themselves of the problem for ever.

Endometriosis

Endometriosis can be a most unpleasant affliction in that it tends to strike thousands of women in their best years (twenty-five to forty-five), producing dysmenorrhoea, infertility and painful sexual intercourse.

What is the cause of endometriosis?

Small pieces of the endometrial lining find their way out through the Fallopian tubes and into the abdomen, where they implant on to the outside of the uterus and tubes, the ovaries, bladder or bowel. In these abnormal sites, the endometrial implants respond to the influence of the cyclic production of oestrogen and progesterone from the ovaries, so that they grow and bleed each month, just as the uterine lining does. However, there is nowhere for the blood to escape to and it just accumulates in the ovaries and on the pelvic organs, provoking scar tissue formation which eventually sticks all the pelvic organs together like cement.

What are the symptoms of endometriosis?

These can vary tremendously from none at all to painful menstruation, continual dull lower abdominal pain, backache, sciatica or irregular heavy periods. Pain during sexual intercourse can be very distressing and affects three out of every four women with endometriosis. This pain occurs as the penis thrusts against the upper vagina and is typically a sharp, knifelike pain. This is because endometrial implants often involve the uterine ligaments which have a rich nerve supply and are stretched by the thrusting penis.

Sometimes, implants on the ovaries grow into large cysts which fill with dark-coloured blood. These have been named 'chocolate cysts'. If the ovaries are extensively involved, their function may be impaired, resulting in lack of ovulation and hormonal imbalance.

Another common sign of endometriosis is infertility and 40 per cent of women with endometriosis have difficulty in falling pregnant. The infertility results for a number of reasons. Scar tissue and endometrial implants sometimes block the Fallopian tubes and, as the tubes are bound down by adhesions, they cannot move to hover over the ovary at the time of ovulation to suck in the released egg. The production of inflammatory prostaglandins from the implants can also reduce the movement of the Fallopian tubes, preventing them from hovering over the ovary at the time of ovulation. Because intercourse is unpleasantly painful, it is often avoided, and this too reduces chances of conception.

Is endometriosis a common problem?

It afflicts 10 to 15 per cent of women and symptoms usually start in the early twenties, reaching a peak incidence between the ages of twenty-five and thirty-five. It is more common in women with regular ovulation and menstruation and in women who delay pregnancy till later years.

How is a definite diagnosis of endometriosis made?

If you suffer from the typical symptoms or infertility, an inspection of the pelvic organs via a laparoscope is made. Laparoscopy is done under a general anaesthetic in hospital and involves having a look around the pelvis with a special telescope (laparoscope) passed through a small puncture wound below the navel. If endometriosis is present, the surgeon will see blisters and cysts containing dark blood implanted on the surface of the uterus and its ligaments and on the ovaries. The disease may be in the early stages or may be found scattered all over the pelvis, and assessment of the extent of the disease by laparoscopy helps to determine the best treatment.

How can you reduce your chances of developing endometriosis?

If you are in your early twenties and are beginning to get symptoms of endometriosis, the best way to halt progression of the disease is to fall pregnant as soon as possible. During pregnancy there is no ovulation and menstruation, and the endometrial implants rapidly shrink and, after childbirth, may never return. If endometriosis does return after childbirth, the best tactic is to have your pregnancies close together, thus not giving the implants time to develop.

The long-term use of the oral contraceptive pill which suppresses ovulation and decreases menstrual blood loss may help to reduce chances of endometriosis developing in susceptible women.

Treatments for endometriosis:

1 Hormone therapy

The aim of hormone therapy is to create in the woman a state similar to pregnancy, in which there are continually high hormone levels and absence of ovulation and menstruation. In this situation, as in pregnancy, implants will shrink with the relief of pain after two to three months. This state of 'false pregnancy' is produced by taking a high dose oral contraceptive pill every day without a break for six to twelve months. Alternatively, some doctors use injections of a long-acting progesterone such as depo provera for six to twelve months.

After such hormone therapy is stopped, more than half of the treated women remain free from pain for three to five years. In the remainder, the endometrial implants will grow again when the hormones are stopped and ovulation and menstruation resume. The high doses of hormones used in treatment may result in such side effects as vomiting, headache, weight gain, fluid retention and blood clots.

In women with 'early endometriosis', the use of the oral progesterone, dydrogesterone, can be very effective and has the great advantage over the oral contraceptive pill in that it will not suppress ovulation. Thus, pregnancy can result during treatment, which in itself usually produces a cure.

What about the powerful new hormone danazol?

Danazol blocks the production of the pituitary chemical messengers, follicle stimulating hormone (FSH) and luteinizing hormone

(LH), thereby preventing ovulation and menstruation. During daily ingestion of danazol, oestrogen production from the ovaries is very low and a menopause-like state is produced. Danazol has a powerful and speedy effect in shrinking the endometrial implants and pain is usually relieved within the first four to six weeks of treatment. When danazol is stopped, the menopause-like state goes away and is replaced by a prompt return of ovulation and menstruation which often enables women to conceive quickly after treatment. Because danazol is a weak male hormone, it may increase acne, oily skin, facial hair and induce weight gain and deepening of the voice. Some women taking danazol notice menopausal-like symptoms such as hot flushes, sweating, vaginal dryness and shrinking of the breasts. Thankfully, these side effects disappear when danazol is stopped; however, in some women the voice changes may be permanent.

If a recurrence of endometriosis occurs when danazol is stopped, the second treatment option, namely that of surgery, may be necessary.

2 Surgery

In cases where endometriosis is diagnosed in relatively young women, 'conservative surgery' which preserves the uterus and ovaries but removes the endometrial implants is preferable.

Endometrial implants are burnt (cauterized) or excised, scar tissues and adhesions divided, and, if the uterus is cemented down by scar tissue, it is freed and suspended in a normal position.

Such conservative surgery is reasonably successful and results in one third to one half of women, so treated, falling pregnant within three to six months. Conservative surgery may be combined with hormone therapy in an attempt to prevent a recurrence, although in around 40 per cent of these cases severe symptoms will return, necessitating further surgery.

'Radical surgery' may be the only effective way to relieve pain in very severe endometriosis, which, thankfully, only occurs in a minority of sufferers. This involves hysterectomy, plus or minus removal of the ovaries. If removal of the ovaries is necessary, hormone replacement therapy can be given as there will be no endometrial tissue remaining to be aggravated by the hormones.

With today's methods of early diagnosis and treatment, the disease can be prevented from becoming widespread and radical surgery is now only necessary in very severe cases.

3 Naturopathic remedies

A comprehensive vitamin and mineral supplementation programme should be followed to reduce inflammation and boost the immune system. This consists of:

1 Zinc plus tablets, one twice daily with food.

2 Vitamin E with pectin, 250 milligrams daily.

3 Pure calcium ascorbate powder, one quarter of a teaspoon four times daily in juices.

Are there any natural pain relievers for endometriosis?

The dietary amino acid D-L phenylalanine, if taken in a dosage of 200 to 400 milligrams three times daily, can produce a gradual pain-relieving effect. It must be taken every day to be effective, is very safe and free from side effects and is available without a prescription. It should not be taken by pregnant women, during lactation, or by people suffering from the rare metabolic disease of phenylketonuria.

Anti-inflammatory herbs such as white willow bark, yucca, devil's claw, golden seal, greater periwinkle, crampbark, black cohosh and false unicorn root may help and can be obtained from a naturopath. These herbs are safe if taken in the dosages recommended in the British Herbal Pharmacopoeia, but they should be avoided during pregnancy. They can be made into herbal infusions and sweetened with honey, just like ordinary tea.

If heavy vaginal bleeding and internal haemorrhage are a problem, some relief may be achieved by taking:

1 A naturopathic preparation containing beta-hydroxy-rutosides 100mg, nicotinic acid 10mg, bioflavonoids 100mg, calcium ascorbate 150mg and the herbs ruscus aculeatus 50mg, aesculus 20mg, hamamelis 20mg, ranunculaceae 10mg. Dosage: two tablets three times daily.

2 Sandocal 1000, one tablet, twice daily, dissolved in water.

As always, an imbalance in prostaglandins in the uterus is a contributing factor to pelvic pain and this can be reduced by taking anti-prostaglandin drugs such as aspirin or indomethacin (available on prescription). Also, you can reduce production of the inflammatory prostaglandin family PG2 and increase the beneficial prostaglandin families PG1 and PG3 by following the dietary recommendations given on page 376. This is a natural way of restoring prostaglandin balance and will often provide a gradual reduction in painful cramps.

Diseases of the ovaries

Mother Nature endows us with two ovaries which not only produce the female hormones and mature eggs, but also have the potential to enlarge because of the development of various types of cysts and tumours. Some of these growths may disappear spontaneously whereas others can grow to enormous size, filling the entire abdomen if left untreated.

Physiological cysts

During the childbearing years, the most common cause of enlargement of the ovaries is the presence of 'physiological cysts'. These cysts develop from either a 'follicle' or a 'corpus luteum' (see page 24) in the ovary. For some unknown reason, a follicle may fail to release its egg at the predicted time of ovulation or one of the competing follicles may continue to enlarge. In these cases, the follicle swells and fills with clear fluid and turns into a 'follicle cyst'.

Likewise, approximately fourteen days after ovulation has occurred, the corpus luteum normally shrinks and turns into a fleck of scar tissue. Occasionally, and for some unknown reason, it fails to shrink and continues to swell with clear fluid, producing a 'corpus luteum cyst'.

What happens to these physiological cysts?

Most physiological cysts do not enlarge beyond the size of a small apple and, therefore, they may not produce any sign of their presence. Usually, follicle cysts gradually shrink and disappear by themselves after one or two menstrual cycles. For this reason, if a small cyst is found on an ovary during pelvic examination, the doctor will usually wait three months and then repeat the pelvic examination, as the cyst may have disappeared.

Corpus luteum cysts may be a little more troublesome in that they can produce a hormonal imbalance and menstrual irregularity and, occasionally, may rupture, causing internal bleeding, which, if severe, necessitates an operation to remove the cyst.

Other cysts and tumours

The ovaries can harbour other types of cyst which differ from the physiological cysts just discussed, in that they usually continue to grow, often to enormous sizes. An example is the 'dermoid cyst', which is a non-cancerous ovarian cyst of a very bizarre nature in that it often contains teeth, hair, oily liquid and bone. A dermoid cyst may be first diagnosed when, for some reason, an X-ray is taken of the abdomen and the radiologist sees teeth and hair in the pelvis – quite a surprise for the uninitiated!

Another common ovarian cyst is called the 'mucinous cystadenoma' which swells with a jelly-like mucus and may grow to an enormous size – some have weighed in around fourteen kilograms (thirty pounds)!

What is the treatment for persistent ovarian cysts and tumours?

Thankfully, only a small percentage of ovarian cysts and tumours are cancerous (malignant). However, it is not possible to tell which ones are by pelvic examination alone. Thus, for any persistent ovarian swelling, surgery with removal of the cyst or tumour for scrutiny under the microscope is necessary, as this is the only sure way of excluding a cancerous cyst or tumour. Another good reason for removing persistent ovarian cysts and tumours is that they are prone to such complications as rupture, internal bleeding, infection or twisting on their stalk. Furthermore, these persistent cysts and tumours, in contrast to physiological cysts, will often grow to a large size and squash the surrounding normal ovary and its blood supply. If growth of such a cyst or tumour is left unchecked, the surrounding ovary may be completely squashed and stop functioning, resulting in loss of a precious ovary. In these cases, it is best not to let sleeping dogs lie.

So, for 'real' ovarian enlargements, in contrast to temporary physiological cysts, the treatment of choice is surgical removal. During surgery, great effort will be made to conserve as much of the surrounding normal ovary as possible.

Cancer of the ovary

The outlook for this type of cancer is not very optimistic if it is first detected only in the late stages, and although it is much less common than cancer of the uterus and cervix, it causes more deaths than any other pelvic cancer.

The major problem is that over half of ovarian cancers are diagnosed at an advanced stage and this gives an overall five year survival rate of only around 30 per cent. Conversely, if the ovarian cancer is detected at an early stage, the five year survival rate can be as good as 85 per cent.

Ovarian cancers are more common in women over fifty years of age, childless women, or those who have had an infertility problem.

The reason why many ovarian cancers are not detected until an advanced stage is because they tend to grow very rapidly and send off malignant cells to seed other organs nearby, such as the bladder, bowel and uterus, and these malignant seeds in turn grow into new cancers. Furthermore, the symptoms of early ovarian cancer may be vague, with only a slight discomfort or heaviness felt in the lower abdomen, or backache. Often the menstrual periods remain regular and normal, and thus the woman may feel that nothing serious is wrong and neglect to have a pelvic examination. However, eventually, the cancer will become large enough to produce swelling of the abdomen and pain, especially if the cancer secretes large amounts of fluid into the abdomen.

Obviously, therefore, ovarian cancer needs to be detected at an early treatable stage. However, this can be difficult as the ovaries lie deeply buried in the pelvic cavity and an enlarged ovary may be easily missed on a routine pelvic examination. Pap smears and X-rays are not helpful in diagnosis, although an ultrasound scan of the pelvic organs is nowadays very good at detecting ovarian enlargement. The best insurance is to see your GP regularly for pelvic examinations, even if you feel well and are free from symptoms. If a suspicious persistent enlargement of an ovary is found, early surgical exploration and diagnosis is the procedure of choice.

What is the treatment for ovarian cancer?

This task falls to the surgeon and it will usually be necessary to remove both ovaries and tubes, the uterus and any obvious cancer that has spread to other organs. In many cases, anti-cancer drugs (chemotherapy) and/or radiation therapy to the abdomen will be advised after surgery to destroy any remaining cancer cells. Occasionally, if a slow-growing, very early cancer is detected in a young woman, surgery can be limited to removal of the affected ovary. Long-term survival rates are influenced by the cellular type of cancer (fast or slow growing), spread of the disease at the time of detection, age of the woman and whether or not the surgeon can remove all the cancer.

Other cancers of the pelvic organs

Cancer of the vulva

The vulva is the part of the female anatomy between the upper ends of the inner thighs and consists of the inner and outer vaginal lips (labia), the vaginal and urethral openings and the clitoris – see Figure 4 on page 18. Any one of these vulval parts may develop a cancer, although it is not particularly common and accounts for only 3 per cent of all pelvic cancers.

What are the symptoms of a vulval cancer?

Chronic itching of the vulva, especially in older women, may be the first sign of a vulval cancer and should be taken seriously. The cancer may appear as a white thickening of the vulval skin, a mole that changes colour or bleeds, or a lump, ulcer or warty mass.

The cancer will eventually spread from the vulva to the vagina and lymph glands deep in the pelvis, and when this occurs the outlook is poor.

Chances of survival depend upon how early the cancer is detected and surgically removed. If you have any suspicious symptoms in your vulval area, do not assume they are merely a little irritation or 'a touch of thrush', as self-diagnosis can be fatal.

Cancer of the vagina

Cancer of the vagina is not common and accounts for only 1 per cent of all pelvic cancers. It is more common in women over fifty-five and may first be noticed when a speculum examination is done by the doctor. Symptoms, if there are any, include vaginal spotting, bleeding or discharge, especially when these occur after the menopause.

Just because a woman has had a hysterectomy, there is no guarantee that a vaginal or vulval cancer cannot develop and even after hysterectomy it is a good idea to have an annual Pap smear of the upper vagina done, even though the cervix may be absent.

In the late 1960s, there was a spate of usually rare vaginal and cervical cancers diagnosed in the adolescent daughters of women who had been given the synthetic oestrogen, diethylstilbestrol (DES) during pregnancy, in the mistaken belief that it could reduce the risk of miscarriage. Out of all the women who were exposed to DES during their mother's pregnancy in the 1940s and 1950s, an estimated 70 to 90 per cent have abnormal glandular tissue in the vagina. This abnormal glandular tissue is not cancerous, but it has an increased potential to develop cancer compared to the normal mucosal lining of the vagina, and women who have been exposed to DES should have regular vaginal examinations. The results of such examinations to date show that the abnormal glandular tissue usually goes away or remains harmless. The actual chance of a DES exposed woman developing cancer of the vagina or cervix is estimated to be around one in a thousand.

The treatment of vaginal cancer is surgery or radiation and depends upon how far the cancer has spread at the time of diagnosis.

Cancer of the Fallopian tubes

This is a rare cancer, afflicting mainly older women, and may remain silent or cause abnormal vaginal bleeding. Treatment is with surgery and radiation, but survival rates are low because of the common delay in diagnosis.

In summary

If all women had a yearly pelvic examination and Pap smear and went to the doctor as soon as any abnormal vaginal bleeding occurred, especially at the time of the menopause or beyond, thousands of lives would be saved. The death rates from cancer of the cervix and uterus would drop to very low levels and many other pelvic cancers would be nipped in the bud.

Urinary tract infections (UTI)

The urinary tract consists of the kidneys, ureters, bladder and urethra. See Figure 1 on page 13. Urine is made from the blood in the kidneys and passes down the ureters to the bladder, where it is stored until a woman feels the desire to pass urine voluntarily.

Normally the urine is free from bacteria (sterile) and it is only when bacteria contaminate and multiply in the urine that a urinary tract infection occurs. If the infection is confined to the bladder, we call it 'cystitis'. However, if the infection passes up the ureters to the kidneys, a more serious infection occurs known as 'pyelonephritis'.

The symptoms of cystitis include a frequent desire to pass urine, burning and pain during the passing of urine and a strong odour of the urine. If the infection passes upwards to the kidneys (pyelonephritis), backache, fever and chills usually occur.

What causes infection of the urinary tract?

Women suffer more commonly from UTI than men because they have a shorter urethra, and this means that bacteria from the vagina or anus have a shorter distance to travel up the urethra to reach the bladder, compared to men.

Sexual intercourse can bring on a UTI because the thrusting

penis in the vagina massages bacteria in the urethra up into the bladder. You can see how this is made easy by looking at Figure 1 on page 13, which shows how close the vagina is to the urethra.

If the frequency of sexual intercourse is high, especially for the first time in a woman's life, an acute episode of cystitis can result thirty-six to forty-eight hours after sex. This is known as 'honeymoon cystitis' but usually settles down as a woman becomes more habituated to sex. In some unfortunate women, sexual intercourse continues to precipitate cystitis and can lead to the avoidance of sexual activity.

Other causes of UTI are poor hygiene leading to excessive numbers of bacteria in the vulval area, stones in the urinary tract or congenital abnormalities of the urinary tract.

During pregnancy, women are vulnerable to serious urinary tract infections because the urinary tract dilates, causing urine to stagnate.

What can be done for UTI?

Firstly, if you suspect you have UTI, see your doctor for a test of a urine specimen, as if you neglect UTI, permanent damage to the kidneys can result.

If you suffer from UTI after sex it is important that you drink three to four glasses of water immediately after sex and empty your bladder completely before going to sleep. Sexual UTI will often respond to this trick alone; however, if it does not, see your doctor for a suitable antibiotic and take one tablet before going to sleep on nights when sexual activity has occurred.

Other handy hints for UTI

1 Good hygiene – wipe your vulva from front to back so as to avoid wiping anal bacteria onto the urethra.

2 Drink five to six glasses of water daily.

3 Drink raw vegetable and fruit juices, especially orange, carrot, celery, cucumber and parsley, every day.

4 Vitamin C, 1000 milligrams three times daily, can act as a urinary antiseptic.

5 A natural antibiotic may be tried, such as garlic capsules, two, three times daily with food.

6 Empty your bladder regularly so there is no reserve of urine for bacteria to contaminate and multiply in.

7 Avoid excessive consumption of analgesic drugs as they can irritate the urinary tract.

8 Avoid the consumption of excessive amounts of sugar, for example, lollies, chocolates and very sweet processed foods, as people with high blood sugars are more susceptible to recurrent infections.

Non-specific urethritis (NSU)

This disorder is an inflammation of the urethra and can be due to several different causes. It is more common in men who complain of burning on urination and of a mucous discharge from the penis. In women, NSU can cause burning and frequency of urination.

A variety of organisms can cause this infection but all can usually be cleared with appropriate antibiotics. However, unfortunately, symptoms can linger on for months. This may be helped by taking raw vegetable juices, especially carrot, and high dose garlic capsules, two capsules, three times daily.

In menopausal women, urethritis will often be cured by hormone replacement therapy or hormone creams.

Hysterectomy

Throughout the Western world, hysterectomy is a very common surgical procedure, and about half of all women can be expected to undergo this operation during their lifetime. In the past, many unnecessary hysterectomies were performed for such minor things as PMS or period pains, but these days a hysterectomy is rarely done without justifiable cause. Valid reasons for a hysterectomy might include heavy bleeding from the uterus which is unable to be controlled by hormone therapy, large fibroids, severe endometriosis, severe pelvic inflammatory disease and various pelvic cancers. The vast majority of women are mentally and physically relieved of their unpleasant symptoms after the hysterectomy and, indeed, are usually pleasantly surprised. They are also free from the fear of pregnancy, monthly bleeding and the possibility of cancer developing in the uterus or cervix at a later date. For menopausal women, being without a uterus can be a great boon because the fear that hormone replacement therapy with synthetic female hormones will increase the risk of uterine cancer no longer applies to them and furthermore, they can take their daily hormone pills without the break that is required in menopausal women with a uterus.

What does the surgeon remove during a hysterectomy?

There are various tyupes of hysterectomy, depending upon how much of the uterus needs to be removed. The most common operation performed today is that of 'total hysterectomy', meaning removal of the uterine body plus the cervix. In a total hysterectomy, the ovaries will be conserved if at all possible and thus a surgically induced premature menopause will not result. In older menopausal women whose ovaries are no longer functioning, it is not so important to conserve them and they will often be removed as well.

In a 'partial hysterectomy', only the body or upper part of the uterus is removed and the cervix is left in place at the upper vagina. This has no advantage over a total hysterectomy and is only rarely performed nowadays as, if the cervix is left, there is always a possibility of cancer developing in it at a later date.

In a 'radical hysterectomy', the uterus, ovaries and cervix are removed, along with the nearby lymph glands in the pelvis. This is a much more extensive operation and is only required for certain cases of pelvic cancer.

If the surgeon needs to remove both ovaries and tubes, this procedure is referred to as a 'bilateral salpingo-oophorectomy'. Bilateral means both sides, salpingo refers to the Fallopian tubes and oophorectomy refers to the ovaries. If only one ovary and Fallopian tube are removed, the procedure is called either a right or left salpingo-oophorectomy.

If you have been advised to have a hysterectomy, make sure

your gynaecologist explains exactly what he intends to remove and why. Do not sign any consent forms for a hysterectomy until you are very clear on both these points, especially where your ovaries are concerned, because if your ovaries are removed before the age of your natural menopause, you will experience a sudden and dramatic drop in oestrogen levels, which can bring on a premature menopause. The reductions in oestrogen levels induced by a surgical menopause are far more immediate and severe than those occurring gradually during a natural menopause. Symptoms of a surgical menopause can be controlled with hormone replacement therapy; however, it is nice to be forewarned and to make your own choice.

How is life after hysterectomy?

Having a hysterectomy in itself will not change the sexuality or femininity of a woman. However, the surgical removal of the ovaries can transform a sexual woman into a non-sexual being. This is particularly so if adequate hormone replacement therapy is not given after removal of the ovaries.

If the ovaries are left inside, having a hysterectomy will not influence a woman's hormonal state, sexual desire and pleasure or ability to lubricate and achieve orgasm.

Some women are under the misconception that after hysterectomy the rate of ageing speeds up, grey hairs suddenly appear, the skin shrivels, sexual libido disappears and weight gain occurs. This is all a load of old wives' tales and indeed, for many women, a hysterectomy can result in sexual liberation as they no longer have to worry about pregnancy and contraception.

It is important to realize that sexual performance is not hampered by a hysterectomy, the vagina is not shortened and vaginal lubrication and orgasm will continue to occur naturally.

If you are faced with the prospect of having a hysterectomy, first of all make sure you really need it and don't be afraid to ask the gynaecologist all your deepest questions. Once you have decided with your gynaecologist that it is necessary, take a positive attitude towards the operation. Pain and suffering will be minimal in hospital with modern drugs and if you get yourself fit before the operation, with diet and exercise, you will make a speedy recovery. If you are significantly overweight, try to lose some before the operation as obese women have a higher incidence of surgical complications.

After the operation do not allow yourself to become inactive. Remember, you are not an invalid or suffering from a debilitating disease and you should continue to exercise regularly and eat a sensible, natural diet high in raw fruits and vegetables. Be optimistic, as life will now be free from painful periods and free from uterine or cervical cancer. In some ways you are far more fortunate than the woman who carries her uterus during her entire life span.

Nutritional protection against cancer

In this book we describe various cancers which are common to women, namely, cancer of the ovaries, uterus, cervix and breast, and yet virtually every cell of the body has the potential to become cancerous. The cause of many cancers is unknown; but the various risk factors which increase the chances of certain types of cancer are well defined, for example, smoking, poor diet, alcohol, virus infections and exposure to pollution and ionizing radiations (X-rays). The end result is irritation and damage to the nucleus of a cell with derangement of the cell's genetic code, causing the cell to act as a cancer cell and multiply and grow uncontrollably, invading normal tissues of the body.

The basic aim in cancer prevention is to protect our cells against this damage and this is done by reducing their exposure to toxins and building up a healthy immune system to defend our normal cells and kill cancer cells. We can afford ourselves this protection by eating a natural, chemical-free, well-balanced diet and by taking special supplements to boost our immune system. We should also avoid excessive exposure to such cellular toxins as cigarette smoke, alcohol, chemical drugs, pollution and processed fats.

The mainstream orthodox medical profession is finally realizing that dietary changes can reduce the risk of cancer and this has been recently backed up by research findings of the National Research Council of the National Academy of Sciences in the

USA. Some of the bigwigs in cancer research have discovered that diet can be implicated in 50 to 60 per cent of all cancers in women and in 33 per cent of cancers in men. A significant number of cancer specialists are now advising their patients to take specific vitamin and mineral supplements, reduce their intake of saturated fats and increase their consumption of fibre, along with the standard programme of radiotherapy, surgery and chemotherapy.

In the United Kingdom one in three people will develop cancer and 22 per cent of the population will die from it. Of those becoming ill with cancer, 30 per cent will be cured. Medical treatments such as chemotherapy and radiation almost always produce unpleasant side effects and yet, despite these shortcomings, some orthodox cancer specialists stubbornly refuse to give any credence to the possible benefits of nutritional therapies.

I feel this is shortsighted and undemocratic, as there are thousands of inspiring anecdotes around which show us that, by using the power of Mother Nature, hope *can* spring eternal.

Take the story of Mary Lee Rork, whose right eye was removed in 1972 to eradicate a highly malignant cancer of the tear duct. At the time of the operation she was twenty-eight. Three years later, when the cancer had invaded her lungs, she was advised to have chemotherapy to give her an extra year of life. Remembering the unpleasant side effects of her last radiation treatment, Mary refused chemotherapy because she felt although her life might be a little longer, the quality of it would be debatable, having to cope with nausea, hair loss, weakness and fatigue. So Mary chose a scientifically unproved nutritional alternative originated by a German physician, Dr Max Gerson. Dr Gerson's diet was a fat-free, meat-free, high-fibre diet with an emphasis on large amounts of the provitamin, beta-carotene. Mary also began taking fresh raw juices of carrots and green vegetables every hour and applying regular enemas to clear 'toxins' from the bowel. Mary is still alive today and considers herself cured, without the use of chemotherapy.

There are many other miraculous anecdotes that survivors of cancer can recount, and these are a testimony to the benefit of nutrition and cleansing programmes in fighting cancer cells. There are stories of failure also, as there are amongst cancer patients treated with chemotherapy. Neither can *promise* a cure. In many cases, best results will be obtained by using both approaches, as surgery, chemotherapy and radiation can be used concurrently with a nutritional programme.

Alternative treatments such as the diet prescribed by Dr Max Gerson still rest unproved in scientific eyes and that must be accepted. However, there are now many dietary factors recognized to be associated with cancer and with these in mind, it is possible to formulate logical nutritional guidelines to reduce your risk of developing cancer.

Cancer prevention diet

1 Reduce daily intake of calories
This will not only keep you slender but, according to large insurance companies, will reduce your risk of cancer. Animal studies have conclusively shown that a low calorie diet can delay the development of cancer in animals exposed to cancer toxins.

A long-term study of almost one million Americans showed a significant increase in the incidence of cancer of the colon, breast, uterus, gall bladder, kidney and stomach in people who were 40 per cent or more overweight.

2 Reduce total fat intake
The National Research Council believes that there is a link between a high fat diet and a higher incidence of cancer. There is no doubt that a high fat diet results in more breast, colon and prostate cancer. This is illustrated by the fact that Japanese women who eat an average of 45 grams of fat per day have an incidence of breast cancer of 15 to 20 cases for every 100,000 women while Australian women, who eat an average of 145 grams of fat per day, have a much higher incidence of breast cancer of around 55 cases for every 100,000 women. If Japanese women adopt a high fat Westernized diet, their risk of breast cancer increases to that of Australian and American women.

At present, fat makes up 40 per cent of the average Western diet and yet the National Research Council recommends that total fat (saturated and polyunsaturated) should make up no more than 30 per cent of the daily calorie intake. Ideally, the fat content of the diet should be reduced to 20 to 25 per cent of the total caloric intake. For the average person, this translates into a total of around 50 grams of fat per day.

We should aim to eat more polyunsaturated fats than saturated fats because polyunsaturated fats result in the production of beneficial prostaglandins which help to promote a healthy circulation and immune system, as well as reducing cellular damage. Excellent sources of polyunsaturated fats are fish, soya beans, cold pressed vegetable oils, raw safflower and sunflower seeds, linseed, wheatgerm, walnuts and cod liver oil.

A high intake of saturated animal fats can result in the production of inflammatory prostaglandins and undesirable bile acids and steroids which can be changed into cancer-producing toxins in the large bowel. A diet high in saturated fats will also increase the synthesis of the female hormone oestrogen which can play a role in the stimulation of breast cancer.

3 Reduce foods treated by smoking or salt preservation

There is a strikingly high incidence of cancer of the stomach and oesophagus in parts of Iceland, China and Japan, where smoked or salt cured foods such as smoked hams and fish and nitrite cured bacon and sausages are consumed regularly. Pickled vegetables and other fermented foods may contain highly carcinogenic moulds, fungi and toxins. Charcoal-grilled foods and smoked meats contain toxins called polycyclic aromatic hydrocarbons which can increase the risk of cancer. This brings home the importance of eating raw, natural, unprocessed foods in preference to these preserved foods.

4 Eat more fibre

High amounts of crude fibre are contained in vegetables, bran, grains, legumes (soya beans, chick peas, beans, lentils) and fruits. Fibre can protect against cancer and cancer of the bowel is uncommon in countries where fibre intake is around 50 grams or more per day. It also seems that a high fibre intake reduces the incidence of breast cancer. Fibre in the diet reduces fat absorption and also has the beneficial effect of satisfying the appetite, resulting in a reduced craving for fatty foods.

5 Eat foods rich in vitamin C

Excellent sources of vitamin C are guava, raw red capsicum, blackcurrants, oranges, lemons, grapefruit, limes, strawberries and broccoli.

Biochemical studies show that ascorbic acid can act as a deterrent to cancer by soaking up toxic nitrites, thereby preventing them from forming cancer-producing chemicals (carcinogens). Vitamin C also stimulates the cells of the immune system which attack and destroy cancer cells.

The cooking of food destroys its vitamin C content, as does long-term storage. It is a good idea to take a supplement of between 1000 to 6000 milligrams a day, depending on your individual need.

6 Increase vitamin A intake

Many population studies have shown a lower incidence of various mucosal cancers, such as cancer of the lung, throat, bladder, oesophagus, stomach, colon, rectum and prostate gland in groups that eat foods with a naturally high content of the provitamin known as beta-carotene. The provitamin beta-carotene is converted in the body into vitamin A which seems to exert a protective effect upon our cells in the face of exposure to carcinogens and it also stimulates the immune system.

Vitamin A must not be taken in *huge* doses, as it can be toxic to the liver. However, vitamin A toxicity does not occur easily and massive doses of over 50,000 international units must be taken daily, over a period of months, to give this effect. The recommended daily allowance of vitamin A is only 5000 international units. However, many cancer and nutritional experts advise daily doses of 30,000 international units in people who are at risk of developing cancer.

Beta-carotene does not cause toxic side effects in overdose and the only sign of an excess ingestion is an orange-yellow colour to the skin called 'carotenemia'. It is a harmless condition and the bronze skin colour fades very quickly after the intake of beta-carotene is reduced.

Good sources of vitamin A are liver, spinach, carrots, turnip greens, pumpkin and rock melon.

7 Increase consumption of cruciferous vegetables

The cruciferous vegetables of the mustard family, namely cabbage, cauliflower, kale, brussels sprouts and broccoli, are so named because their flowers have four leaves in the shape of a cross. These cruciferous vegetables are eaten in large amounts by groups which demonstrate a lower cancer incidence, especially of the gastrointestinal and respiratory tracts. They are very useful dietary items in people wanting to reduce their risk of cancer. However, this family of vegetables contains substances called goitrogens, which can interfere with the utilization of iodine by the thyroid gland, resulting in an underactive thyroid gland. Therefore, it is a good idea to take a dietary source of iodine such as iodized salt, seafood or seaweed at a time different from that of your ingestion of these cruciferous vegetables.

8 Ensure a sufficient intake of vitamin E and the minerals zinc and selenium

The National Research Council recommends that sufficient vitamin E, zinc and selenium be obtained from the diet. Foods high in these substances are:

Vitamin E	Selenium	Zinc
Eggs	Wheatgerm	Wheatgerm
Wheatgerm	Bran	Bran
Sweet potato	Lobster	Oysters
Leafy vegetables	Flounder	Crabmeat
	Sole	Turkey
	Scallops	Dark meat
	Prawns	

However, it is not uncommon to find that soils are deficient in zinc and selenium, resulting in a lower content of these minerals in foods. Vitamin E may also be destroyed by the exposure of foods to air and long-term storage.

Several cancer and nutritional experts recommend a selenium supplement of between 100 to 300 micrograms per day.

A worthwhile supplement of vitamin E is 100 to 250 milligrams daily. Both vitamin E and selenium are protectors of the cells, as they scavenge toxic-free radicals that have the potential to damage the nucleus of the cell. Zinc should be taken in a supplemental dosage of 50 to 100 milligrams daily, as it optimizes the function of the immune system.

In summary, there is no doubt that by following a few basic principles, you can reduce your risk of developing many types of cancer. These principles are that the diet should be 'low' in fat, 'high' in fibre, raw natural foods and vegetables, and that a significant percentage of your protein intake should be obtained from grains, nuts, seeds and legumes.

A suitable diet for cancer patients

For those of you already suffering from cancer, there is no harm and possibly great benefit, in following a dietary treatment for cancer similar to the one devised by the late Dr Max Gerson.

If you do decide to follow a dietary programme as part of your treatment for cancer, you should do so only under the supervision of your own cancer specialist. Your specialist can monitor the effect of the diet on the growth of the cancer and also check for any specific nutritional deficiencies that may be induced by the cancer or the diet itself.

As a prerequisite, you should eliminate all toxic substances from your life-style, including cigarettes, alcohol, polluted water and processed chemically treated foods.

If you have sufficient strength and weight according to your doctor's assessment, it is beneficial to drink only raw fruit and vegetable juices every fifth day of the dietary programme and eliminate all other foods on this day. These juices should be made at home with a juice extracting machine and if you can obtain organically grown fruit and vegetables, all the better.

Suitable vegetables for juicing are beetroot, carrots, celery, cucumbers, green and red capsicums, alfalfa, comfrey, wheat grass, string beans, radishes, tomatoes, parsley, kale, turnip tops, lettuces, dandelion and common nettle.

Suitable fruits for juicing are apples, pears, oranges, grapefruit, pineapples, guavas, peaches and apricots.

In general, it is best not to mix the fruit and vegetable juices in the same drink if you have a sensitive digestive system, as it may result in stomach gas and belching. If the juices are too sweet or bitter tasting, you can dilute them fifty-fifty with water.

Some people think they can make enough juice for the whole day and store it in the refrigerator. This is not a good policy, as raw juices when exposed to the air, even in a refrigerator, oxidize quickly and lose some of their medicinal value. Thus the juices should be prepared *immediately* before drinking.

On every fifth day, the day on which only juices are taken, the patient should aim to drink one glass of 250 millilitres volume, every hour, on the hour, during the sixteen-hour waking period. If you have heart or lung problems, you may need to be on a fluid restriction diet and you should seek the advice of your doctor regarding the maximum volume of fluid that you can drink in any twenty-four-hour period. People on fluid restriction requirements can drink smaller volumes of juices every hour according to their doctor's orders. You should drink twice as many vegetable juices as fruit juices.

The juices are extremely beneficial for cancer patients because they are very high in minerals, vitamins, trace elements, natural carbohydrates and enzymes which can be easily absorbed without straining the digestive system. They reduce acidity in the body tissues and contain valuable vegetable hormones and antibiotics. If you are not robust enough to restrict yourself to only raw juices every fifth day, you should still drink them in between meals every day.

Basic meal plan for cancer patients:

Upon rising	– two glasses of spring water
Breakfast	– one small glass (100 millilitres) of raw fruit or vegetable juices
	– one or two pieces of fruit, especially bananas
	– one small bowl of unprocessed muesli with soya bean milk and added wheatgerm and lecithin
Mid morning	– one large glass (250 millilitres) of raw vegetable juices

Lunch	– vegetable salad with a dressing of cold pressed vegetable oils and apple cider vinegar or lemon
	– steamed vegetables
	– two free range eggs or grilled fish
Mid afternoon	– one large glass (250 millilitres) of raw fruit juices
	– one piece of whole fruit and low fat yoghurt (if desired)
Dinner	– Entrée – low fat yoghurt with honey or dried fruit (if desired)
	– one vegetable salad or steamed vegetables
	– grilled seafood or a cooked combination of three of the following: millet, whole rice, buck wheat, soya beans, lentils, chick peas, barley or oats
One hour after dinner	– one or two pieces of whole fruit or a handful of raw almonds, seeds, walnuts, or sun-dried fruits
Two and a half hours after dinner	– one large glass (250 millilitres) of raw vegetable juices.

Seasoning and dressings for the meals may be made with cold pressed vegetable oils, natural herbs, seaweed and small amounts of macrobiotic soya sauce or natural homemade tomato sauce free from sugar and preservatives.

You will see in this meal plan that there is an emphasis on natural raw foods which have not been processed and, ideally, have been organically grown without toxic pesticides and preservatives. There is a total absence of dairy products (except for low fat yoghurt) and red meats and chicken. This will not lead to malnutrition as grilled seafoods and free range eggs are allowed. Furthermore, if you combine any three of the following – nuts, seeds, grains and legumes – at the same meal, you will obtain first class protein.

It is preferable to eat small frequent meals interspersed with raw juices so as not to strain the digestive system, and if any discomfort occurs with meals, a complete enzyme digestive tablet containing pancreatic enzymes, pepsin and hydrochloric acid, should be taken with the main meals. If hunger occurs between meals, you should restrict yourself to raw juice (250 millilitres), a piece of fresh fruit or a handful of raw or sprouted seeds with sun-dried fruits.

Constipation should be avoided at all costs, as otherwise the cleansing effect of this diet will be limited. You should take raw bran, half a cupful daily, and if constipation is a real problem, have an enema every day to clean the lower bowel.

This basic meal planner is only a guide and you can discuss various modifications with your own doctor. Further information and help can be had from the Marie Curie Memorial Foundation, 28 Belgrave Square, London SW1X 8QG (071-235 3325). The Bristol Cancer Help Centre, Grove House, Cornwallis Gardens, Clifton, Bristol BS8 4PG (0272 743216) offers advice on diet and meditation. BACUP is also a cancer help agency, which is committed mainly to conventional medicine but will give callers advice on alternative agencies. Address: 121/123 Charterhouse Street, London EC1M 6AA (071-608 1661).

8 Diseases of the breast

The breasts are organs of great beauty but, alas, they are the organs in which cancer will develop most commonly in the female. And despite modern cancer therapy, the chances of survival with breast cancer have not changed in forty years. Women can play a vital role in maintaining the health of their breasts and screening themselves against cancer, with just a little education. It is important for you to understand the anatomy of the breast and how it is drained by lymphatic vessels, similar to small blood vessels, which travel to small glands in the armpits and neck. These small glands are called 'lymph nodes' or 'lymph glands' and it is to these glands that a breast cancer will usually first spread. See Figure 29.

In this chapter we will look at the different types of disease which can attack these uniquely female organs.

Painful lumpy breasts (benign breast disease)

The word benign means non-cancerous and, in this disorder, there is non-cancerous inflammation of the glandular, ductal and fibrous tissues of the breast. The disorder is also known as 'mammary dysplasia' and 'fibrocystic disease'. It is a very common disorder and, in general, affects 40 per cent of all women to some degree, although it tends to be most common in the age group thirty to fifty years and improves after the menopause.

What are the symptoms of painful lumpy breasts?

1 Painful, usually multiple small lumps in both breasts, although one breast may be worse.

2 Swelling and change in the size of the breasts. There may also be cysts.

3 The armpits may be painful.

4 The symptoms are exaggerated premenstrually and by strongly oestrogenic contraceptive pills.

5 There may be a discharge from the nipple.

What is the treatment for painful lumpy breasts?

1 Conventional
  (a) Cysts – these should have the fluid aspirated with a needle.
  (b) Wear a strong firm-fitting supportive brassière.
  (c) Hormonal therapy using oestrogen and progesterone is not usually advisable as it is not known whether the use of oestrogen and progesterone increases or decreases the risk of breast cancer. In extreme cases, the hormone 'danazol', which is an anti-oestrogen, may be used.
  (d) In severe cases, especially if a nipple discharge is present and where there are excessive prolactin levels in the blood, the drug bromocriptine is very effective. This is only obtainable from a specialist gynaecologist and must be given under careful supervision.
  (e) Diuretic drugs may be used to reduce fluid retention in the breast, although on a long-term basis they may have side effects.

2 Naturopathic
This is usually very successful although it may take two to three months to bring significant relief. It is much safer than treatment with the hormones, oestrogen and progesterone, and is free from side effects. The programme consists of:

  (a) Vitamin E, 250 milligrams daily, especially if cystic lumps are present.
  (b) A preparation containing vitamins B1, B3, B6, zinc and manganese.
  (c) Diuretic herbs such as uva ursi, parsley, juniper, crampbark, rutosides, ruscus aculeatus, aesculus and hamamelis.
  (d) High dose, cold processed, high allicin, high selenium garlic

capsules, containing at least 270 milligrams of garlic per capsule. Dosage is two capsules, three times daily with food, and they are available in odourless form.

I have seen some truly amazing results with this type of garlic in severe fibrocystic disease of the breast. It probably works because selenium is a free radical scavenger and protects against cellular damage and inflammation. A New Zealand breast surgeon has had some very encouraging results using pure selenium; however, I find the garlic source just as effective as selenium tablets.

(e) Vitamin C in the form of pure calcium ascorbate powder in a dosage of a quarter of a teaspoon, four times daily, in raw fruit and vegetable juices.

(f) Diet is very important, especially to reduce the formation of destructive free radicals and inflammatory prostaglandins in the body. To do these things, I recommend the following:

i Drink three to four glasses of raw vegetable juices daily; carrot juice is excellent for its high content of beta-carotene which is a cell protector.

ii Increase fish (unfried), fresh salads and fruit, raw seeds and nuts, cold pressed vegetable oils and whole grains.

iii Avoid excessive caffeine beverages, saturated animal fats, red meats, white sugar and white flour, salt, alcohol and cigarettes.

iv Massage the breasts gently with a herbal cream containing the herb 'phytolacca' which is said to be beneficial for the lymphatic tissue in the breasts and armpits.

Is the risk of breast cancer increased in women suffering from benign breast disease?

Yes. The risk of cancer is slightly higher than in that of women in general, and regular six-monthly check-ups should be done by your doctor. You should also practise monthly self-examination of the breasts as described on page 198.

Breast lumps (non-cancerous)

Finding a breast lump is no reason to panic as only one in ten lumps is cancerous.

What are the causes of a lump in the breast?

1 Fibroadenoma

This type of breast lump is common, and usually occurs in women under forty years of age. Typically, the lump is round, firm, non-tender, measures one to five centimetres (half to two inches) in size and is mobile, such that it may slip out of the examiner's hand during a physical examination. For this reason it has been called a 'breast mouse'. It is not a cancerous lump and can easily be surgically removed.

2 Fat degeneration

In some women, trauma to the breast, such as a hard blow, will result in death of a section of fatty tissue in the breast and this area will turn into a 'lump'. Bruising may be present near the lump. Treatment is to remove the 'lump' surgically to rule out cancer.

3 Breast abscess

Infection of the breast with bacteria is common during breast-feeding, when an area of redness, heat, thickening and tenderness may develop in the breast. If this is not treated early with antibiotics and expression of the milk, pus may form and accumulate in a lump which is called an abscess. An abscess is treated by surgical incision and drainage of the pus.

Breast cancer

At present breast cancer is the commonest cancer in women. However, it will soon be overtaken by lung cancer as women are beginning to smoke more heavily. Breast cancer is also the commonest cause of death in women aged between thirty-five and fifty-four years. It is estimated that a woman has a one in fourteen chance of developing breast cancer at some time in her life.

What are the risk factors that will increase your chances of developing breast cancer?

1 A family history of breast cancer, especially in a mother or sister before the menopause.

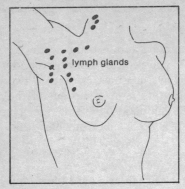

lymph glands

Figure 29

2 A previous breast cancer – if there has been a cancer in one breast, then the other breast has a greater than average risk of developing a cancer.

3 Childless women or women having their first child late (after thirty years of age), especially if the first child is born when they are over thirty-five years old, have a higher risk. A full-term pregnancy at an early age protects against breast cancer. The popular belief that breastfeeding protects against breast cancer is unproved.

4 Hormonal state – both early onset of menstruation and late menopause increase the risk. Prolonged use of oral contraceptives may also increase the risk and further studies are needed to disprove this.

5 Benign breast disease, as previously discussed, appears to increase the risk.

6 Radiation to the breast – this is a dose-related effect.

7 Nutrition – population studies show that higher consumption of saturated fat is associated with an increased risk. This is supported by the fact that breast cancer is mainly a disease of Western countries.

8 If a woman has previously had a cancer of the uterus, her risk of breast cancer is doubled.

9 Social class is important and breast cancer appears to be more common in upper social classes.

Diagnosing breast cancer

1 Mammography

This is a special X-ray of the breast and these days it is quite effective in detecting small cancers and is, perhaps, the only method of diagnosing very early breast cancer. It can detect tiny cancers only two to three millimetres ($^1/_{16}$ to $^1/_8$ inch) in size, thus enabling a breast cancer to be diagnosed long before it becomes big enough to be felt by the human hand.

Who should have mammography?

Ideally, all women aged forty and over should have mammography as a screening test, and also women who are at an increased risk for breast cancer, for example, women with a family history of breast cancer, generally lumpy breasts or benign breast disease.

How accurate is mammography?

Although false positive and false negative results are occasionally obtained, the experienced radiologist can interpret mammograms correctly in 90 per cent or more of cases. Mammography is less sensitive, and therefore less accurate, in women under twenty-five years of age, as their breast tissue is generally more dense and may conceal a very small cancer from the X-rays.

How often should mammography be done?

Mammography should be done once a year if a woman has a high risk profile for developing breast cancer.

Is mammography safe?

The radiation doses are very small and a woman would need several hundred mammograms to receive a total toxic dose of radiation which could be capable of causing new cancers. Nevertheless, it should not be abused.

2 Ultrasound

Ultrasound involves the passing of very high frequency sound waves through the breast tissue, and is particularly useful in distinguishing a solid lump from a fluid-filled cyst. It is best combined with mammography as, by itself, ultrasound will not pick up tiny breast cancers.

3 Breast self-examination

You will get to know the unique feel of your own breasts by regular breast self-examination, and will be much more likely to detect breast cancer in the early treatable stages.

If you are aged twenty or over, you should begin examining your breasts and do it regularly after each menstrual period. If you are past the menopause, you should select a particular day of the month, say the first, and examine your breasts on that day every month.

What will you feel?

You may find some irregularity or inconsistency in the tissues of your breast and one breast may differ from the other; these things are normal. Every woman is different and you should be thoroughly familiar with your own unique type of breast.

If you note any new changes or an obvious thickening or lump, you should see your doctor immediately.

How do you perform self-examination of the breasts?

There are two ways – in the shower or lying down, and you should check the breast appearance in a mirror as well.

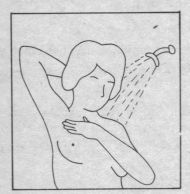

Figure 30

In the shower – see Figure 30.
- Wet, soapy skin makes it easier to feel your breast structure.
- First, lift your elbow and place your hand behind your head, as illustrated.
- Keep your fingers flat and together. Use the flat surface of the fingers, not your fingertips.
- Now mentally divide your breast into segments and feel each segment carefully. Be gentle and relaxed.
- Alternatively, examine each breast in widening circles, starting from the nipple. Choose the method that is easiest for you.
- And with each breast examine right up to the armpit. Do not forget to feel around the nipple.

Lying down – see Figure 31.
- This method can be better for women with large breasts and older women whose breast structure has relaxed.
- To examine your right breast place a pillow or folded towel under your right shoulder and put your right hand behind your head to flatten the breast on the chest wall.
- With the other hand, fingers flat and together, thoroughly examine the breast – either in segments or by the expanding circles method described above.

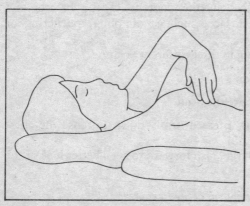

Figure 31

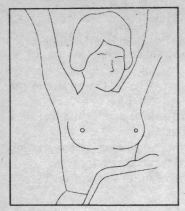

Figure 32

● For the left breast, do the opposite, putting the pillow or towel under the left shoulder and the left hand behind the head.
● Lying down you can feel your ribs beneath the breast. Don't mistake them for lumps. Also a ridge of firm tissue at the lower curve of the breast is normal.

In the mirror – see Figure 32.

● Looking in the mirror you may notice something you could not feel with your hands – by either method.
● Look for differences in the contour of the breasts and irregularities of the surface, such as dimpling, puckering or retraction of the nipple.
● This is done standing in three different postures:

1 With arms by the side

2 With arms raised above the head

3 With palms on hips, pressed firmly down to tense the chest muscles.

● If your breasts are large, lean forward to get a better look at the contours.

What are the possible symptoms of breast cancer?

1 A breast lump, often irregular in shape and sometimes painless.

2 Nipple discharge and/or nipple itching.

3 Erosion of the cancer into the skin, producing an ulcer or sore.

4 Puckering of the skin or nipple or asymmetry of the nipples.

5 Swelling of the breasts.

6 Back pain or pain in other bones.

7 Weight loss.

8 Swollen lymph glands in the armpit and neck.

9 Pain in the breast.

How is a definite diagnosis made?

Any breast lump should be removed entirely and examined under the microscope for cancer cells. This procedure is called a breast biopsy. If the lump is not too large, this can be done under a local anaesthetic in the doctor's rooms and a general anesthetic is not necessary. If cancer is found on biopsy, then a mastectomy (removal of the breast) can be done soon after. This is the preferred two-step approach of biopsy-mastectomy as it gives the patient time to adjust to the diagnosis of cancer, to seek a second opinion, or consider alternative forms of therapy.

Only about 35 per cent of breast biopsies are found to be malignant. However, if the surgeon is almost certain that a breast cancer exists before he does the biopsy, it is usually best, after consultation with the patient, to do a biopsy under a general anaesthetic and immediately freeze the removed lump and examine it under the microscope. If it is positive for cancer cells the surgeon can then proceed straight to mastectomy under the same general anaesthetic.

Treatment of breast cancer

This will depend on how widespread the cancer is at the time of discovery and surgeons have classified this as stages 1, 2, 3 and 4, with 4 being the most advanced stage. For each stage, there is given such a morbid thing as a woman's statistical chances of surviving five years beyond the time of discovery of the cancer.

However, miracles do occur, and some women survive much longer than the average statistics, especially if they have a strong immune system.

Table D shows the various stages of breast cancer and their associated five-year survival rates:

Table D

Stage of Breast Cancer	Percentage of women surviving five years
Stage 1 – Cancer less than two centimetres (¾ inch) in size. Lymph glands free of cancer. No distant spread to other parts of the body.	85 per cent
Stage 2 – Cancer less than five centimetres (two inches) in size. Lymph glands only slightly involved and not fixed to surrounding tissues. No distant spread to other parts of the body.	66 per cent
Stage 3 – Cancer larger than five centimetres (two inches) in size or invasion of skin or chest wall. Lymph glands in the neck involved. No distant spread to other parts of the body.	41 per cent
Stage 4 – Cancer accompanied by distant spread to other parts of the body.	10 per cent

With very small cancers that have not spread to other parts of the body, 95 per cent of patients will live ten years or more. The above chart brings home to us in a rather shocking way that a reasonable chance of survival is possible only with early diagnosis. In stage 4 and some cases of stage 3 breast cancer, treatment can never be considered curative. In these cases, the best that treatment can offer is to prolong life for a limited time and, hopefully, improve the quality of that life.

What are the treatment options?

1 Radical mastectomy
In this operation, the breast, its underlying chest muscles and

lymph glands in the armpit are removed. This was the standard 'curative' procedure for breast cancer from the turn of the century until about 1975. Radical mastectomy may be modified so that only the superficial covering of the underlying chest muscle is removed, instead of the whole muscle – this is called a 'modified radical mastectomy'. Modified radical mastectomy results in a better cosmetic result and preserves the mobility of the arm as compared to radical mastectomy.

2 Simple mastectomy
This consists of removing only the breast.

3 Segmental mastectomy
This consists of removing only a segment of the breast and is becoming more popular for small cancers.

The most significant recent breakthrough in the treatment of breast cancer has been the realization that less than total mastectomy, for example a segmental or partial mastectomy combined with radiotherapy, may be as effective as the more radical operation alone, especially for patients with small cancers.

Nowadays, for most patients with a possibility of cure, the operation of choice is a modified radical mastectomy in which the whole breast is removed along with the lymph glands in the armpit. Radical mastectomy is no longer advisable for the average breast cancer patient.

4 Irradiation
This has proved efficient in killing cancer cells in the breast and surrounding lymph glands and is often used *with* mastectomy, but is not effective when used alone.

5 Chemotherapy
Anti-cancer drugs are sometimes recommended along with mastectomy where the lymph glands in the armpit are invaded with cancer cells at the time of diagnosis.

The object of chemotherapy is to kill the breast cancer cells which may have silently spread to distant sites such as the bones, liver and brain, while they are still small enough (microscopic) to be vulnerable to chemotherapy. Some breast cancers have chemical receptors on their surface for the female hormone oestrogen and we call them 'oestrogen dependent tumours', in that the presence of oestrogen will make them grow faster. In these cases, the use of 'anti-oestrogen' hormones such as tamoxifen can enhance the effects of chemotherapy.

What happens after mastectomy?

Great advances have been made in reconstructive surgery of the breast and a relatively good final appearance after mastectomy is now possible. Breast prosthesis, as it is called, also enables a totally normal appearance when dressed, so fortunately, today, the imagined fear of mutilation is not so prevalent. This should remove the anxiety factor that previously prevented many women from going to a doctor when the breast cancer was small enough to offer some hope of cure.

What about the immune system and nutrition?

A healthy immune system is your greatest asset in overcoming cancer as the immune cells and certain antibodies attack and kill cancer cells. Cancer researchers are now utilizing the immune system to develop new antibodies which can selectively transport anti-cancer drugs to cancer cells while sparing the normal cells of the body, and perhaps in the future this will greatly increase the chances of survival.

In the meantime, you can do a great deal to build up your immune system by taking special supplements and cell protector vitamins.

This is especially important as surgery, radiation and chemotherapy put a great amount of stress on your immune system, which is already trying to fight cancer. Also, cancer patients frequently suffer from loss of appetite and nausea and therefore their diet is often inadequate in providing nutrition for the immune system. The following supplements should be taken:

The protector anti-oxidant vitamins, C, E and A.

1 *Vitamin C* should be taken. I recommend pure calcium ascorbate powder, 2000 milligrams four times daily. It is necessary to drink at least two to three litres of clear fluid daily while on this high dose of vitamin C.

2 *Vitamin E* (D-alpha tocopheryl succinate), 500 milligrams daily.

3 *Vitamin A*, 10,000 international units daily. However, this dose can be safely doubled. Carrot juice is a good source of vitamin A.

4 *Vitamin B12*, 25 micrograms daily.

5 *Selenium*, in a dosage of 50 micrograms daily. Selenium tablets should not be taken at the same time as zinc supplements.

6 A 50-milligram *zinc supplement*, also containing the co-factors which improve the efficiency of zinc (manganese, magnesium, vitamin B6 and vitamin A) should be taken and the dosage is one tablet with every meal, i.e. three times daily.

7 If lack of appetite is a problem, a good alternative is to invest in a juice extracting machine and make yourself raw *vegetable and fruit juices*. It is a good medium in which to dissolve your vitamin C powder and provides an easily digestible source of living vitamins, minerals and carbohydrates. Drink as much as possible of these juices.

Disorders of the nipples

During self-examination of the breasts, careful attention should be paid to the nipples. They should have the same appearance, be symmetrical in size and shape and be situated at the same level. Some women are born with inverted nipples which do not protrude during adolescent development and this can cause problems during breastfeeding. However, if a previously normal nipple becomes inverted, pulled to one side or puckered, then this can be a sign of breast cancer.

You should also check your nipples for discharge by gently squeezing them between your thumb and forefinger. If you manage to squeeze out a discharge of a bloody or yellowish nature, this should be checked by your doctor, because a nipple discharge can be the first sign of a hidden cancer in the breast duct. This type of nipple discharge can also occur without cancer being present in some cases of painful lumpy breasts (benign breast disease) and in cases of inflammation or infection of the ducts. A milky discharge similar to lactation should never be ignored, especially if associated with absence of menstruation, as it may be a sign of a pituitary tumour.

There is one particular type of breast cancer which affects the nipples, known as Paget's disease of the breast. A woman with Paget's disease will notice that the nipple area becomes painful, itchy and burns and this is followed by cracking of the nipples which ooze to form a crust over the nipple area. Some women may ignore these signs and confuse them with a skin disorder of the nipple such as eczema. As I have said before, never self-diagnose, visit your doctor early. Treatment for Paget's disease is removal of the nipple or mastectomy.

In summary

Legislation initiated in several states of the USA requires physicians to inform patients of alternative treatment methods in the management of breast cancer. This is because the standard orthodox forms of treatment, already described, have not increased the chances of survival in forty years. One should keep an open mind and look at all possible types of help.

Always be guided by your doctor but feel free to seek several opinions and keep a positive attitude. There is no doubt that an optimistic will to live and relaxation skills are helpful in overcoming any cancer. The famous psychiatrist Dr Ainsley Meares helped to prolong and improve the quality of life for victims of many types of cancer with his profound meditation techniques.

9 Sexually transmitted diseases

These days, the implications of the occasional amorous indiscretion or fling are far greater than fifty years ago. Imagine the scene . . . a young woman in Paris or Rome, alone on holiday, is approached by several charming men. The temptation is there, the atmosphere is just right and spring is in the air – one hopes that she will think of sexually transmitted diseases (STD) before making any impulsive moves but, alas, her heart acts before her head. These days it is more important than ever not to lose your head in the face of turbulent desires and feelings. It could hurt you deeply and bitterly for the rest of your life.

In the course of my practice of medicine, where people disclose their deepest feelings and regrets to me, I have encountered many young women who have become bitter and scarred because of catching a sexually transmitted disease from a careless and selfish man. Of course, these women were not forewarned by the man and, in most cases, they were just very unlucky and naïve.

Many of these women suffer from the dreaded herpes virus and are afflicted with recurrent outbreaks of painful genital blisters, swollen glands and the prospect of a potentially complicated pregnancy and labour after conceiving a child. They come to see me regularly to try to exorcize the guilt and stigma from their minds and to discuss various methods of telling their prospective boyfriends or husbands about their chronic carrier state. Not a happy story! That is, unless modern medicine can come up with a miracle cure, which is certainly not on the doorstep.

Do not assume that sexually transmitted diseases are reserved for the sexually promiscuous or socially disadvantaged, as this is no longer correct. Regardless of social background, education or age, more and more women, including those who limit their sexual activity to one partner, are running the risk of possible infection. In this chapter we will cover all the common and well-known sexually transmitted diseases from harmless vaginal infections to the notorious AIDS.

Herpes – the epidemic

The word 'herpes' has become an emotive one and sufferers often feel stigmatized, ashamed and unclean, especially because of their potential to infect those most dear to them. It must be said at the outset that the only real danger of genital herpes lies in its potential to infect and damage permanently the developing foetus or the new-born child. It has another less serious association: that of an increased risk of cancer of the cervix. In rare instances, herpes may cause serious infection of the spinal cord and brain.

Apart from the above, herpes is really of nuisance value only, in that it causes discomfort and inhibition of sexual activity. Indeed, it is far more threatening to your health to contract the venereal diseases syphilis and gonorrhoea or serum hepatitis. Except in so far as the unborn child is concerned, the dangers of herpes have been over-sensationalized.

It may surprise you to learn that almost every human being is a carrier of the 'herpes virus'. This is because when we refer to the 'herpes virus' we don't mean exclusively the herpes virus that infects the genital organs. There are three very common herpes viruses that infect human beings:

1 *Herpes simplex type II:* this type causes ulcers on the genitals, for example, the penis and vagina.

2 *Herpes simplex type I:* this type usually causes cold sores on the lips, face and eyes but may, in rare instances, cause an ulcer on the genitals.

3 *Herpes zoster:* this type causes chicken-pox on first contact, and shingles in later life or after reactivation.

Why do these viruses stay in the human body for life?

After initial infection, the herpes virus retires to the roots of the spinal nerves and lies there dormant most of the time, much like a bear hibernates for the winter. Under times of reduced general health and of stress, the virus leaves its resting place and travels down the nerves to the skin. When it reaches the skin it breaks out as painful blisters. Once the blisters heal, the virus again becomes dormant in the nerve roots until it gets its next opportunity to break out in the skin. As time goes on, the herpes attacks become less frequent and less severe. Factors which may precipitate a recurrence are alcohol, heavy smoking, drug abuse, poor diet and sexual activity. Outbreaks also often occur premenstrually.

Let us take a look at the features of the most notorious of the herpes viruses, type II or genital herpes.

Herpes simplex type II (genital herpes)

The incidence figures from venereal disease clinics at present show a steady rise of around eight per cent each year of infection with this virus. It is sexually transmitted, occurs worldwide and is less common in circumcised men.

What are the symptoms of genital herpes?

They begin with an irritation in the genital area such as itching and tenderness and sexual intercourse is uncomfortable. The earliest signs in women are small red spots on the vulva, vagina, urethra, cervix and perhaps around the anus. These spots turn into blisters which break quickly to form painful ulcers. It is often very, very painful to urinate, sit down or walk and, in really severe cases, the ulcers may spread widely over the buttocks. The first attack is always the most severe and the entire vulva and anal area may be just a mass of red ulcers.

These ulcers last one to four weeks and there may be swelling of the lymph glands in the groin; the ulcers will heal without scarring. If there is secondary infection with bacteria, the ulcers have a yellow discharge and foul odour. The patient may have a fever, weakness and mental depression.

Lesions in the male are similar in appearance and usually occur on the glans and shaft of the penis.

Recurrent attacks may occur at variable intervals, from every few weeks to many months or several years apart. Because the sufferer will have developed some antibodies, a recurrence is usually less severe and the blisters are smaller and usually localized to a single area. Some lucky people, following their first attack, will never have another one – this puzzling fact cannot be explained but it is probably due to a better immune system in certain individuals.

How does your doctor make a diagnosis of herpes?

1 The physical appearance of the ulcers is quite characteristic and swabs are taken from them with the aim of growing the herpes virus in a laboratory in order to confirm the diagnosis.

2 To clarify matters further, blood tests for antibodies against the virus are taken to determine:

(a) If the infection is herpes I or herpes II. Although herpes I usually confines itself to the face it may, on occasions, infect the genitals and some confusion can arise as to which type of herpes is present.

(b) If the infection is *new* or *old*. If new, antibodies in the blood will be of the large-sized variety, whereas in a chronic old infection, the antibodies will be of the small-sized variety. By this means you may be able to pinpoint more accurately the time at which you caught the infection.

Your doctor should also do other blood tests and swabs to rule out co-existing syphilis or gonorrhoea which may have been contracted at the same time as herpes.

How does a herpes sufferer transmit the virus to others?

Ordinary sexual intercourse, foreplay with fingers or oral sex can transmit infection with both types I and II herpes virus. The infection may occur on the genitals, mouth, fingers or anus. It is best to avoid all sexual activity when either you or your partner has an active outbreak of herpes of the lip (cold sores) or the genitals.

After an attack of herpes, it is not certain how long a sufferer remains infectious. A sufferer is probably also infectious during the incubation period of two to seven days between catching the virus and developing symptoms. The open sores are very infectious and it is risking a lot to have sexual contact if there is even a slight soreness from an initial infection or recurrence. Sufferers are probably decreasingly infectious for up to six weeks after the sores have disappeared. It also seems possible that herpes can be transmitted to a sexual partner even between attacks when a herpes carrier is entirely free from ulcers and symptoms. It seems highly unlikely that the virus can be transmitted by shared towels, clothing and toilet seats, since the virus is very delicate and cannot survive outside living cells. However, the possibility may exist, so it is best to be careful about this.

Can transmission of this widespread virus be prevented?

Knowing how to prevent catching herpes would be wonderful for the many people who have now curtailed their sexual activity because of it. Unfortunately, nothing is looming on the horizon and although vaccines against herpes have been used in continental Europe and the United States of America for several years, they cannot be recommended for general use. Controlled studies have failed to substantiate the vaccine claims, and, as they contain herpes DNA genes, they may have some potential to produce cancer. A safe vaccine against herpes is still several years away.

At present we recommend that you use condoms which provide an excellent way of preventing transmission of herpes.

What are the complications of genital herpes?

1 If the infection is caused by herpes type II virus, then there may be a higher risk of cancer of the cervix. This risk is not present if the infection is due to herpes type I virus. Herpes sufferers should have a Pap smear of the cervix every six months to detect early signs of cervical cancer.

2 During pregnancy, herpes is potentially dangerous and can produce a miscarriage, premature labour or stillbirth. It is also very dangerous to the new-born.

If a woman has an active case of vaginal herpes around the time of labour, the baby must be delivered by caesarean section. This will prevent infection of the new-born, which is extremely important as there is no effective treatment for herpes in new-borns and, at this stage, the disease is life-threatening. Once infected, 50 per cent of new-borns die. Amongst those who survive, a large percentage have permanent brain damage and severe widespread skin lesions.

During the first week of life the new-born should not be touched by an individual with any type of herpes infection, even the common herpes type I cold sore of the lips.

The treatment of genital herpes

There is currently no treatment that can promise a permanent eradication of the herpes virus from the body, although two things can be achieved:

1 Relief of acute symptoms.

2 Boosting of the immune system to increase one's resistance to recurrent attacks.

1 Relief of acute symptoms
There are several things that may be tried and some sufferers find that one particular thing works better for them.

(a) The solution 'idoxuridine' can inhibit replication of the virus but is only effective if applied to the earliest lesions, for example, the tiny red lumps that precede the blisters. If it is applied to fully developed lesions, it will only be of limited help as the virus has already had ample time to multiply in the skin. The idoxuridine solution must be used for three days and should be applied hourly to the lesions. The solution is available on prescription under the trade name of Herpid. It should not be used by pregnant women.

(b) Cold compresses of milk or aloe vera may be applied to the vulva to relieve burning.

(c) Local anaesthetic creams containing lignocaine may dull the pain from angry ulcers, especially if they occur near the urinary opening in which case the passing of urine can be excruciatingly painful. These creams are available on prescription. Also, spraying cold water on to the lesions with a small plastic spray bottle can reduce pain, especially during the passing of urine.

(d) Cotton wool balls soaked in ether can be applied directly on to the ulcers to relieve pain and some sufferers have found this shortens the duration of the attack. Be careful as ether is highly inflammable.

(e) Vaginal tampons soaked in zinc sulphate solution and changed three times daily can be inserted during an acute attack and for two weeks after. Some studies have shown that zinc sulphate may speed up healing and reduce recurrence rates. Zinc sulphate is available without a prescription.

(f) Beware of a new technique in which special dyes are applied to the lesions in association with radiation from fluorescent lighting. This photodye technique did seem to bring excellent relief; however, it has now been rejected because animal studies have shown that it may cause cancer.

(g) There has been a recent breakthrough in the fight against herpes with the development of an anti-herpes tablet called 'acyclovir'. This will be a great boon to the estimated 20,000 people in the UK who seek treatment for herpes each year. Acyclovir, which is available on prescription, is a highly specific tablet which breaks the genetic code in the virus and prevents its multiplication. The drug inhibits the virus while leaving the normal body cells undamaged and, for this reason, at this stage, it appears fairly safe with side effects being mainly limited to an upset stomach. The research company which has developed this new drug has spent three hundred million dollars on it and likens acyclovir to 'the penicillin of the virus world', saying that it is a brand-new type of molecule. Unfortunately it is still very expensive.

In an acute attack of herpes, acyclovir will speed up the healing of the lesions. It is particularly good for the first attack which is often severe.

In a person who is suffering from severe and frequent attacks, it can be given for six months to suppress these.

Longer courses of treatment are not currently recommended because of possible long-term unknown side effects.

Acyclovir will *not cure* herpes and is only effective while the herpes virus is actively multiplying and causing an attack. Long-term therapy *may suppress attacks* but it will not eradicate the virus from its resting place in the spinal nerves. For this reason, reactivation and further attacks may occur when acyclovir is stopped.

Another disappointing fact is that acyclovir will not stop shedding of the virus from the genital skin, even when the virus is not active and there are no symptoms, and thus patients taking acyclovir, although free from symptoms, may still be able to transmit the disease to their sexual partner.

Acyclovir should not be taken by pregnant women.

2 Boosting the immune system

Many of my herpes patients prefer to use nutritional and naturopathic medicines to prime their immune system, rather than take drugs, especially when there is no promise of cure. I have several patients who find that, by doing this, they can greatly reduce the frequency and severity of their attacks, providing they stick rigidly to the programme. If they forget, an acute attack arrives, which serves as a salutary reminder to recommence their supplements.

The programme is simple and consists of:

(a) Zinc chelate tablets, one, three times daily with food. Zinc has been shown in laboratory studies to inhibit the genetic material of the herpes virus and reduce its multiplication. Not only is zinc 'virostatic', it is also essential for an optimal function of cellular and humoral immunity.

(b) Pure calcium ascorbate powder in a dosage of a quarter of a teaspoon four times daily, in raw vegetable and fruit juices.

(c) The amino acid 'lysine' in a dosage of 1200 milligrams daily has been found to reduce herpes attacks in some carriers. Maintenance doses vary and should be determined by your doctor.

(d) The diet should be high in polyunsaturated fats which improve prostaglandin control of the immune system. Good sources of polyunsaturated fats are fish, cold pressed vegetable oils, raw seeds, primrose oil and fish liver oils. There should also be an abundance of raw and living foods in the diet.

(e) Herpes sufferers should avoid stress, heavy smoking, excessive alcohol intake and recreational drugs.

Chlamydia – the new epidemic

The incidence of most sexually transmitted diseases appears to have increased dramatically over the past decade but the largest increase has been in diseases caused by the sexually transmitted organism, chlamydia. I first heard of chlamydia at medical school when the organism was still poorly understood and its significance in sexually transmitted diseases was not appreciated. In those days it was very difficult to detect chlamydia in laboratory specimens.

We now know that chlamydia plays an enormous role in infection of the eyes, urethra, cervix and pelvic organs. Indeed, it has a 50 per cent greater prevalence than gonorrhoea.

What kind of organism is chlamydia?

It is actually a very small bacterium, yet at one time it was thought to be a virus because, in contrast to other bacteria, it grows *inside* the body's cells, using the cell's energy processes for its sustenance.

What are the symptoms of chlamydia infection?

Infection with chlamydia can occur in a silent fashion with no outward symptoms of disease. Up to 70 per cent of carriers are normal on physical examination. For this reason, unless special screening tests are done, the infection can at first go unnoticed, but in the long term it can cause severe damage. In the early stages, some infected men will complain of a penile discharge and discomfort (urethritis) and women may notice an offensive vaginal discharge coming from the cervix, and lower abdominal pain. However, as the infection may smoulder on silently, the first sign is often infertility or ectopic pregnancy. Women in the age bracket fifteen to thirty-five years are at the highest risk, and in this group chlamydia is the leading cause of pelvic inflammatory disease and infertility.

How can this insidious disease be detected?

Previously this was very difficult, as chlamydia is an elusive bacterium and difficult to grow in conventional culture dishes in the laboratory. Also, blood tests were not helpful as most sexually active people have antibodies from way back and their presence does not necessarily mean an active infection.

The diagnosis might be made easier in the future by use of a new diagnostic test for detecting the protein of the chlamydia which simply involves taking a special swab of the cells lining the urethra and inner cervix. This test is not yet widely available on the NHS.

Can the chlamydia epidemic be halted?

Yes indeed, with the antibiotic tetracycline, or erythromycin if the patient is allergic to tetracycline. The recommended course of treatment takes fourteen to twenty-one days and is well tolerated, especially if the tablets are taken with food and liquid. This treatment has the ability to cure the infection. Of course, regular check-ups of sufferers and their sexual contacts are essential, with repeated swabs being taken to ensure total eradication of the chlamydia.

The most frequently sexually transmitted disease in Western countries, including Australia, isn't AIDS, herpes, syphilis or gonorrhoea. It is chlamydia and it is probably more common than all the others put together. Be aware, take precautions and see your doctor for regular check-ups.

Gonorrhoea

In the last decade it seems that AIDS and herpes have stolen the limelight, yet this should not detract from the fact that sexually transmitted disease due to the bacterium 'neisseria gonorrhoeae' (gonococcus) is still as prevalent as ever.

Gonorrhoea is a highly infectious disease acquired by sexual intercourse or other intimate sexual activity. Homosexuals often acquire the infection in the back passage (rectum) or throat. Very occasionally, some unfortunate people acquire it from infected hand towels or soiled bed clothes.

How long is the incubation period of gonorrhoea?

On average, it will take two to seven days for symptoms of infection to appear after initial sexual contact with an infected person. However, in women, the infection may linger in the body for up to one year before symptoms develop, and in this respect it can be compared to infection with chlamydia. A large percentage of infected women never develop symptoms but remain silent carriers, unknowingly transmitting the infection to others.

If symptoms do develop, what will they be?

Typically, the organism of gonorrhoea attacks the urinary opening in front of the vaginal opening and this results in a pus-like discharge and burning and frequency of urination. These symptoms may be mild and many sufferers mistake them for a passing bladder irritation. Gonorrhoea may then attack the inner cervix, resulting in a copious yellow vaginal discharge. The glands at the sides of the vaginal opening may also become infected, resulting in painful abscesses. If gonorrhoea invades the uterine cavity and passes up into the Fallopian tubes, inflammation and pus will form inside the tubes and this will usually cause lower abdominal pain, heavy offensive vaginal discharge, fever and chills.

What are the complications of infection with gonorrhoea?

1 Abscesses full of pus may form in the ovaries and tubes. Rupture of one of these may result in life-threatening infection in the abdominal cavity or blood stream. If this occurs, the only possible treatment is to remove the reproductive organs, including the uterus, ovaries and tubes.

2 Recurrent pelvic inflammatory disease (PID) caused by gonorrhoea can result in repeated stays in hospital for severe

abdominal pain, abnormal bleeding and period pains. Once again, often the only possible treatment is pelvic surgery.

3 Of women in whom there is a delay in treating tubal infection, approximately 15 per cent subsequently become sterile as a result of tubal scarring and blockage.

4 In one to three per cent of women, gonorrhoea will spread from the reproductive organs, through the blood stream to involve the skin, heart valves, brain, liver or joints, and this is particularly so if a woman is pregnant at the time of infection. If the disease causes arthritis, it may affect the knees, wrists and ankles, causing pain and fluid accumulation in these joints.

How does the doctor diagnose gonorrhoea?

The doctor takes a swab and smear of the discharge from the urinary opening, anus and cervix, and this is spread out on to a glass slide and stained with a purple dye before being checked under the microscope. If infection is present, the bacteria will be seen as an intracellular organism occurring in a double form. The discharge should also be grown on culture dishes in the laboratory, as the glass slide test may be falsely negative.

If your sexual partner tells you he has recently been treated for gonorrhoea, see your doctor immediately. Your doctor will take swabs but will probably treat you straightaway without waiting for the results, as this is a much safer process.

The treatment of gonorrhoea

The standard treatment in non-allergic sufferers is two deep intra-muscular penicillin injections, given at the same time and divided between the two buttocks. The dosage is high and is usually given with a tablet called probenecid which enables the body to keep the penicillin levels high for a longer period. Some doctors may use a penicillin equivalent in tablet form called 'ampicillin', but treatment failures are more frequent with this and the injections are to be preferred. For individuals allergic to penicillin, the second drug of choice is tetracycline which is taken in tablet form for seven days.

If the gonorrhoea is resistant to these standard drugs,
what treatment is left?

In the past few years, some strains of gonorrhoea have developed enzymes which enable them to break down penicillin and tetracycline and thus these strains are resistant to the standard antibiotics. Fortunately, there is another antibiotic called 'spectinomycin' which can kill most resistant strains. It is expensive and must be given by intra-muscular injection; however, it is a life-saver in these resistant cases.

Follow-up after an infection is very important. Three swabs should be taken at one-week intervals after the course of antibiotic treatment is finished. If all three swabs are negative for gonorrhoea, a cure has occurred. However, having had one episode of gonorrhoea does not confer immunity against reinfection from another sexual partner. It is necessary to abstain strictly from sexual intercourse for eight weeks after an infection with gonorrhoea. If you are worried about a prospective sexual encounter, ask the man to wear a condom as this provides a reasonable degree of protection from reinfection.

Syphilis – the sexually transmitted disease of ancient times

This disease has been described in many ancient history books as infecting kings, queens and emperors, as well as the lowly people, and it used to be treated with the toxic metal arsenic.

Until the arrival of AIDS, syphilis was by far the most awesome of the sexually transmitted diseases, as early symptoms can disappear by themselves, only to return years later with horrifying consequences if they should be left untreated. The incidence of syphilis has been increasing rapidly since 1950 and early recognition is imperative.

What causes syphilis?

A highly infectious bacterium with the exotic name of 'treponema pallidum' causes syphilis. It has a corkscrew shape which enables it to dig and twist through small breaks in the skin and mucous membranes into the body. It is transmitted by intimate sexual contact with a partner who has an infected syphilitic sore.

The incubation period varies from ten to ninety days after contact and thus the first syphilitic sore may be a long time coming.

The stages of infection with syphilis

1 Early syphilis (primary and secondary stages)
The primary stage is signified by a painless hard sore called a 'chancre', which heals itself in six to ten weeks. This chancre may be on the genitals, the cervix, the anus, the lips or throat, and is associated with enlargement of the surrounding lymph glands. This stage may pass unnoticed by the patient.

The secondary stage is due to the bacteria entering the blood stream and manifests itself as a widespread non-itchy skin rash and eruptions on the mucous membranes. This rash may involve many areas, such as the scalp, soles of the feet and palms of the hands. Syphilitic warts may also develop on the genitals. All these skin lesions are highly infectious and teeming with bacteria. The patient may feel generally unwell, with fever, general aching and patchy loss of hair. Some people with these early stages of syphilis may have very few symptoms and thus the disease may not be diagnosed. If a patient with early syphilis does not receive treatment, the skin lesions will heal themselves in three to six weeks and the disease will enter the next phase which is known as the latent phase.

2 Latent syphilis
During this stage there are no signs or symptoms of the disease and the patient is not infectious to others. A diagnosis can only be made by doing a specific blood test. If the patient still remains untreated during this silent stage, there is a one in three chance that the disease will progress to the final or late stage. This transition may take from ten to fifteen years.

3 Late syphilis (tertiary stage)
By this stage, the bacteria of syphilis are deeply entrenched in the body and can attack any organ. The manifestations vary between

individuals but often syphilis will attack the brain, heart, bones, blood vessels, spine and skin. If the brain becomes infected, the patient becomes demented and may have delusions of grandeur.

How can early syphilis be diagnosed?

There are two ways:

1 By identifying the syphilis bacteria in the skin lesions.

2 By a blood test – it may take four weeks after the appearance of the chancre for blood tests to become positive. Thus, if the test is initially negative, it should be repeated six and twelve weeks later to be on the safe side. In secondary syphilis, blood tests are always positive. The most common blood test used to screen for syphilis is known as the VDRL.

The treatment of syphilis

Thankfully, the bacterium is still sensitive to good old penicillin which is given in the form of intra-muscular injections for ten to fifteen days. If the patient is allergic to penicillin, tetracycline tablets are a suitable alternative. Even at the tertiary stage, syphilis can still be cured, but by this stage some damage, especially damage to the brain, may be permanent.

If treatment is curative, follow-up blood tests will be negative, unless the disease is not treated until a very late stage, in which case blood tests will always remain weakly positive even though the infection has been cleared. After treatment regular blood tests should be done for two years in order to check for a recurrence.

Pelvic inflammatory disease (PID)

PID is a general term meaning inflammation of the female organs in the pelvis, in particular the uterus, Fallopian tubes and ovaries.

What is the cause of PID?

Infection with various bacteria causes PID, and in Western countries, these sexually transmitted infections are most commonly due to chlamydia, gonorrhoea and mycoplasma. In the Third

World, tuberculosis also commonly infects the pelvic organs, but this is only rarely seen in the developed world.

What will increase the risk of PID?

A woman who has multiple sexual partners will have an increased risk of PID. Also, the use of the intra-uterine contraceptive device is associated with a significantly higher risk of PID.

What will decrease the risk of PID?

1 Women on the oral contraceptive pill have less PID because the hormones in the pill thicken the mucous plug in the cervix, making it difficult for bacteria to pass through into the uterus.

2 Barrier methods of contraception such as condoms and diaphragms reduce the risk.

3 Regular check-ups – if you have multiple sexual partners or have recently acquired a new partner with an uncertain past history see your doctor regularly for screening tests to detect commonly transmitted sexual diseases.

What symptoms does the woman feel when she has an infection deep inside her pelvic organs?

There may be no symptoms or just a feeling of being generally unwell with tiredness, fever and lack of appetite. Some women have constant or recurrent lower abdominal pains, vaginal discharge and odour or backache. They may also experience pain during sexual intercourse.

How can the doctor diagnose PID?

Sometimes a pelvic examination will reveal deep tenderness and enlarged lumpy tubes and ovaries. The most accurate way to assess the severity and extent of the damage is by laparoscopy in which the doctor has a direct look at the pelvic organs by means of a telescope passed through the wall of the lower abdomen.

What are the complications of PID?

1 For every ten women with PID one will become infertile due to blockage, scarring and twisting of the delicate Fallopian tubes.

The risk of infertility increases with each subsequent attack of PID, and after a third attack, one in two women will become infertile.

2 The risk of ectopic pregnancy is increased seven times after PID. Ectopic pregnancy is a pregnancy occurring in an abnormal position, such as in the Fallopian tube, and this is a very dangerous condition as the tube will eventually rupture, causing heavy internal bleeding. If a woman with a past history of PID becomes pregnant, it is advisable for her to undergo an ultrasound scan to check that the pregnancy is in a normal position inside the uterine cavity.

The treatment of PID

A long course of antibiotics to eradicate the bacteria will be necessary. Pain relief can be provided by analgesic drugs and anti-inflammatory, anti-prostaglandin drugs. Microwave heat to the lower abdomen and acupuncture have been found effective by some sufferers of chronic low abdominal pain.

In patients where medication fails to bring relief, surgery will be necessary to remove infected and inflamed ovaries and tubes and to divide scar tissue. In extreme cases, the pelvic organs may be just a mass of pus-filled abscesses and scar tissue and a radical hysterectomy may be required.

What about naturopathic treatments for PID?

1 Garlic has been proved in the laboratory to inhibit growth of bacteria and fungi and, in contrast to antibiotic drugs, the bacteria do not develop resistance to garlic. Dosage of garlic capsules is two capsules, three times daily with food, and I recommend the high allicin cold processed type which are odourless.

2 A good quality vitamin C powder (calcium ascorbate) should be taken in a dosage of a quarter of a teaspoon three or four times daily in juices, as this will improve the immune system.

3 Zinc chelate, 50 milligrams daily with food, and vitamin A, 5000 international units daily, will boost immune functions.

4 Anti-prostaglandins – to reduce the production of inflammatory prostaglandins which may cause pain and inflammation in the pelvis, doctors often prescribe anti-prostaglandin drugs and these can be quite effective. You can also reduce the production of inflammatory prostaglandins naturally by dietary means:

(a) Increase fish, raw seeds, raw nuts, cold pressed vegetable oils and raw vegetable juices.

(b) Reduce saturated animal fats and processed fatty meats.

See page 376 for a complete diet table.

Vaginal infections and discharges

The Victorian era of the Western world left a veil of prejudice and embarrassment upon the outward signs of female sexuality. Although, ostensibly, we are full swing into the age of permissiveness, vestiges of this taboo still persist and many doctors are surprised at the amount of fear and confusion remaining in the minds of some women concerning the health and function of their sexual organs. In this section we will discuss the nature of the vagina and ways in which you can prevent and treat its medical maladies.

The vagina is a hollow muscular tube sitting at the bottom of the uterus. Its roof is formed by the cervix which is the portal of entry into the womb – see Figure 33.

The cervix and vagina are lined with scale-like (squamous) cells which are normally hardy little cells that ward off germs and viruses. Also contained in the vagina are mucus-secreting cells which maintain the acid-alkaline balance of the vagina – ideally the vagina is on the acidic side – and provide lubrication of the tissues. The mucus secreted by these cells is normally not offensive to smell. This mucus and acid balance function is under the control of the female hormone oestrogen. Thus, during the menopause and beyond, when there is a deficiency of oestrogen, the vagina becomes dry, alkaline and more susceptible to infection.

Many people think that the normal vagina is a sterile and totally pure organ which contains no bacteria at all. This is a fallacy and,

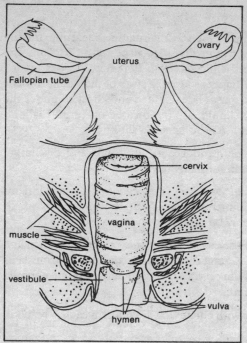

Figure 33

in the normal vagina, several different species of bacteria are usually found. Indeed, it is highly desirable that there are lactobacilli present in the vagina as these help to keep it acidic. These friendly lactobacilli also ward off other undesirable bacteria and viruses which have no place in the normal vagina.

Many women also think that a normal vagina should have no discharge. This is also a fallacy but there is a large normal variation between women in the amount of vaginal discharge. The normal vaginal discharge is milky or yellowish white. The oral contraceptive pill may increase and thicken the vaginal discharge and, in some women, may slightly increase the chance of vaginal infections, in particular candida or thrush.

What are the causes of excessive vaginal discharge?

1 *Infections of the vagina* – the most common organisms causing infection are: gardnerella vaginalis (40 to 50 per cent), trichomonas (30 per cent) and candida albicans (20 to 30 per cent).

These infections are diagnosed from a swab of the vaginal mucus which is spread on to a glass slide, stained and checked under the microscope. The swab should also be smeared on various laboratory culture dishes to try to grow bacteria and fungi.

2 *Retained tampon* – this produces a foul odour and discharge, especially if it is forgotten for many days.

3 *Vaginal deodorants and spermicides* may cause a chemical inflammation of the vaginal lining resulting in irritation and discharge. In some cases, a woman may be allergic to these preparations.

4 A pouting mouth of the cervix is known as a *cervical erosion* and may result in a heavy vaginal discharge because the mucous cells lining the inner part of the cervix are turned outwards and exposed to the vaginal atmosphere.

5 *Infection of the cervix* with chlamydia or gonorrhoea may result in discharge.

Types of vaginal infection

1 Gardnerella vaginalis
This sexually transmitted disease has often been called 'non-specific vaginitis' although the term is not helpful. Infection with gardnerella bacteria results in a foul fishy odour and watery grey discharge which may contain bubbles. If the acid-alkaline balance of the vagina is measured in cases of this infection, it is usually found to be alkaline (pH greater than 5). Various treatments may be used, such as vaginal sulphur antibiotic creams, oral antibiotics or flagyl type antibiotics. These are obtainable on prescription.

2 Trichomonas vaginalis
The sexually transmitted disease trichomonas is caused by a parasite which has a flagellated tail that beats from side to side and enables the parasite to swim actively in the vaginal mucus. With

trichomonas the vagina is usually too alkaline with a pH greater than 5. The vaginal discharge in this infection is usually a yellow-green colour, copious in amount and may contain bubbles. The vulva is usually sore and red, with irritation during sexual intercourse and burning on urination. There may be an unpleasant odour but it is not usually as pungent as infection with gardnerella. Effective treatment is usually achieved with a single dose of a flagyl type antibiotic taken with food. This antibiotic is obtainable on prescription.

3 Candida albicans

This is colloquially known as 'thrush' and is due to overgrowth of the fungus, candida albicans, which results in a white cottage-cheese type vaginal discharge. This causes redness and itching of the vulva. In contrast to the other infections, the vagina is usually not too alkaline, with a pH of less than 4.5.

Candida is not always a sexually transmitted disease and its main significance is that of nuisance value as it tends to keep recurring. It is more common in pregnancy or women on the oral contraceptive pill. It is important to avoid antibiotics and a high sugar diet when trying to overcome thrush.

Specific treatment involves the use of antifungal vaginal creams and pessaries obtained by prescription. In severe cases, there are special antifungal tablets such as nystatin or the new drug keto-conazole.

In rare cases, candida, if present in the small intestine, can grow little tentacles called 'pseudohyphae' which burrow into the inner lining of the intestine. This can open up small channels from the bowel to the blood and may result in the absorption into the blood of partially digested food. This can cause allergic reactions to these foods, especially proteins, and has been claimed to result in many different symptoms such as headaches, eczema, fatigue, dizziness, depression, arthritis and so on. Indeed, whole books have been written on this subject. But in the vast majority of cases of candida infection, only the mouth, vagina or skin is disturbed.

Recurrent vaginal infections

Many women suffer from recurrent 'vaginal infections'. However, this label is not always strictly correct. Often the problem begins with a slight vaginal irritation for which inappropriately strong antibiotic drugs are prescribed. Inevitably, these drugs destroy not only the bad bacteria but also the good, and subsequently there is an overgrowth of unfavourable bacteria and fungi. Obviously, this will just keep the vicious circle of vaginal infection and irritation going. Often another antibiotic is prescribed, and this, again, only serves to make matters worse. Many women become frustrated because, although they are seeking constant medical advice and taking regular courses of antibiotics, their condition does not improve. In these women the use of a douche containing the friendly lactobacilli, such as yoghurt, will prove very helpful and may be curative. In women who have severe vaginal infections for which antibiotics will definitely be required, I recommend that they use a lactobacilli-containing douche for two weeks subsequent to the completion of the course of antibiotics. This will encourage the regrowth of normal friendly bacteria after the antibiotic has done its job.

Some ways of alleviating chronic vaginal discharge and odour

If you have a vaginal irritation and discharge which keeps on coming back and seems to be resistant to all the usual treatments offered by your doctor, you may find the following suggestions helpful.

1 It is best to avoid recurrent prescriptions for antibiotic drugs as these will cause overgrowth of resistant bacteria and fungi.

2 Always treat your sexual partner at the same time as yourself, using the same medication from your doctor. Otherwise, your partner will reinfect you.

3 Try to avoid sexual frustration and get adequate rest and relaxation.

4 Lead a healthy, active life-style, avoid smoking, and eat an abundance of raw foods such as fresh fruit and vegetables to

provide adequate amounts of vitamins C and A, which are essential to maintain a healthy vagina. Avoid a high carbohydrate diet which contains refined sugar and flour and eat yoghurt regularly, as this will help to maintain the normal lactobacilli in the bowel and vagina.

5 Avoid the use of tights and nylon underpants – wear cotton underpants instead or, indeed, none at all, under loose skirts. It is best to avoid wearing tight jeans as these perpetuate a case of chronic thrush.

6 Avoid irritating soaps, bath salts and vaginal deodorants and use pure soap to wash your underpants and vulva.

7 Wipe yourself from front to back so that infection is not carried into the vagina from your bowels. Keep your vulva clean by sponging with warm sterile saline. A good trick for drying the vulva area after washing is to use an electric hair dryer.

8 If you are a menopausal woman suffering from vaginal discharge or irritation, try a vaginal oestrogen cream to strengthen the mucous membrane lining the vagina.

9 Try a natural antibiotic. The best one is a high allicin, cold processed garlic capsule, with each capsule containing 300 milligrams of garlic. The dosage required is high – two or three capsules, three times daily with food, to overcome chronic vaginal infection. Garlic is an effective antibiotic against many strains of bacteria and fungi and one of its big advantages is that organisms do not develop resistance to its action.

10 It is most important to improve your immune function when trying to overcome a chronic vaginal infection and this is easily done by taking the following supplements:

(a) Pure calcium ascorbate powder, a quarter of a teaspoon, four times daily in raw juices.

(b) Zinc chelate three times daily with food.

(c) Raw carrot juice, one to two glasses daily.

11 Measure your vaginal acidity with a pH stick which can be obtained from your local pharmacy. If your pH is greater than 4.5,

take measures to restore vaginal acidity so that the pH becomes less than 4.5. Vaginal acidity can be restored by:

(a) Vaginal douching with a dilute solution of apple cider vinegar or lemon, once daily.

(b) Inserting a tampon soaked in yoghurt.

(c) Vaginal douching, twice weekly, with a solution of sterile water and yoghurt in a ratio of five parts water to one part yoghurt. This contains a culture of lactobacilli and once the lactobacilli are introduced into the vagina, they grow and maintain vaginal acidity for a long time, thereby preventing overgrowth of unfriendly bacteria. An excellent douche can be made with acidophilus powder mixed in sterile water, in a dilution of one teaspoon of powder to one litre of water.

The flushing effect of vaginal douching has the added advantage of removing excessive accumulated vaginal secretions which might otherwise develop a bad odour and act as a culture medium for the growth of unfriendly bacteria. Douching will also remove sperm and sexual secretions from the vagina, which is of benefit as these fluids are highly alkaline and therefore reduce vaginal acidity.

How is a douche used?

Douching can be done most efficiently by squatting in the bath or sitting on the toilet and takes no more than three minutes. Compress the vaginal lips together around the douche nozzle while administering the douche solution and the vagina will fill to the top. Then release the vaginal lips to allow the solution to gush back out into the toilet bowl. Repeat this three times or until the douche solution is finished.

Are there any dangers in vaginal douching?

For the woman who has just delivered a child, douching can be dangerous and it is recommended that vaginal douching not be done for at least ten weeks after giving birth. The use of unsterile water can be dangerous, as it may introduce infection from the outside. Therefore any water used should be boiled beforehand or bought in sterile bottles from the chemist. In some commercially available douches there are irritating perfumes, colourings and preservatives added to the douche solution and these should be avoided as after recurrent use the development of allergies to these ingredients is surprisingly common. It is best to stick to natural douche solutions such as lemon, cider vinegar or yoghurt. Douching is forbidden during pregnancy as it may introduce infection into the uterus. Apart from these factors, vaginal douching is extremely safe and indeed, it is practised regularly in European countries, especially in France.

Vaginal tampons

These are a convenient and safe way of absorbing menstrual blood flow, provided the tampon is changed every six hours. It is recommended that women alternate the use of tampons with absorbent pads, using the pads at night. It is not advisable to use vaginal tampons on a regular basis for absorbing excess vaginal discharge at times other than menstruation. This is because the daily use of tampons can irritate and rub the vaginal mucosa and increase the chances of vaginal infection.

The toxic shock syndrome

The toxic shock syndrome (TSS) is a serious illness with the following symptoms:

Muscular aching;
Nausea and vomiting;
Fever;
Low blood pressure leading to dizziness;
Generalized rash and peeling of the skin on the hands and feet;
Mental confusion;
Diarrhoea;
Abnormal liver and kidney function.

This syndrome became infamous in 1980 in the USA when healthy menstruating women using certain brands of tampons suddenly developed TSS. By 1981, there had been 941 cases of TSS and 73 of these were fatal. Now that women are aware of this dangerous disease and are using tampons more hygienically, the incidence of TSS has dropped to very low levels and is around 6.2 cases for every 100,000 menstruating women, each year.

What increases the risk of developing TSS?

Continuous tampon use increases the risk. It is recommended that women alternate the use of tampons with absorbent napkin pads. The pads are best used at night and tampons can be used during the day, provided they are changed at least every six hours.

It is thought that TSS is due to bacteria entering the blood stream from the vagina but, in many cases, this has not yet been proved. Poor general health and the presence of vaginal or pelvic infections increase the risk of TSS and tampons should be avoided in women with pelvic infection. You should be aware of the symptoms of TSS and if you develop any of them while using tampons during menstruation, remove the tampon immediately and see your doctor.

Genital warts

Warts are bad enough when they grow on the fingers and feet, but when they begin to spread on the genitals they are truly horrifying for a woman. They begin as a tiny pinkish pimple-like growth around the vaginal opening and anus and often spread up into the vagina and the cervix. In the moist and warm vagina, they can flourish into large cauliflower-like protuberances which may entirely cover the vaginal lips. They are caused by a papilloma virus which is usually transmitted from an infected sexual partner.

Can genital warts be serious?

They are usually painless, unless scratched excessively, in which case bacterial infection may occur around them. Women with genital warts have an increased risk of irritative changes in the cells of the cervix, vulva and vagina, and this can increase the risk of cancer of the cervix, vulva and vagina. Women with genital warts should have regular six-monthly Pap smears of the cervix to detect early changes.

During pregnancy, warts tend to grow rapidly and may become traumatized and bleed during childbirth; thus it is best to have vaginal warts treated and cleared before pregnancy occurs.

The treatment of genital warts

Firstly, excessive vaginal secretions should be cleared up and small warts may then disappear by themselves simply because the vagina is not so moist and warm. The oral contraceptive pill can speed up the growth of warts and it may be necessary to stop taking this until the warts are eradicated.

If the warts are small and separate, topical application of a caustic substance known as 'podophyllin' can be performed by your doctor to each individual wart, two to three times a week for one month. Only a few warts can be treated with podophyllin at any one time as if it is absorbed through the skin and mucous membranes, a toxic reaction can result. For this reason it must not be used during pregnancy.

In women who are suffering from warts during pregnancy, it is best to delay treatment until after childbirth as a spontaneous cure may result in the post-natal period.

Large warts are best treated by burning (cauterization), freezing (cryotherapy) or surgical removal with scissors and a curette. If the number of warts is small, this can be done under local anaesthetic; however, if they are widespread, especially inside the vagina, these procedures should be done under a general anaesthetic in hospital. There may be some temporary pain post-operatively but healing will be excellent in this area as it has a rich blood supply.

AIDS

What is AIDS?

Acquired immune deficiency syndrome (AIDS) is a disease in which there is destruction of the body's normal immune defence system. The immune system defends the body against infections and cancers and it consists of blood proteins called antibodies and white blood cells. The antibodies attach to and neutralize viruses and bacteria, while the white blood cells attack viruses, bacteria and some cancer cells with the aim of destroying them.

The AIDS virus destroys one particular type of white blood cell called the 'helper inducer T4+ lymphocyte'. These T4+ lymphocytes are needed to protect against viruses and cancer and thus, in AIDS-infected people, this protection is lost. Indeed, the AIDS virus so completely incapacitates the immune system that the AIDS sufferer becomes prey to common environmental organisms that are usually harmless to healthy people.

What causes AIDS?

This immune destruction is caused by infection with a virus known as the AIDS virus. The AIDS virus has also been given names such as the ARV virus, LAV virus and HTLV III virus. The AIDS virus, unlike other viruses such as the common cold or influenza, inserts a copy of its own genetic code into the cell it infects so that this infected cell is permanently controlled by the AIDS virus.

Where did AIDS originate?

Increasing evidence suggests that AIDS first affected remote rural populations in Central Africa and was possibly derived from the African green monkey.

From there it spread to cities of Central Africa where it was then spread as a heterosexually transmitted disease. Caribbean nations which had interaction with Central Africa were affected next, and the mobility and sexual behaviour of American homosexual men subsequently took AIDS into the large gay communities of the United States of America.

Intravenous drug users in New York then contracted the virus and also the American supply of donors' blood became contaminated. Spread to other Western countries followed, usually by homosexual contacts. The first cases of AIDS in the USA occurred in 1981 and the first case in the UK occurred in 1982.

Who is at risk of developing AIDS?

AIDS has not been transmitted through casual contact with blood, sneezing, coughing, touching, social interaction or casual kissing. The AIDS virus is removed by normal washing of cutlery and dishes and is not transmitted in households where people share common dishes. You cannot get AIDS from public toilets or transport, telephones or drinking fountains.

People at risk used to fall into well-defined categories:

1 Sexually active homosexual or bisexual men.

2 Recipients of multiple blood transfusions before 1985, as this was prior to antibody testing of blood donors.

3 Intravenous drug users and prostitutes.

4 Haemophiliacs.

An infected pregnant woman has a high chance of transmitting AIDS to her baby during pregnancy or soon after birth.

Since AIDS was first identified, it has remained mainly in these high risk groups. AIDS can be spread by heterosexual contact and this is beginning to occur in Western countries, so AIDS should no longer be considered as a plague confined to homosexual men. Although only a small number of women have so far been infected with HIV, this seems likely to increase in the future. No longer can AIDS be considered exclusively a disease of the homosexual population. If Western countries do not recognize the threat of heterosexual transmission of AIDS, they could see a situation similar to the African one developing in their own countries.

What is the AIDS situation in Africa?

This is very different from the AIDS problem in the Western world where the risk is still mainly confined to homosexual men, prostitutes and drug addicts. In Central Africa, the AIDS virus infects mainly young heterosexually active men and women, with up to 15 per cent of the population carrying the virus. In Africa, it is currently estimated that up to six million people are infected with AIDS. The reasons for this are not entirely clear, but it is thought that endemic malnutrition there has led to poor immune function and thus increased susceptibility to the virus. These countries are too poor to screen blood donors and so 15 to 20 per cent of blood transfusions are contaminated with AIDS. Medical needles for injections are reused and thus also help to spread the disease.

In Western (Saharan) Africa there is a glimmer of hope, as a new type of AIDS virus called the HTLV IV virus has been discovered. This virus does not cause disease in humans and thus could possibly be used to develop a vaccine against the real AIDS virus, HTLV III. Trials are currently being done in mice to see if vaccination with HTLV IV virus can provide protection against infection with HTLV III virus. If it can, such a vaccine would only protect people who have had no previous contact with AIDS and could do nothing for those who are already antibody positive.

What is the incubation period for AIDS?

The majority of people infected with the AIDS virus for the first time will have an acute viral illness within a few weeks of initial infection. This may consist of a sore throat, fever, cough, runny nose, aches and pains, sweating, diarrhoea and a rash. This first illness lasts from three to fourteen days.

Most of these cases settle down to normal health and, after that, the only sign of contact with AIDS becomes the presence of the AIDS antibody in the blood.

With new diseases one can never be sure of the future. However, at present, the majority of those infected with the AIDS virus have not developed the AIDS disease.

Is there a test for AIDS?

When a virus attacks the body, the body's immune system produces antibodies to fight and neutralize the virus. The blood test for AIDS shows if there are any antibodies against the AIDS virus present and does not test for the virus itself. If a person has the antibody against the AIDS virus in their blood (antibody positive), he or she has been infected at some time and is potentially able to transmit AIDS to others.

Blood tests are available on the NHS mainly at Sexually Transmitted Disease (STD) clinics at departments of genito-urinary medicine in hospitals, and counselling by hospital staff is available. Tests can be carried out privately but counselling is not so readily available. If you are in a high risk group, you should consider taking a test, but it must be thought through first. This is where pre-test counselling can help.

Stages of infection with AIDS

Stage C

These people are only known to be infected through laboratory tests on their blood which show that they are positive for the AIDS virus antibody. They are otherwise quite well. Of all stage C patients, only 10 to 20 per cent will progress to stage A within five years.

As AIDS is only a new disease, it is not yet known if all antibody positive, but otherwise well AIDS carriers, harbour a viral time bomb with biological fuses of different lengths – this is the Nobel Prize winning question. One hopes that the answer is no, and it seems that most people with stage C AIDS (AIDS carriers) will remain well indefinitely.

Stage B

These people have developed a mild chronic form of the disease consisting of swollen lymph glands in the neck, armpits and groin. They may have intermittent fever, sweating and fatigue.

Stage A

These people have fully developed or 'full-blown' AIDS symptoms which will lead to death within two to three years. The symptoms are due to the multiple infections and specific cancers which attack them because their immune systems are so inefficient. These symptoms may be similar to those everyone feels occasionally, but in people with AIDS, the symptoms are more severe and persistent. The symptoms may include:

Extreme tiredness, depression and irritability;
Headaches or visual problems;
Weight loss of more than five kilograms (eleven pounds) without dieting;
Purple reddish growths on the skin or the mucous membranes inside the mouth, nose or anus;
A heavy persistent cough;

Severe continual diarrhoea;

Thrush in the mouth or throat;

Ulcers on the tongue and infections of the gums;

Persistent fever;

Anaemia and enlarged spleen;

Excessive bleeding from any body opening or from mucous
   membranes, such as those inside the mouth or nose, and easy
   bruising;

Shortness of breath;

Fungal skin infections;

Genital warts and severe recurrent genital herpes;

Chronic sores lasting more than one month and recurrent
   shingles;

Bacterial skin infections such as impetigo, boils and abscesses of a
   severe degree.

These symptoms may represent a lung infection with rare organisms, infection of the intestine or a rare type of cancer which occurs
on the skin or in the mouth and looks like a round bluish, raised
patch. This cancer is called 'Kaposi's sarcoma'. In severely affected
patients, there may be symptoms of brain or spinal cord infection
such as dementia, meningitis, convulsions and muscular weakness.

The treatment of AIDS

For the millions of people who are antibody positive, there is no
promise or hope of cure on the horizon.

The main aim should be to *prevent progression* of stage C and B
AIDS to stage A, as once a patient has arrived at stage A, death is
almost certain within three years.

The best protection against this progression of the disease is very
simple – maintain a strong healthy body and efficient immune
system while we wait for a possible cure. Life-style should be
puritanical, minimizing stress and ingestion of drugs, cigarettes,
sperm, alcohol and unnecessary antibiotics.

The diet should be high in living raw foods (salads and fruits),
whole grains and polyunsaturated fats (fish, seeds, primrose oil and
cold pressed vegetable oils). An excess of saturated animal fats
should be avoided.

It is advisable for AIDS sufferers to avoid vaccinations such as travel inoculations or against hepatitis. This is because vaccines stimulate the immune system's T cells and may cause multiplication of the AIDS virus living inside those cells.

The development of anti-AIDS drugs is still in the experimental stage and no definite signs of hope have yet emerged. Most drugs tried so far have caused unacceptable side effects. Clinical trials using the anti-cancer drug 'Interferon' have produced improvements in about half of the AIDS patients with the bluish skin cancers of Kaposi's sarcoma.

Drugs commonly used to treat cancer cannot be used successfully in AIDS patients because they weaken further the already damaged immune system of the AIDS sufferer and thus increase the risk of infections. Interferon, however, is a safe anti-cancer drug for AIDS patients.

The drug 'Cyclosporine', if given in the early stages of the disease, may reduce AIDS from a lethal to a chronic, grumbling disease, perhaps allowing AIDS victims to buy time until a real cure is found. Other so-called wonder drugs, such as Suramin and Ribavirin, have been tried to stop multiplication of the virus in the body but have resulted in only a temporary halting of the progress of the disease, and at the price of severe side effects.

A new genetically engineered protein known as 'methione enkaphalin' has been shown to boost the flagging immune system of AIDS and cancer patients. This drug cannot provide a cure, but it can reduce the terrible infections which attack the AIDS patient and so far has proved to be free of toxic side effects.

There is no effective treatment which enables us to restore the T4 lymphocytes of the immune system that have been destroyed by the AIDS virus. Bone marrow transplants or the giving of healthy lymphocytes have not proved to be effective treatments. Therapy should be directed at trying to overcome the numerous infections with antibiotics and good hygiene.

The prevention of AIDS

1 Vaccination

Researchers are working on a vaccine to protect against contracting AIDS. However, the AIDS virus has an uncanny ability to mutate and thus escape a specific antibody of the immune system and this could make a vaccine useless in the long term. Similar slight mutations in the cold and flu viruses have made truly effective vaccination against them impossible, and the AIDS virus has so far proved even cleverer.

2 Screening donors of blood and semen

The institution of effective nationwide blood screening tests together with the heat treatment of blood have greatly reduced the threat of transmission through donor blood. All blood collected since April 1985 has been screened for antibodies to the AIDS virus and this test is very accurate in identifying infected blood. Any blood that indicates AIDS infection is not used for transfusion. Blood transfusion services are now as secure as they possibly can be, and the risk of contracting AIDS from an emergency blood transfusion is now less than one in a million.

Donations to sperm banks for artificial insemination and to organ banks for transplantation are subjected to the same screening test as blood.

3 Sexual practices

If you or your partner have homosexual or heterosexual contact outside your regular relationship, make sure it is safe and avoid exchanging risky body fluids. The following is a list of safe and unsafe sexual practices:

Safe

Mutual masturbation
Social kissing (dry kissing)
Body massage and hugging
Frottage (body to body rubbing including genitals)
Mild sadomasochism (excluding bleeding)
Use of own sex toys

Possibly safe
Anal intercourse using a condom
Fellatio interruptus
Mouth to mouth kissing (wet kissing)
Vaginal intercourse using a condom
Oral vaginal contact

Unsafe
Receptive insertive anal sex without a condom
Receptive insertive vaginal sex without a condom
Manual anal sex (fisting)
Fellatio with ejaculation
Oral anal contact (rimming)

Condoms are effective in blocking the transmission of disease but it is important that they do not break, which can happen during anal intercourse. They are not 100 per cent foolproof in preventing pregnancy and were not designed to prevent disease, so they cannot give complete security. The Terrence Higgins Trust suggests using two condoms for added protection.

4 Drug addicts
Drug addicts should not share needles and syringes and should indulge only in safe sexual practices.

5 Isolation or quarantine of AIDS cases
There is no evidence that casual contact with a person who has AIDS poses any risk whatsoever of contamination. AIDS is not spread by air, food, touching or handling the same things, but only by direct blood to blood contact or unprotected sexual intercourse.

Human rights issues

People with AIDS should not be ostracized and treated as lepers as they do not pose a risk to the general public. There is no need for the everyday AIDS carrier to wear a special warning badge alarming those with whom he or she works or has social contact. There is no need to ban AIDS carriers from working in people-contact jobs such as banks, buses, restaurants and bars. All AIDS sufferers should be allowed to work unless their job poses a risk of direct blood to blood contact with others.

When it comes to promiscuity and free sex, AIDS sufferers do not have unlimited human rights. They should take precautions and tell any prospective sexual partner that they carry the AIDS virus before they indulge in unprotected sexual intercourse. Quite obviously, no one has the right to go around spreading a potentially fatal disease.

The current projection for AIDS is that 270,000 people, in the USA alone, will have contracted AIDS by the tenth anniversary of the disease in 1991. We can only hope that the brilliant medical research which has been undertaken so far will continue, and that before 1991 we will have stopped this formidable enemy, the AIDS virus, in its evolution. Let us stick together and all take responsibility in this challenge.

Help for victims of AIDS

There are a number of charities in the United Kingdom specifically supporting those whose lives have been afflicted by AIDS.

The best known is the Terrence Higgins Trust which has a comprehensive support and information network. The Trust undertakes counselling among its services. The Trust is at 52–54 Grays Inn Road, London WC1X 8LT. Its helpline is on 071-242 1010 between 3 p.m. and 10 p.m. daily and on 071-405 2463 for the deaf and hard of hearing between 7 p.m. and 10 p.m. daily. The Trust will also give information on a caller's nearest STD clinic.

Frontliners is a self-help group for PWAs (people with AIDS). It is open 11 a.m. to 5 p.m. daily on 071-831 0330.

Body Positive, a self-help group for HIV antibody positive homosexual men. Contact through the Terrence Higgins Trust.

Positively Women, for antibody positive women. Tel 081-671 4469.

Women's Reproductive Rights and Information Centre (for information on donor insemination) 52–54 Featherstone Street, London EC1Y 8RT. 071-251 6332.

Haemophilia Society, which helps its members who have been infected through transfusions or blood products. 123 Westminster Bridge Road, London SE1 7HR. 071-928 2020.

Scottish AIDS Monitor, PO Box 169, Edinburgh EH1 3UU. Helpline 031-558 1167. Monday to Friday 7.30 p.m. to 10 p.m.

10 Pregnancy

The topic of pregnancy and childbirth is a vast one, and to cover all its facets would require a whole book. This chapter does not intend to cover all aspects of pregnancy but is designed to provide you with practical facts on the most common disorders of pregnancy. You will find a comprehensive table of nutritional requirements during pregnancy and helpful hints to cope with minor disorders.

New techniques for the diagnosis of hereditary diseases during pregnancy are described and the personal biography of a remarkable woman and mother is included which will give you insights into the experience of pregnancy.

For women requiring more detailed information on pregnancy and childbirth, I recommend them to read the book entitled *Everywoman* by Derek Llewellyn-Jones.

Nutritional requirements during pregnancy

A pregnant woman requires an average of 2500 to 2800 calories daily which is 500 calories above the usual daily calorie quota necessary to maintain body weight during the non-pregnant state. This number of calories can be obtained by eating the amounts of the five food groups given in Table E every day.

Table E

Food group	Servings (1 serving = half large cup)
1 Dairy (Milk, cheese, yoghurt, ice-cream)	4 servings
2 First class protein (a) Animal (chicken, red meats, fish, seafoods, organ meats) (b) Vegetable Combine three of the following at one meal: nuts, seeds, grains, legumes.	3 to 4 servings (65 to 80 grams each serving)
3 Fruit and vegetables, especially raw and of green leafy variety. Citrus fruits are particularly beneficial.	3 servings of fruit, 2 servings of vegetables, salads may be taken freely.
4 Bread and cereals (preferably whole grain)	4 slices or 4 servings
5 Butter and oils	15 to 30 grams daily

The servings described in Table E also provide for the daily requirement of vitamins and minerals during pregnancy. These requirements can be found in Table F.

Table F

Nutrient	Daily requirement	Function
Calcium	1.2 grams	Manufacture of baby's skeleton and teeth, breast milk and essential for muscular contraction and coagulation of blood.
B Complex Vitamins		
B3 niacin	15 milligrams	Necessary for the manufacture of
B2 riboflavin	1.8 milligrams	blood, and the metabolism of
B1 thiamine	2 milligrams	carbohydrate and protein. Essential
B6		for the development of the baby's
pyridoxine	2.5 milligrams	brain and spinal cord.
B12	5 micrograms	
Folic acid	0.4 milligrams	There is an increased demand for folic acid during pregnancy, especially multiple pregnancy. It is necessary for the manufacture of blood and development of the baby's vital organs.
Vitamin C	100 to 500 milligrams. The requirement is controversial and some women need more, especially if they smoke. A vitamin C supplement in tablet form is worthwhile.	Necessary for production of blood and connective tissues in the skin, bones, cartilage, teeth and muscles. Increases resistance against infection.
Iron	60 milligrams	Necessary for production of blood and to build up maternal stores of iron in preparation for breastfeeding.

Nutrient	Daily requirement	Function
Vitamin A	6000 international units	Necessary for the function of the skin, mucous membranes and immune system.
Vitamin D	400 international units	Necessary for the absorption and utilization of calcium and phosphorus. Thus it is essential in the formation of the baby's skeleton and teeth.
Vitamin E	100 international units	Necessary for the manufacture of blood and maintenance of a healthy circulation.
Iodine	125 milligrams	Necessary for the production of thyroid hormone which is involved in determining the metabolic rate and development of the baby's nervous system.
Zinc	15 to 30 milligrams	Necessary for the manufacture of genetic material and protein. Involved in the metabolism of hormones and carbohydrates. Zinc deficiency can cause intra-uterine growth retardation, birth defects and underdeveloped sex glands.

Minor problems of pregnancy

1 Nausea and vomiting

The high levels of female hormones during pregnancy act on the liver and the vomiting centre in the brain to stimulate nausea.

Helpful hints:

(a) On rising in the morning eat one or two dry biscuits and move about slowly. Always eat something for breakfast.
(b) Avoid acidic or fatty foods or highly spiced foods.

(c) If you have cravings for unusual combinations of foods, it is all right to indulge them, as they may be nature's way of overcoming nutritional deficiencies.

(d) Eat small frequent meals, four to six daily.

(e) If you cannot tolerate any food try sucking barley sugar to maintain blood sugar levels.

(f) Homoeopathic drops – these may be taken in a dosage of ten drops every hour in a half glass of water. The following drops are useful: cocculus, ipecacuanha, aethusa cynapium, tabacum, ignatia, nux vomica.

(g) Vitamin B6 (pyridoxine), 50 milligrams daily with food.

2 Fatigue and drowsiness

Your body's energy is being utilized to maintain the growth and nutrition of the foetus.

Helpful hints:

(a) Nutritional supplements such as iron, folic acid, B complex and vitamins C and E.

(b) Sleep an extra hour in the afternoon and go to bed early.

(c) During the first twenty weeks of pregnancy you may rest flat on your back if you desire. After the twentieth week it is best to rest and sleep on your side as blood return to the heart is more efficient in this position. If you feel breathless or faint, lying on your side will also ease these symptoms.

3 Constipation and haemorrhoids

The enlarged uterus presses on the bowels and the pelvic veins. The high levels of the hormone progesterone produce relaxation of the intestinal muscles. Thus the bowels become sluggish and if straining occurs during a bowel action the possibility of haemorrhoids will be increased.

Helpful hints:

(a) Eat high fibre cereals and lots of raw fruit and vegetables. Avoid greasy and processed foods.

(b) Bulk laxatives such as metamucil, raw bran or normacol are safe to take and will make the bowel action softer and larger.

(c) Increase water and raw vegetable juices to four to eight glasses daily.

(d) Exercise regularly.

(e) Apply a local ointment to the haemorrhoids if they are painful during the passing of a bowel action, for example, a local anaesthetic ointment such as lignocaine.

(f) If you find iron tablets cause constipation, try taking a slow release variety of iron tablets.

4 Heartburn and reflux

During the last three months the large uterus compresses the stomach, reducing its capacity and increasing reflux of stomach acid back up into the chest and throat.

Helpful hints:

(a) Do not drink with meals.

(b) Take small frequent meals and do not eat late at night. Go for a walk after eating.

(c) Avoid aspirin, painkilling drugs, coffee, alcohol, cigarettes.

(d) You may take certain antacids which are low in sodium (salt), for example, Titralac. If reflux is a big problem, Gaviscon granules may be tried after meals, but not in women with high blood pressure or on low salt diets.

(e) Certain herbal teas such as marshmallow, chamomile and peppermint may be beneficial, and slippery elm tablets in a dosage of two, four times daily, can also help.

(f) Elevate the head of the bed with two bricks and use extra pillows to elevate the head.

5 Cramps in the legs

These commonly occur in the last three months of pregnancy and are worse after retiring to bed at night. They are probably due to the reduction in blood circulation to the muscles of the legs and the change in the mineral concentration of the blood during pregnancy.

Helpful hints:

(a) Stretch the leg muscles by sitting up and pulling the toes upward towards the head. Have someone massage your leg muscles and feet and, if this fails, go for a walk.

(b) Mineral supplements:
  i Sandocal 1000, one or two dissolved in water daily.

ii Mineral supplement containing potassium aspartate 250mg, magnesium aspartate 250mg, one tablet three times daily.

(c) Vitamin E and vitamin C. Also garlic, two capsules, three times daily with food.

6 Varicose veins and clots in the superficial veins (thrombophlebitis), swollen feet

The high levels of female hormones cause relaxation and swelling of the veins. The large uterus compresses the pelvic veins, increasing pressure in the leg veins.

Helpful hints:

(a) Before rising from bed put on maternity tights or support stockings.

(b) Take regular physical exercise, especially swimming, and elevate the legs on two pillows when resting.

(c) Supplements of vitamin C, bioflavonoids, vitamin E. Also garlic, two capsules, three times daily with food. Apple cider vinegar from a health food store in a dosage of two tablespoons daily.

(d) Massage the areas of thrombophlebitis where the veins are hard, red and painful with a cream called Lasonil.

7 Skin disorders, such as stretch marks and patches of darkened skin (chloasma)

Weight gain causes stretching of the skin. The female hormones stimulate melanin production in the pigment-producing cells of the skin which results in brown patches.

Helpful hints:

(a) Avoid the sun or wear a large brimmed hat and use a strong sunscreen.

(b) Avoid excessive weight gain and massage stretch marks as soon as they appear with vitamin E and collagen cream.

8 Sciatica, backache and pelvic aches

The increased abdominal weight tends to increase the curve of the lumbar spine putting extra strain on this area. The high levels of female hormones cause stretching and softening of the ligaments of the back and pelvis. Occasionally the pubic bones may separate causing sharp pains over the pubic area when walking.

Helpful hints:

(a) Posture is important. Stand tall and straight and tuck in your tummy. When sitting use a straight-backed chair and place both feet on the floor and sit tall.

(b) Avoid standing for long periods and avoid bending from the waist. When bending keep the back straight and bend at the knees. Avoid jogging in late pregnancy. Also, avoid jarring exercises.

(c) The best exercises for women with back problems during pregnancy are swimming and yoga.

(d) A daily pelvic rock is beneficial – to do this kneel down on all fours and arch the back upwards by pulling in the buttocks and contracting the abdominal muscles inwards. Stay in this position for one or two minutes and breathe in slowly and deeply. Practise the pelvic rock exercise for ten minutes, twice daily.

(e) Massage, acupuncture and physiotherapy to the back can relieve pain.

(f) Homoeopathic drops – ten drops, four times daily in half a glass of water. Suitable drops are symphytum, arnica, hammamelis, ruta graveolins.

(g) When lifting, keep the weight close to the body, the feet wide apart, the back straight and bend only at the knees.

Anaemia

Anaemia during pregnancy is not rare and is definitely a danger to watch out for. If you are anaemic you will probably feel tired, irritable, short of breath on exercise and notice that you look very pale. The test that a doctor does to check for anaemia is called a haemoglobin (HB) measurement. The HB measurement is an indication of the amount of iron-containing red blood cells in your blood. A low HB measurement means a low number of iron-containing red blood cells and this is the condition of anaemia.

In developed countries, a woman during pregnancy is classified as being anaemic if her haemoglobin is below 12 grams/100 millilitres during the first twelve weeks of pregnancy, or below 10 grams/100 millilitres in later pregnancy.

What are the risks of anaemia during pregnancy?

If your doctor finds you are very anaemic, you will be more at risk of infection and heart strain during your pregnancy. Furthermore, you will be less able to tolerate heavy bleeding should it occur during or after childbirth.

The risks to your baby include a poor oxygen supply as the iron-containing red blood cells carry oxygen to the placenta and vital organs. If your placenta is not particularly healthy, the poor placental function will be exaggerated by the poor quality of your anaemic blood. This could make your baby more susceptible to poor intra-uterine growth. Another risk to the baby, if your anaemia is severe, is a higher incidence of premature labour.

What are the types of anaemia?

1 Iron deficiency anaemia

This is the most common type of anaemia and is due to lack of iron in the body. The mineral iron is required to manufacture healthy red blood cells and, when there is not enough iron, the red blood cells are not only insufficient in number but are also small, pale and oddly shaped. These small red blood cells also have a decreased ability to carry oxygen.

The factors which increase a woman's risk of iron deficiency anaemia are a diet low in iron, poor absorption of iron from the intestines or excessive loss of blood from the body due to heavy menstruation, bleeding during pregnancy or bleeding from haemorrhoids. The treatment of iron deficiency anaemia involves an iron supplement such as ferrous sulphate, 200 to 300 milligrams, three times daily. If upset of the intestine and stomach occurs you may find that the organic salts of iron such as iron gluconate or iron succinate are better tolerated. If you experience nausea, diarrhoea or constipation from iron tablets you should try slow release preparations of iron as these have a lower incidence of such side effects. It is best to take your iron tablet between meals with a vitamin C supplement or citrus fruits, as vitamin C improves the absorption of iron to a very significant degree. Also, you should avoid drinking beverages containing tannic acid, such as tea, as these will drastically reduce the absorption of iron from the intestine into the blood.

Remember that iron tablets are poisonous to small children so keep them hidden away in a cupboard that is high up on the wall, in a child-resistant container.

Some women, late in pregnancy, have severe iron deficiency anaemia and there is no time to wait for iron tablets to work. In this situation, it is best to give the iron as an intra-muscular injection.

All pregnant women, whether anaemic or not, should eat foods high in iron as pregnancy and breastfeeding both require large amounts of iron and rapidly use up the iron stored in the body.

The minimum amount of iron required daily is eighteen milligrams. Foods that are high in iron are: liver, kidney, lean red meats, eggs, cereals, whole grains, dried nuts, dried fruits, legumes, beetroot and green leafy vegetables. Iron from animal sources is more easily absorbed than iron from plant sources; therefore during pregnancy if you have low iron stores, it is best to make sure you do get some red meat in the diet.

By eating organ meats, shellfish, nuts, legumes and a wide range of vegetables, one also ensures adequate supplies of the minerals copper and zinc, which are also required for production of red blood cells.

2 Folic acid deficiency anaemia

Folic acid is a vitamin required for the division of cells and for the growth of red blood cells and white blood cells in the bone marrow in the bones. A deficiency of folic acid results in insufficient numbers of red blood cells being formed in the bone marrow and, therefore, a deficient number of red cells in the blood. A lack of folic acid can also result in a miscarriage or foetal abnormalities and, therefore, this vitamin should be treated seriously during pregnancy, as much larger amounts are needed.

A deficiency of folic acid can result in anaemia, especially in the second half of pregnancy when the demands of the foetus increase.

Causes of folic acid deficiency are: poor diet; overcooking of food; storing of food, especially of fresh leafy vegetables; poor absorption from the gut; multiple pregnancy; some anti-convulsant drugs. The level of folic acid can easily be measured in your blood and red blood cells to exclude a deficiency. It is recommended that all pregnant women take a supplement of folic acid of between 100 to 500 micrograms three times daily. Your doctor will work out the dosage required for you as women with multiple pregnancy require much more.

During pregnancy foods high in folic acid should be eaten, namely raw green leafy vegetables, liver, kidney, nuts, yeast, legumes, soya beans, soya flour, wheat, rice germ and dried peas.

3 Vitamin B12 deficiency anaemia

Deficiency of vitamin B12 can result in poor production of red blood cells in the bone marrow leading to insufficient red blood cells in the blood. This type of anaemia is not rare in complete vegetarians, such as vegans, who avoid all animal products, because B12 is only found in significant amounts in animal and dairy products. Other causes of B12 deficiency are diseases of the stomach and small intestine which reduce the capacity of the intestine to absorb B12 into the blood. In these disorders the patient requires regular injections of vitamin B12.

Human beings need only small amounts of B12 every day, but it is an extremely important vitamin as deficiency can result not only in anaemia, but nervous depression and degeneration of the spinal cord with numbness and tingling of the feet, poor balance, painful legs and eventually paralysis.

It is particularly dangerous to take folic acid by itself in a case of non-specific anaemia in which B12 deficiency may exist, as the folic acid, if taken without B12, may precipitate degeneration of the spinal cord and paralysis.

Foods high in B12 which should be eaten during pregnancy are: liver, kidney, meat, fish, dairy products and eggs.

4 Congenital anaemias

In this type of hereditary anaemia, the haemoglobin protein and pigment in the red blood cells is abnormal in structure and function. The most common type of congenital anaemia is thalassaemia minor which is common in people from the Mediterranean, such as Italians and Greeks. It can be easily diagnosed with a blood test.

Because the haemoglobin of the red blood cells is abnormal the red blood cells are destroyed more rapidly and live only 40 days instead of their usual 120 days. Most people with the minor form of thalassaemia manage to pass through pregnancy with a haemoglobin count of 8 to 10 grams per 100 millilitres. There is not much that can be done about this, other than to supply extra amounts of folic acid to keep up with the more rapid division of cells in the bone marrow; however, it is best that these people avoid iron as they usually have excessive storage of iron in the body.

The major form of thalassaemia is thankfully very rare. It requires many blood transfusions and often results in an early death. Other congenital anaemias are spherocytosis and sickle cell anaemia.

Vaginal bleeding in the first half of pregnancy

Abortion

An abortion is the loss of a pregnancy before the time that the foetus is able to survive in the outside world. This time of foetal viability has been defined, somewhat arbitrarily by the medical and legal professions, as being at twenty-eight weeks of pregnancy. If a foetus is born after twenty-eight weeks of pregnancy it is considered, theoretically, as being able to survive and thus is no longer considered as an abortion.

There are three different types of abortion:

1 Spontaneous abortion (miscarriage) which is an abortion occurring without outside provocation.

2 Criminal abortion – an abortion procured by outside methods that are not medically safe and are not considered legal.

3 Therapeutic abortion – an abortion that is procured by outside methods to protect the mental and physical health of the woman, and using techniques which are medically safe and legally recognized.

Miscarriage (spontaneous abortion)

A miscarriage is said to occur when the foetus and placenta are spontaneously expelled from the uterus before the twenty-eighth week of pregnancy. It comes as a shock for many women to learn that around 10 to 15 per cent of all pregnancies under twenty weeks end in a miscarriage. Most threatened miscarriages occur during the first twelve weeks of pregnancy and once you have passed the milestone of the first three months, your chances of having a miscarriage become very much smaller.

Why are miscarriages so common?

The high rate of miscarriages is due to the many possible conditions that can result in rejection and loss of the early foetus.

The most common cause is an abnormal foetus or placenta caused by abnormal genetic material. In other words, the chromosomes or genes of the baby are abnormal. In such cases the miscarriage is just Mother Nature's way of getting rid of a deformed baby before it really gets a hold on life, and this type of miscarriage is really a blessing in disguise.

Another condition which increases the chance of a miscarriage is a hormonal imbalance in the mother, particularly a deficiency of progesterone.

Psychological stress and emotional illness in the mother can have a negative effect on the nervous system and circulation which can result in a miscarriage.

If the mother takes toxic drugs or suffers from an infection or other medical disorder in early pregnancy, this may result in an unfavourable environment for the foetus and lead to a miscarriage.

The muscular uterus forms the walls of the house of the foetus and, if the uterus is irritated, malformed or diseased this can make it an unsuitable environment for the foetus and result in a miscarriage. The uterus may be irritated by trauma after an accident, a rough pelvic examination or very vigorous sexual intercourse. The uterus may be malformed by fibroids or may be resting in a position of extreme retroversion. See page 15.

If a miscarriage occurs after the twelfth week of pregnancy the doctor will usually test for an incompetent cervix. An incompetent cervix is due to weakness and damage of the circular muscular fibres in the cervix, making the cervix incapable of holding the foetus and placenta inside the uterus as they grow in size. An incompetent cervix is responsible for 1 per cent of all miscarriages and 20 per cent of recurrent miscarriages.

When the cervix is incompetent, the bag of water surrounding the foetus tends to bulge through the slack cervix and is more likely to rupture prematurely. A woman with an incompetent cervix often first realizes she is miscarrying because of water leaking out of her vagina due to premature rupture of the membranes. This is later followed by vaginal bleeding and painful uterine contractions. Once the membranes have been ruptured the pregnancy cannot be saved and the doctor will encourage the uterus to expel the foetus with intravenous drugs or a curette. Factors which may give rise to an incompetent cervix are an excessive number of surgical terminations of pregnancy, especially if the terminations were performed at a fairly advanced stage of pregnancy, and surgical procedures performed on the cervix such as a large cone biopsy to treat early cancer of the cervix.

In the woman with cervical incompetence, the aim of the doctor is to detect the problem in early pregnancy before the cervix begins to stretch and dilate and allow the membranes to bulge through it. The doctor may be suspicious of the existence of cervical incompetence because of a pre-existing history of recurrent miscarriages occurring after the twelfth week of pregnancy. If the doctor discovers cervical incompetence in a woman, he will place a strong firm stitch around the cervix to pull it tight, at the fourteenth week of pregnancy. This will stop the cervix dilating and prevent the membranes from bulging through it. Statistics have shown that such a stitch can prevent miscarriage or premature labour in 70 per cent of women with cervical incompetence, provided the stitch is placed early enough in the cervix.

How do you know if you are going to have a miscarriage?

The first sign of a miscarriage is usually vaginal bleeding. Most miscarriages only threaten to occur and do not proceed to the death or expulsion of the foetus. Indeed, in the majority of threatened miscarriages, the vaginal bleeding gradually settles down, is not associated with significant abdominal pain and pregnancy continues normally.

Conversely, if the vaginal bleeding is heavy, bright red in colour or associated with clots and continues to increase, it is likely that the foetus will be expelled or die inside the uterus. In these cases, the woman usually experiences period-type pains due to the dilatation of the cervix which occurs to allow the passage of the foetus and placenta into the vagina.

A miscarriage is said to have definitely occurred once the bleeding has so disturbed the pregnancy that the foetus is unable to survive. This type of miscarriage cannot be arrested and is called an inevitable abortion. An inevitable abortion may be complete, meaning that the entire foetus and placenta are spontaneously expelled by the contractions of the uterus leaving an empty uterus behind.

More commonly, during an inevitable abortion, the uterine contractions only partially expel the foetus and placenta so that the uterus still contains part of the products of pregnancy in a non-living state. Such a miscarriage is called incomplete and, in these cases, the doctor will need to perform a dilatation and curettage of the uterus to ensure that the uterus is empty.

In general, women who may be going to have a miscarriage should be admitted to hospital for rest and investigation of the possible cause. An ultrasound test may be done to see if the foetus is still alive and normal in form and position. A pregnancy test will also be done to see if the foetus is still alive.

It is reassuring to know that the majority of threatened miscarriages settle down with bed rest. After this the pregnancy usually continues normally and there is no significant increase in malformation of the foetus or interference with its growth. After a threatened miscarriage has settled down, the patient can go home as long as she takes it easy and avoids sexual intercourse for three weeks. If a miscarriage progresses and becomes inevitable, blood loss and pain may be severe. In such cases a dilatation and curettage to empty the uterus and stop bleeding will be required.

In a small percentage of early pregnancies, death of the foetus may occur without any external warning to the mother. This type of abortion is called a missed abortion as no one is aware it has occurred. There may be some slight vaginal bleeding but this does not always happen and the possibility that something has gone wrong is usually brought to the doctor's attention when the woman says that her symptoms of pregnancy, such as nausea and breast pain, have diminished and that her uterus and abdomen are becoming smaller. In cases of a missed abortion an ultrasound scan will show that the foetal heart is no longer beating. If the uterus does not spontaneously expel the dead foetus and placenta, a dilatation and curettage will be required, or if the pregnancy is more advanced, a miniature labour can be induced with an intravenous drip.

What is the outlook for a woman who has had a miscarriage?

Spontaneous abortion is quite common and if a woman has had one miscarriage this does not mean she is likely to keep miscarrying with her subsequent pregnancies. Statistics show that:

1 If a woman has had one miscarriage the chances of her next pregnancy being totally normal and advancing to full maturity are the same as a normal woman's, meaning a woman who has never had a miscarriage. If you have had a miscarriage and are feeling particularly depressed about it, the best way to overcome this feeling of depression and loss is to fall pregnant again as soon as possible. This strong maternal instinct is very common and many women become pregnant quickly after their first abortion.

2 After two successive miscarriages there is a 75 per cent chance that the next pregnancy will be normal.

3 After three successive miscarriages there is a 70 per cent chance that the next pregnancy will be normal.

Thus it is clear that having one or several spontaneous abortions does not cast a bleak cloud over the success of your future pregnancies.

If a woman has three or more successive spontaneous abortions she is said to be a recurrent or habitual aborter. Such a woman should have a thorough examination, blood tests and ultrasound scans. An X-ray of the uterus may be required using oily dyes to see if there is any underlying cause which can be corrected.

Ectopic pregnancy

Another cause of vaginal bleeding in the first half of pregnancy is ectopic pregnancy. This is a very dangerous condition in which the fertilized egg implants outside its normal position in the uterine cavity. In an ectopic pregnancy, implantation usually occurs inside the Fallopian tube, although very occasionally it may occur in the ovary, cervix or abdominal cavity. As the embryo begins to grow in these abnormal sites it becomes too large to be supported by the surrounding structures and rupture of the tube, ovary or cervix will occur, producing heavy internal bleeding. If the problem is not recognized, the patient may die without timely treatment and an abdominal operation.

Ectopic pregnancy is not rare and occurs in about 1 in 200 pregnancies. Previous factors which increase your chances of having an ectopic pregnancy are pelvic inflammatory disease with infection in the Fallopian tubes, severe appendicitis, endometriosis, previous tubal surgery and the use of an intra-uterine contraceptive device.

What are the signs of an ectopic pregnancy?

If you notice that your period is late and you are suffering from symptoms of lower abdominal pain, pain in the tips of the shoulders, vaginal bleeding, faintness or dizziness, you should see your doctor immediately so that tests can be done to rule out an ectopic pregnancy.

A pregnancy test may be negative or positive in ectopic pregnancy and the most reliable means of diagnosis is an ultrasound scan of the pelvis or a laparoscopy which will enable the doctor to directly visualize the embryo and blood clot sited outside the uterine cavity.

An abdominal operation is required. The surgeon may be able to conserve the swollen Fallopian tube, if that is where the pregnancy has occurred, by milking out the dead embryo and blood clot; however, in many cases, it is necessary to remove the whole tube as it is damaged beyond repair.

After one ectopic pregnancy there is a 30 per cent infertility rate and a 10 per cent risk of another ectopic pregnancy occurring.

Vaginal bleeding in the second half of pregnancy

Significant bleeding from the vagina occurring after the twentieth week of pregnancy and before birth, is defined as antepartum haemorrhage. The most important causes of antepartum haemorrhage are:

1 Accidental haemorrhage (placental abruption)

2 Placenta praevia

Accidental haemorrhage

In this condition bleeding occurs between the placenta and its attachment to the uterine wall, thus causing premature separation of some or all of the placenta. If the haemorrhage is large, this can interfere with the blood supply to the foetus and result in its death. Thankfully, this serious condition is not common and occurs in only about one per cent of pregnancies.

Signs of an accidental haemorrhage include a variable amount of vaginal bleeding, from none at all to very heavy with large clots. Pain is usually felt in the uterus which may be mild or severe and there is cramping. If the haemorrhage is mild the placenta and baby remain healthy and, after a stay in hospital, the mother can be sent home when everything settles down. In these cases labour will be induced around the thirty-seventh or thirty-eighth week of pregnancy, to ensure that placental function does not deteriorate.

If the haemorrhage is severe, the doctor may decide to do an urgent caesarean section if the foetus appears alive, or labour may be induced with a drip and rupture of the membranes if the foetus is dead.

Placenta praevia

Another cause of bleeding during the second half of pregnancy is placenta praevia. In placenta praevia the placenta is implanted too low in the uterus. The condition is divided into four different grades, from the first grade where only part of the placenta lies in the lower segment of the uterus, up to the fourth or most severe

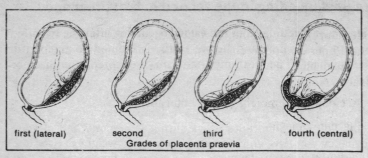

first (lateral)   second   third   fourth (central)
Grades of placenta praevia

Figure 34

grade where the placenta is wholly contained within the lower segment and is centrally placed over the cervical canal. See Figure 34.

Placenta praevia complicates a half to one per cent of pregnancies. In the second half of pregnancy the lower segment of the uterus expands and stretches and this results in the shearing off of a low situated placenta. As you can see from the diagram, the grades 3 and 4 will be separated more from the lower segment as it is expanding and so produce greater haemorrhage than the lower grades of placenta praevia, 1 and 2.

The patient with placenta praevia will usually notice vaginal bleeding without any pain. The colour of the blood is usually bright red and the bleeding tends to be recurrent. The bleeding may be brought on by sexual intercourse, coughing or straining, although in many cases it occurs by itself.

The presence of placenta praevia can be confirmed by ultrasound scan of the uterus which will show the placenta lying too far down in the lower segment of the uterus.

If placenta praevia is found the patient is made to rest in bed in hospital until the foetus is mature, which usually means up to the thirty-seventh or thirty-eighth week of pregnancy. This reduces the risk of a sudden and fatal haemorrhage.

In over 70 per cent of cases of placenta praevia, a caesarean section will be done at thirty-seven or thirty-eight weeks before labour commences.

Pre-eclampsia

Pre-eclampsia only occurs during pregnancy and affects between 5 and 15 per cent of pregnancies, being more common during the first pregnancy. The old-fashioned term for pre-eclampsia was 'toxaemia of pregnancy' and these days it is also known as pregnancy-induced hypertension, meaning high blood pressure.

If you are going to develop pre-eclampsia during your pregnancy, you will often notice that during the second half of your pregnancy you have an excessive gain in body weight of over one kilogram (two pounds) a week. This is due to fluid retention and you may also notice swelling of the legs and puffiness of the hands and face. Your shoes and rings may become too tight.

Your doctor will find that your blood pressure increases beyond the levels of early pregnancy and, indeed, may reach very high levels if medical supervision is neglected.

Another sign of pre-eclampsia that your doctor may find is excessive quantities of protein in your urine. This last sign is indicative of severe pre-eclampsia. In severe pre-eclampsia, the blood vessels go into spasm and the circulation to your vital organs and your baby may be reduced to critical levels. If this spasm is not relieved, severe headaches, visual problems, vomiting, epileptic fits, liver and kidney problems and placental damage may occur. If placental damage is too great the foetus may grow poorly, become distressed or die inside the uterus.

If you develop pre-eclampsia your doctor will not only pay careful attention to your health but will also keep a close watch on the growth of your baby by measuring placental hormones, such as oestriol, recording the foetal heart beat and measuring the growth of the baby's head by ultrasound.

What is the treatment for pre-eclampsia?

If the pre-eclampsia is only mild, blood pressure and fluid retention can often be controlled by a diet low in salt and refined carbohydrates. The diet should be high in raw foods, such as fruit and vegetables, as well as seeds, grains and legumes. Polyunsaturated fats such as fish and vegetables should be increased. Saturated animal fat and red meat should be reduced. Useful supplements for pre-eclampsia are vitamin C, 1000 milligrams twice daily; garlic capsules, two, three times daily with food; and primrose oil capsules, two daily with food. Bed rest is important and the mother should rest every afternoon in bed on her side. This will increase bloodflow to the placenta and therefore to the baby. Bed rest also reduces fluid retention and blood pressure. It is most important that a woman with pre-eclampsia accepts treatment and tries to relax, as frustration will only lead to an increase in blood pressure and a worsening of symptoms. Conventional diuretic drugs are not helpful in pre-eclampsia.

This treatment is continued until the baby is mature, with labour being induced at thirty-seven to forty weeks of pregnancy, if labour has not started spontaneously beforehand. Labour is induced because, in pre-eclampsia, the placenta is likely to have sustained some areas of damage due to poor circulation, and it is not considered safe to let it deteriorate further with age.

If the blood pressure continues to rise despite the above treatment, drugs to reduce it must be given. Other drugs such as sedatives and anti-convulsants may also be required if the risk of brain irritation and fits is present.

If protein appears in the urine, the pre-eclampsia is considered to be of a severe degree and it is unlikely that the baby will continue to grow in such an unfavourable environment. In severe pre-eclampsia, the doctor will induce labour or perform a caesarean section as the chances of intra-uterine foetal death are greater than the risks of prematurity.

Breastfeeding

The vast majority of women can breastfeed effectively and offer their baby its great advantages, even if only for a few months. Breastfeeding provides your baby with optimum nutrition and factors to boost the immune system against infection, as well as increasing your maternal bond to the child. Another great boon of breastfeeding is that it will speed up your weight loss after pregnancy and increase your chances of regaining your shapely pre-pregnancy figure.

If you want to breastfeed, it is best to begin preparing the breasts from the sixth month of pregnancy onwards. To do this, stand under the shower and gently squeeze your breast from behind the nipple with the thumb and forefinger to release early milk (colostrum). Then wash the nipples under the shower with warm water and rub them dry with a towel to unblock the nipple ducts. If your nipples are dry and sensitive you should apply wool fat or vitamin E cream three times daily to keep them moist and supple. Some women like the sensation of their partner stimulating their nipples during love play. By gently sucking the nipples your partner can encourage them to produce and release colostrum.

After the birth put the baby to the nipple as soon as possible and continue to do this every two hours, especially during the first few weeks, as this will encourage an adequate and early milk supply. During the early weeks you should not feed the baby for more than ten minutes on each nipple at any one feed, and make sure you rotate the baby from one nipple to the other, always beginning a feed on the nipple you finished on at the last feed; for example, left to right, right to left, left to right in strict order. Most babies obtain nearly all the milk from the breast in the first four or five minutes. In general, no child needs more than about ten minutes actual sucking on each nipple. Beyond ten minutes, the baby is merely using the nipple as a dummy and is likely to swallow air which could contribute to colic. Usually the baby can be fed on one breast until he slows down in his sucking and then fed on the second breast until he stops sucking or goes to sleep.

Do not give your baby supplementary bottle feeds at the hospital, except distilled water, as this will reduce enthusiasm for sucking on your nipples.

Your milk supply will be influenced by your diet and you should drink water, fruit and vegetable juices and milk regularly during the day. You should also eat large amounts of raw fruit and vegetables, although citrus fruit should only be eaten in moderation as excessive amounts can upset the baby's stomach. Useful additions to your diet are alfalfa tablets and raw bean sprouts. Think of the good old cow who spends all day eating lots of raw fresh green fodder and try to act likewise.

It is important to relax and let Mother Nature take over so that your milk supply can come in. Milk supplies naturally go up and down during the first two months of breastfeeding, so try to ignore these slight changes. Weigh your baby weekly at the local baby health centre to double-check that your milk supply is adequate. After the first fortnight the average child gains 170 to 200 grams (6 to 7 ounces) a week, although some normal children gain significantly more or less. There is less risk of overfeeding in a breastfed child.

A lower weight gain of say 140 grams (5 ounces) a week is acceptable provided the baby is happy, looks healthy, has soft yellow stools and maintains a weight gain around this level.

Problems with breastfeeding

Inverted nipples
In this condition the nipples are turned inwards and may not protrude adequately for effective breastfeeding. If you have inverted nipples at the sixteenth week of pregnancy and you want to breastfeed, you should commence doing two things:

1 Draw the entire nipple, including the areola which is the coloured area containing small pimple-like protrusions surrounding the nipple bud, outwards between your thumb and forefinger. Do this on all four sides, gently stretching the nipple area outwards until it will come no further. This will break down adhesions which tend to tether the nipple inwards inside the breast. Another good technique is to get your partner to suck the nipples two or three times a day to help draw them outwards.

2 You may begin to wear plastic breast shells from the sixteenth week of pregnancy on. You can obtain these through your GP or the National Childbirth Trust. The hole in the centre of the shell should cover your nipples and it is best to wear a bra over the top to keep them in the correct position. Commence by wearing the shell for one or two hours a day during the first few weeks and gradually increase the time until, by the thirtieth week of pregnancy, you are able to wear them right through the day. There is no need to wear the breast shells during the night.

If the breast shells encourage the leakage of milk you can put some absorbent pads over the top of the nipple.

Mastitis

Mastitis is also known as milk fever. The first symptom is often a small tender blister on the nipple which may begin to ooze yellow pus. An adjacent area of the breast then becomes lumpy, swollen and tender.

If this happens to you, do not panic, as this problem can be overcome. It is important to keep the affected breast empty by regular breastfeeding if possible or by expressing the milk with a suction apparatus. Hot compresses can be applied to the swollen area, and it is also beneficial to gently massage the lumpy area towards the nipple under a warm shower as this will encourage the nipple ducts to become unblocked.

A gentle antibiotic and pain-relieving drug may be required but breastfeeding can be safely continued under the supervision of your doctor while you are taking these medications.

Some women find that by drinking fresh pineapple juice and taking odourless garlic capsules in a dosage of two, four times daily with food, they are able to obtain a natural antibiotic effect which reduces the severity and duration of their mastitis. Some women have told me they have gained benefit by using homoeopathic medicine to overcome mastitis and the most useful remedies are: rosmarinus in a dosage of ten drops every two hours in water and hepar sulphuris in a dosage of ten drops, also every two hours in water. Homoeopathic remedies are harmless to the mother and baby and may be taken with other medication.

Care of the nipples

If you take care of your nipples you can prevent many early problems such as cracking of the nipples and mastitis. The best position for the nipples during breastfeeding is when the mother leans forward or lies on her side. It is important to clean the nipples daily but only using water. A portable hair dryer is a very good way of drying them. If the nipples become dry you can use a cleansing cream obtainable from the pharmacy to clean them. It is important to keep the nipples moist and supple in between feeds and you can use either wool fat, vitamin E cream or sorbolene and glycerine. Exposure to the sun can be very beneficial for your nipples but be careful not to burn them.

If dermatitis of the nipples develops you will notice that they become red, itchy and may develop very small cracks and superficial scales. This can be helped by using a half per cent hydrocortisone cream for several days.

If a definite crack develops on the nipple and becomes painful it is usually best to stop breastfeeding and express milk from this breast at the usual feeding times. This milk should be put in a bottle and given to the baby at regular feeding times. The cracked nipple will benefit from exposure to an infra-red lamp, twice daily, or the sun. If any sign of infection develops in the cracked nipple, an antibiotic cream should be applied three times daily.

The secret of overcoming these early problems of breastfeeding is to act at the first sign of any discomfort. There is no need to abandon breastfeeding, as milk can easily be expressed and given to the baby while treatment is being carried out. Usually after a few days the problem will settle down and the baby can be returned to the nipple. Ideally, you should try to breastfeed your baby for at least three months to provide the best nutritional and emotional beginning for childhood.

Exercise during pregnancy

As soon as you know you are pregnant you should arrange for enrolment in an antenatal class. These are offered by the National Childbirth Trust at its 450 branches in the United Kingdom. Your GP can put you in touch with your local branch, or alternatively, if you are having a hospital delivery, the hospital your GP refers you to is likely to offer antenatal classes. They may also be held in the local health authority clinic. Antenatal groups are run by a midwife and physiotherapist and provide education regarding the physical and emotional aspects of your pregnancy as well as specific exercises to make you fit for labour. You will attend regular weekly classes and learn to use the respiratory, abdominal and pelvic muscles required during the second stage of labour. Book in before the twentieth week of pregnancy as the classes are very popular and they may become overbooked. Make sure to take your partner along with you to these classes so that he can actively participate in your labour.

During pregnancy your ligaments and joints become softer and more flexible and thus are more easily strained, so do not begin any new type of vigorous exercise, to which you are unaccustomed, during pregnancy. In other words, don't take up weightlifting, squash, competitive sports and so on, if you have never done them before.

In general, it is best to go slowly and gradually build up your exercise programme beginning with long walks, yoga and swimming.

Over the last few years it has become recognized that a sustained elevation of body temperature above normal can be harmful to the developing foetus. This is because your baby is insulated by the amniotic fluid surrounding it and it is not easy for the baby to cool down once your body temperature becomes elevated. If you are engaging in vigorous aerobic or sporty exercise, take your temperature every half hour, preferably with a modern digital thermometer. If your temperature goes above 101°F (38.4°C) stop exercising and relax in a cool environment, sipping an iced beverage. You can resume exercise when your body temperature has returned to normal, 98°F (36.7°C).

During vigorous exercise, also monitor your pulse at the wrist every half hour, and if it rises above 140 beats per minute sit down, rest and breathe slowly. You should avoid very hot environments such as jacuzzis, steam rooms and saunas.

Before and during strenuous exercise, you should drink adequate amounts of fluids such as water and fruit juice to avoid dehydration, faintness and hypoglycaemia (low blood sugar).

Competitive sports involving balls and rackets carry a danger of injury to your protuberant abdomen and also require a good sense of balance which may be difficult to maintain in late pregnancy when your centre of gravity shifts, thus making you more susceptible to falls.

All pregnant women should practise the pelvic floor exercises described on page 41. These will tone up the muscles which support your uterus and bowel, and also reduce the chance of prolapse of the bowel or bladder after birth. They also help you to expel and control the baby's head during the second stage of labour.

Sexual activity during pregnancy

It is quite normal to enjoy some type of sexual activity during pregnancy and, indeed, some women feel very sexy during the middle three months. If your pregnancy is completely normal you can enjoy sexual intercourse throughout pregnancy, as well as normal foreplay and afterplay.

During the latter weeks of pregnancy, the missionary position in which the woman lies on her back during intercourse may be uncomfortable but coital positions can be varied as desired or other forms of sexual enjoyment can be indulged in. During the last six weeks of pregnancy it is best to keep penile thrusting as gentle and slow as possible, as extremely vigorous penile thrusting may stimulate premature rupture of the membranes or premature labour. If you notice any pain or cramping during intercourse stop immediately and do not have further intercourse until you have checked with your doctor.

Semen contains prostaglandins and this, combined with local trauma due to vigorous penile thrusting, may stimulate uterine contractions in a pregnancy which is unstable, especially during the first and last three months. It may be safer to avoid penile thrusting and restrict yourself to gentle foreplay:

1 If you have a past history of recurrent miscarriages or cervical incompetence.

2 If your present pregnancy is complicated by cervical incompetence, vaginal bleeding (threatened miscarriage or bleeding after the twentieth week of pregnancy) or threatened premature labour.

Certain sexual practices should be avoided during pregnancy, namely anal intercourse and blowing air into the vagina.

Congenital abnormalities of the new-born

If one takes the average normal couple, statistics show that their chance of producing a child with a birth defect (congenital abnormality) is one in thirty. Two to three per cent of all new-borns have significant birth defects which may be due to an abnormality of their hereditary material (genes and chromosomes) or to an unfavourable environment during pregnancy.

An unfavourable environment may be produced if the mother contracts a viral infection during pregnancy or takes toxic drugs or excessive alcohol. Another environmental factor which may operate is the formation of fibrous bands of tissue in the amniotic fluid. This causes shortening of the foetal limbs because the bands constrict the limbs, thereby reducing their vital circulation.

The risk of hereditary birth defects can be assessed by compiling an accurate family history going back as far as possible with the help of a doctor who specializes in genetic medicine. This is called a genetic family tree and traces back diseases in both parental families. It also looks at the possibility of the parents being blood relatives as this is associated with an increased chance of hereditary diseases.

Sometimes it is clear whether a particular birth defect is due to hereditary factors or environmental factors, and this makes an accurate assessment of the risk of recurrence of the same birth defect in future pregnancies much easier. For example, if a baby is born with heart and ear defects due to infection during pregnancy with the German measles virus, these defects will not recur as the mother will now have acquired immunity against German measles to protect her next pregnancy.

Conversely, if a baby is born with cystic fibrosis, it is known that in this hereditary disease there is a one in four chance of recurrence in a future pregnancy.

In a significant number of birth defects, both hereditary and environmental factors work together to create the abnormality and, in such cases, an accurate assessment of the risk of recurrence is much more difficult.

Genetic diseases of the new-born

These are passed on to the new-born from the parents and are due to an abnormality of the genetic material (chromosomes and genes) in the nucleus of the body cells. The genetic material of an individual determines a person's physical and mental abilities, and normal individuals have a set of forty-six individual chromosomes, each chromosome holding thousands of powerful genes. Each parent donates twenty-three chromosomes at fertilization so that the child will have a complete set of forty-six chromosomes, forty-four of which are known as autosomal and determine general body characteristics and two of which are known as the sex chromosomes. In a female the sex chromosomes are XX, in a male they are XY.

Genetic disease occurs in one in every hundred births and may result from one of two possible genetic abnormalities:

1 Abnormality of the chromosomes

There may be too many chromosomes, such as in Down's syndrome where the baby has forty-seven chromosomes, or too few chromosomes, such as in Turner's syndrome where the female child will only have one X chromosome instead of two. Abnormalities of the chromosomes can occur sporadically and are often unpredictable. Some chromosomal abnormalities are more common with advancing age and this is illustrated by the instance of Down's syndrome which occurs in one in a thousand births in women aged thirty, but increases to one in every hundred births in women aged forty.

Severe abnormalities of chromosomes usually result in a spontaneous abortion in early pregnancy or early death of the severely deformed baby.

2 Abnormality of the genes

The genes are like beads threaded on to the chromosomes and regulate the building blocks in the tissues of the body. One can trace hereditary disease due to abnormality of the genes by the construction of a genetic family tree. One or both parents may need to be a carrier of the abnormal gene in order for it to be expressed in their child. If only one parent is required to be a carrier, the disorder is known as a dominant disorder, whereas if both parents are required to be carriers of the abnormal gene, the disorder is known as a recessive disorder. Examples of these types of genetic diseases are Mediterranean anaemia (thalassaemia), cystic fibrosis and haemophilia.

Diagnosis of genetic diseases during pregnancy

The technique of amniocentesis is used to screen for abnormalities of foetal chromosomes, genes and cell function, and also enables determination of the sex of the foetus. Amniocentesis is performed in pregnancies where a higher risk of genetic disease exists, such as in women aged thirty-three years or more, and in women with a past history or family history of genetic diseases or defects of the spinal cord and brain, such as spina bifida.

A normal result from an amniocentesis test can only exclude certain genetic diseases and will not prove that a foetus is absolutely normal in all other respects.

An amniocentesis test is done between the fourteenth and sixteenth weeks of pregnancy, after the placenta and foetus have been visualized by the doctor using an ultrasound video picture. The doctor passes a needle through the wall of the abdomen and uterus into the amniotic fluid in which the baby is floating and takes a sample of this fluid up through the needle. This fluid is then examined for foetal cells, and these are collected and grown. These foetal cells can be tested for abnormalities of genetic material and function. They will also show the sex of the baby.

Amniocentesis is not very painful although it is associated with some risk and one per cent of women who undergo it will have a subsequent miscarriage. In very rare instances, other complications such as intra-uterine infection or foetal trauma and bleeding may occur after amniocentesis.

The main drawback of amniocentesis is that it takes some time to culture and test the foetal cells, and thus results may not be available for three to four weeks. This means that the decision to have a termination of pregnancy must be made at 17 to 20 weeks of pregnancy, and this is emotionally and physically traumatic for a woman.

For this reason, the new technique for diagnosing genetic diseases called chorionic villus sampling or chorionic villus biopsy is becoming more popular and more widely available. In the procedure of chorionic villus sampling (CVS), a hollow tube is passed through the vagina and cervix into the uterus to sample cells from the membrane surrounding the foetus, called the chorionic membrane. Because the technique of CVS is still relatively new, there is a slightly greater risk of complications such as miscarriage occurring after the procedure as compared to amniocentesis. The great advantage of CVS, however, is that it can be done earlier than amniocentesis, usually at the beginning of the third month of pregnancy. Furthermore, results are available after only several days, meaning that the parental decision to continue with the pregnancy or have an abortion can be made much earlier, thus involving less stress and also being much safer for the physical well-being of the woman.

The story of Madeleine

Twenty-three-year-old blonde Madeleine felt unusually tired and noticed her menstrual period was overdue by several days. Over the next few days food began to smell ghastly and she completely lost her appetite. Her usually relished morning cup of tea and cigarette tasted repugnant, and she began to crave Coca Cola, ice-cream, mashed potatoes and corn, all foods she had never liked before.

Madeleine suspected she might be pregnant and she visited her doctor nine weeks after her last menstrual period which meant she was around seven weeks pregnant, as her cycle had always been twenty-eight days on the dot. Her doctor confirmed her suspicions of pregnancy by finding the presence of the pregnancy hormone B-HCG in her urine. Madeleine was delighted with her diagnosis and told her doctor that the first day of her last period had been 25 January. The doctor told her that if she added seven days and nine months to this date she would come up with the estimated date of arrival of the baby. Together they worked out this date by adding seven days to 25 January, which gave them 1 February, and then by adding nine months to this, which put the estimated date of birth at 1 November. Madeleine was amazed to be told that, although her baby at seven weeks of age was less than two centimetres (one inch) long, all of its features such as its limbs, head, eyes and sex were already formed.

Madeleine complained that her morning sickness was severe and lasted all day and her doctor suggested an antihistamine tablet to quell the nausea. She refused this, but accepted vitamin B6 as a natural alternative as she wanted to keep her pregnancy as pure and natural as possible. She knew a drug-free and healthy life-style was important during the first twelve weeks of pregnancy as the baby's organs were forming at this time. The doctor thought this was very commendable and told Madeleine to check with him before she accepted any medication.

The doctor also told Madeleine to give up her quota of ten cigarettes a day as statistics have shown that women who smoke fifteen or more cigarettes a day during pregnancy have babies with a lower birth weight and a higher incidence of poor school performance in later childhood.

Madeleine's blood was taken to determine her blood group and to see if her red blood cells were RH positive or negative. Madeleine's red blood cells were RH negative which meant a protective injection of gamma globulin would be needed after the birth if the baby was RH positive. Her blood was also checked for anaemia, for infection with syphilis and several viruses and for immunity against the virus of German measles (rubella). Madeleine's blood proved to be negative for antibodies to German measles which meant that she had no protective immunity against this virus. Her doctor therefore strongly advised her to avoid places which were crowded with young children and to stay well away from people suffering from 'flu-like symptoms' or feverish illness or rashes, especially during the first four months of her pregnancy. This would greatly reduce the risk of Madeleine's contracting German measles during her pregnancy, a disease which can cause congenital abnormalities and brain damage in the baby.

Madeleine kicked herself mentally for not having received the vaccination against German measles prior to falling pregnant, and the doctor recommended she be vaccinated immediately after the birth of her child. The doctor also warned Madeleine of the dangers of other infections such as toxoplasmosis which may be acquired from strange dogs, cats and birds and she was advised to avoid close contact with her cat and its excreta.

Her urine was checked for diabetes, protein and infection and the doctor did a gentle pelvic examination to determine if her bony pelvis was going to be large enough to accommodate the baby's head during the second stage of labour. A Pap smear, breast check and blood pressure check completed the long initial visit with her doctor and Madeleine was very impressed by his thorough attention to detail.

As Madeleine stood up to leave she suddenly felt dizzy and faint and the doctor told her that her blood pressure reading had been a little low which can cause these feelings of faintness. Low blood pressure is common during the early stages of pregnancy because the high levels of the hormone progesterone in the blood cause relaxation of the muscle in the blood vessel walls. The doctor suggested that Madeleine get more rest in the horizontal position, drink adequate fluids and take a vitamin E supplement of 100 milligrams daily as this helps to maintain blood pressure. She had also heard on the grapevine from some of her friends that spirulina, which is a nutritional supplement, and seaweed are helpful for dizziness secondary to low blood pressure and she made a mental note to try these natural supplements.

Poor Madeleine remained hideously nauseated for three months and the first third of her pregnancy passed very slowly indeed. If her sickness had not eventually passed she would have accepted medical treatment as she was losing weight.

At exactly sixteen weeks of pregnancy, Madeleine felt the baby move for the first time and found this an incredibly beautiful and cosmic experience. Finally, all the months of sickness, fatigue and breast pain seemed worthwhile!

Madeleine found the second third of pregnancy a breeze. She felt and looked wonderful and enjoyed her new glossy skin, feminine breasts and shapely stomach. She ate enormous amounts of raw foods and exercised regularly, enjoying yoga and swimming. Her weight gain was a little less than the desirable amount and the doctor thought this was probably due to the fact that

Madeleine was almost a vegan, meaning that she did not eat animal products. For this reason, the doctor checked her vitamin B12 levels in the blood. These proved to be marginal and she was given a course of B12 injections. This is most important as B12 deficiency is not uncommon in people avoiding meat and dairy products and B12 deficiency can cause spinal cord damage in the infant. Severe deficiency may cause mental impairment.

Total weight gain in pregnancy is normally between 9 and 12.5 kilograms (20 and 28 pounds) with around 3.5 kilograms (8 pounds) being gained in the first twenty weeks and 9 kilograms (20 pounds) being gained in the last twenty weeks. Madeleine was falling way behind this goal, so the doctor decided to do an ultrasound of her uterus to check if the baby's size was consistent with its age. Madeleine did not like the idea of an ultrasound test as she wanted a totally natural pregnancy with no invasive procedures. However, once the doctor had assured her that an ultrasound scan was a very safe procedure, working in a similar way to radar and being entirely free from X-rays or damaging ionizing radiation, she agreed to the test, as she was in fact worried that the baby might be too small.

Madeleine thought it incredible that the high frequency sound waves from the ultrasound scanner could show a video picture (echogram) of the size, structure and sometimes the sex of the developing embryo. One thing was sure, she knew her ultrasound would not show twins hiding in her small abdomen. She found the ultrasound test very comfortable as she lay still for fifteen minutes face downwards on her tummy, on a liquid filled type of bed, while her abdomen was gently rubbed with the ultrasound scanner.

Madeleine was extremely relieved to see her baby moving normally and to learn that it had a normal head size and length for its age. Madeleine thought that many women must be tempted to have an ultrasound scan just to have 'a peek' at their baby and satisfy their curiosity. However, her doctor had told her that the effects of over-exposure to high energy emissions such as ultrasound were not fully understood, and such procedures should only be done for specific reasons, for example poor weight gain, possible congenital abnormalities, the determination of twins or triplets, suspicion of poor foetal growth or heavy bleeding during pregnancy.

Because of her poor weight gain, Madeleine was also required to collect all her urine during a twenty-four-hour period on several occasions to measure the amount of the hormone oestriol in the urine. The measurement of oestriol gives a measure of the health of the placenta and baby and, thankfully, Madeleine's oestriol measurements were within normal limits. She was also asked to measure the number of times her baby kicked during a twelve-hour period. Her baby kicked only five to six times in twelve hours which is less than the accepted healthy number of ten kicks in twelve hours. This prompted her doctor to put her in hospital for a day to connect her abdomen up to an electronic recording machine called a cardiotocograph to record the pattern of her baby's heart beat. Thankfully, the heart beat pattern was normal so the pregnancy was allowed to progress naturally. Madeleine was thirty weeks pregnant at this stage and three more ultrasound scans were done over the next six weeks, at two-week intervals, to measure the diameter of the baby's head in order to check that it was growing at the normal rate.

At thirty-six weeks things seemed to drag on incredibly. At thirty-seven weeks all the weight in her abdomen seemed to descend into her pelvis and she noticed frequency of passing urine. This was because the baby's head was now pressing on her bladder and bowel. Her varicose veins enlarged and her legs and back ached. She found sleeping difficult as she had irregular and slightly painful contractions of the uterus at night and her doctor suggested sleeping tablets. However, Madeleine was intent on doing things the natural way and decided to stick it out without drugs. She knew her painful contractions were only a sign of false labour, as they were totally irregular in their timing and duration and gradually reduced after several hours. She was waiting for them to become regular and increase in frequency and strength before she would pack her bags for the birth centre.

It really seemed as if Mother Nature had forgotten this woman who wanted to do it all so naturally. However, one evening when she was five days over her expected due date, she noticed clear warm fluid dripping down her legs as she was sitting quietly on the couch. She had a feeling of panic as she realized that her membranes must have ruptured and she also noticed a small amount of pink mucus (a show) on her pants. As her husband excitedly began to pack her bags she felt her contractions starting to come regularly every ten minutes, each one lasting for thirty seconds. At last her labour had started and she noted the time as 8 p.m. At 10 p.m. the uterine contractions had increased in frequency to every five minutes and were lasting sixty seconds and Madeleine decided to go to the birth centre.

Ideally Madeleine should have gone to the birth centre as soon as her membranes ruptured as there is always a slight chance that rupture of the membranes will be accompanied by the falling down of the umbilical cord into the vagina (prolapse of the umbilical cord). Thus a vaginal examination should be done at the time of rupture of the membranes. In general, if labour does not commence by twelve to sixteen hours after rupture of the membranes in a mature pregnancy, an intravenous drip of a drug called oxytocin is necessary to initiate uterine contractions. Otherwise, prolonged labour may result in infection ascending into the fluid surrounding the baby.

On arrival at the birth centre, everything seemed homely and Madeleine was glad that she and her husband had visited the centre several times before to accustom themselves to the environment. Madeleine took a hot shower and she was offered an enema and pubic shave which she refused, as she hated the idea of this intrusion upon her personal privacy.

Madeleine's doctor arrived at the birth centre and did a gentle vaginal examination during which he found her cervix was four centimetres dilated. He told her that she was well into the first stage of labour as her cervix was thin and stretched tightly over the baby's head. During the first stage of labour the cervix dilates completely to a maximum of ten centimetres which opens up the birthing canal. During the first half of the first stage, the cervix dilates slowly up to three centimetres, whereas in the second half (active phase) of the first stage of labour, the cervix dilates more rapidly and dilatation usually exceeds one centimetre per hour.

Madeleine asked her doctor rather anxiously if there was anything wrong and the doctor replied that although she should have had a vaginal examination at the time of rupture of the membranes, there was no sign of prolapse of the cord and everything was in order. Furthermore, because the baby's head was well down and tightly applied to the cervix it was safe for her to walk about as there was now no danger of prolapse of the cord. Madeleine was allowed to move around freely provided she did not eat or drink anything. Madeleine and her husband sat on the couch and played their favourite tune while her husband massaged her legs, back and abdomen and helped her to time her contractions. He also encouraged her to concentrate on her slow deep breathing pattern. With the encouragement of the midwife Madeleine walked around from time to time, as this can often speed up the first stage of labour.

Madeleine and her husband were relaxed as they knew that the first stage of labour took on average eight to twelve hours, especially with a first baby, and that there was nothing much more they could do to speed it up.

At 4 a.m., approximately eight hours after labour had commenced, Madeleine's contractions started to become more painful and frequent. She lay on her left side and breathed deeply while her husband massaged her back. This ensured that the blood supply to her uterus was not reduced, which can occur if a woman lies flat on her back on a hard surface during labour. She was also allowed to sit propped up with a cushion behind her, so that her back was at an angle of forty-five degrees to the horizontal, as this is another safe position for the baby and its blood supply.

Madeleine began to approach full dilatation of the cervix which is the most intensely painful time of labour and her contractions became excruciatingly painful. She began screaming and her husband panicked, so the doctor was called. Madeleine's doctor was very cool and calm, and his reassuring voice immediately relaxed her. He examined her vaginally and found her cervix was fully dilated, in good condition and that the baby's heart was beating healthily. It was 8 a.m. and the first stage of her labour had lasted twelve hours. Her husband kissed her passionately and told her that she could do it. The doctor told Madeleine she could now start pushing, which was easy as she had an irresistible urge to force the baby down into the vagina and out into the world.

Madeleine took two deep breaths, holding the air in her lungs with the second breath to make her diaphragm hard and rigid so that she could use it with the muscles of her lower chest and abdomen to push the baby down. She found that she could push more efficiently if her husband held her head with her chin on her chest while she clasped her legs with her hands, drawing them up on to her tummy. Pushing during contractions was hard work, and she had to relax completely in between while her husband would rub her face with a cold moistened towel. The nurse offered her a gas called trilene to breathe to ease the contraction pains, but she declined as she did not want to be drowsy when the baby's head passed through the vulva.

This did not take long and, after thirty minutes of pushing, the baby's head appeared at the vulva, known as the crowning of the head. The thin tissue of her vulva was stretched tightly as the baby's head descended lower. Her doctor suggested he do an episiotomy which is a small cut extending out from the vaginal opening to enlarge the vaginal opening in a neat controlled fashion, thus avoiding a ragged tear of the vagina which is untidy and difficult to repair. Madeleine refused this as she felt she could manage without an episiotomy, and the doctor said perhaps she could if she went slowly and panted in between contractions instead of pushing. By panting she could control the rate of the descent of the baby's head as it passed through the vaginal opening, thus avoiding any sudden tearing. With one final gentle push the baby's head now passed out of the vaginal opening in the normal position with the back of the baby's head (occiput) facing upwards to her pubic bone. Mucus was streaming from the baby's nose and mouth and this was gently sucked out with a soft plastic sucker. The doctor then helped the baby's shoulders and hips to slide out of the vagina and, lo and behold, the baby had arrived. As the shoulders passed out of the vaginal opening the midwife gave Madeleine an injection of oxytocin which would reduce postpartum blood loss when the placenta separated from the uterus.

The baby was immediately given to Madeleine and as she held the slippery, warm, wet creature close to her breast, it began breathing regularly. She felt that this immediate contact with her skin was more intimate and natural than the 'Leboyer technique' which several of her friends had tried, in which the baby is floated in a bath of warm water immediately after delivery. The lights were not too bright and everything seemed tranquil and romantic as Madeleine gazed at her fragile and perfect new acquisition. The umbilical cord stopped pulsating after approximately four minutes, at which time it was cut and cord blood collected for testing of the baby's blood group. The nurses wanted to take the baby away to wash it and weigh it; however, Madeleine refused this as she did not want to be separated from her baby for one second.

The third stage of her labour now began. During the third stage of labour the placenta separates from the uterus and is expelled into the vagina. The third stage usually lasts around twenty minutes and is not painful. Madeleine's doctor assisted the expulsion of her placenta and, once he felt her uterus contract, he put gentle and steady pressure in an upwards direction upon her uterus and pulled down on the umbilical cord. The placenta came out and was accompanied by a loss of blood of only 200 millilitres. Madeleine's blood loss was slight because the oxytocic injection had promoted a strong contraction of the uterus which had squeezed the blood vessels in the raw area where the placenta had been attached to the uterine wall.

Madeleine gave the baby to its father who washed and dressed it, and she could not help but feel contented and proud of her efforts and endurance. She then put the baby to her breast where it began sucking quite vigorously as her husband stroked its tiny back. They decided to all their new little boy Isaac. Isaac was 52 centimetres long and only 3 kilograms in weight. Thus, he was lean and tall, and the doctor told Madeleine that Isaac definitely fell below the average birth weight of 3.3 kilograms (7 pounds 4 ounces). The doctor told Madeleine that full term babies weighed between 2.5 kilograms (5½ pounds) and 4.5 kilograms (10 pounds) and that Isaac obviously took after his lean lanky parents.

Madeleine's retrospective thoughts

Subsequent to the birth of Isaac, Madeleine had five further pregnancies and only two of these resulted in the birth of full term babies. During the three years after the birth of Isaac, she had three successive first-three-month miscarriages and felt so desperate to have another child that she applied to adopt an Asian child. No cause could be found by her doctors for these recurrent miscarriages and it was presumed that she had a hormonal imbalance, probably a deficiency of progesterone. When she fell unexpectedly pregnant for the fifth time, she rushed off to the doctor and asked him to do everything and anything to help her sustain the pregnancy. Her doctor gave her injections of progesterone to enhance her appetite and weight gain and hopefully to increase the health of the placenta. These injections seemed to give her new strength and this fifth pregnancy passed peacefully and terminated at full term in a spontaneous vaginal delivery of her second son Thorry. The birth was quick and natural and Madeleine did it only with the moral support of her midwife, her doctor being really just an observer.

After the birth of Thorry, Madeleine was found, by means of a Pap smear, to have abnormal cells in her cervix. These abnormal cells were treated with a cone biopsy in which a sizeable cone of tissue was cut out of her inner cervix.

After this traumatic experience, Madeleine did not expect to fall pregnant again and, indeed, her doctor advised her against it in view of her past history of recurrent miscarriages and the large scar remaining in her cervix from the cone biopsy.

However, deep inside, Madeleine felt that another soul was meant to come through her body and so she discouraged her husband from having a vasectomy.

To the surprise of all, she fell pregnant for a sixth time. She rushed off to her doctor every week, although he told her this was not necessary. However, Madeleine was very anxious regarding the possibility that her cervix might be incompetent and weak, resulting in the birth of a premature infant.

She was determined to keep this baby and so she did and the pregnancy progressed to full term. Indeed, a cervical stitch was not even considered necessary and Madeleine's cervix was probably held together tightly by the sheer force of her will-power and personality.

When she finally came into labour the birth proved traumatic and long as she had considerable scarring in her cervix as a result of the previous cone biopsy. This scarring retarded the dilatation of her cervix during the first stage of labour and, indeed, when the second stage arrived, her cervix literally tore open. She was given pethidine to reduce the pain of this tearing and was very grateful for the small relief it afforded her.

In retrospect she said to me, 'Many women like myself get to a point in their labour where they believe they cannot do it, it becomes unbearable. I know that at this point the worst is over, or at least the labour is about to shift gear. When it does move on you seem to gain new strength and the force to carry on. It is extremely important to have an optimistic and supportive midwife or doctor with you at this most difficult time.' Madeleine had experienced the difference between a normal labour and a prolonged and difficult one, and she told me that this had tempered her original idealistic concept that all women should prefer a natural drugless birth. Even she, who was an ardent and courageous naturalist, had welcomed the moderate relief brought by pethidine when it was really required.

She had realized that 'natural' is not the only way and that some women just cannot make it by themselves. Madeleine's final statement to me was that she felt that the woman approaching labour should not be too attached to her preconceived ideas of how her labour would be, and that it was more realistic to be flexible so that one could accept whatever was necessary to get through the labour and produce a healthy baby.

Madeleine felt that the chances of having a normal and uncomplicated labour were definitely increased if the woman took measures to remain healthy and fit, and if she was well-educated regarding the breathing techniques which can be used during labour to reduce pain.

11 Infertility

Until recently infertility tests have been more an art than a science – one could say they have been the result of inexact investigation leading to imprecise conclusions and debatable treatments. Recently, however, diagnostic accuracy and treatments have greatly improved, so that in some conditions it is now possible to increase an infertile couple's chances of pregnancy to almost normal. This is due mainly to the use of drugs which stimulate ovulation and the development of techniques which enable fertilization of the egg to occur outside the body, bypassing diseased Fallopian tubes.

In the United Kingdom, one in ten couples experience infertility which may or may not be treated. The number of infertile couples coming to doctors for help is increasing. This is not to suggest that the incidence of infertility is on the increase, rather, that social attitudes and stigmas have changed, allowing couples to express their needs more readily.

Infertility is most often due to a malfunction of the body and should be considered as such, clinically not emotively, just like any other malfunction.

As long ago as 1949, the Declaration of Human Rights at Geneva stated the right of a couple to have children: doctors should facilitate this right and keep in mind the Hippocratic oath which is to relieve suffering. Society as a whole should also support this right.

The rendezvous of sperm and egg

Medical history has never documented a case of immaculate conception and the mechanics of conception are very basic – a male must have an erection and ejaculate sperm in or around the vagina. It is not absolutely necessary that the penis enter the vagina and sperm placed around the vaginal opening can sometimes still find their way up through the cervix so that fertilization occurs. That is why the contraceptive technique of coitus interruptus, meaning the withdrawal of the penis from the vagina just before ejaculation, is a very risky business.

The ejaculated sperm are dedicated to their purpose of meeting with the egg and do not easily become distracted. In fact, it has been found that healthy sperm can swim upwards from the cervix into the outer part of the Fallopian tube for fertilization in less than five minutes!

In a healthy couple what are the chances of conception?

If you are very fertile you may fall pregnant the very first time you have intercourse. In a young couple having sex every second day, 25 per cent will have conceived after only one month. By the end of six months, 60 per cent will have conceived, by the end of twelve months, 80 per cent and by the end of eighteen months, 90 per cent will have conceived. For the 10 per cent of couples who have not fallen pregnant after eighteen months of trying, the chances begin to decline regardless of the frequency of sexual intercourse. Investigation should be started after twelve months of unsuccessful trying if the desire for a baby is strong.

How can a couple increase their chances of conception?

Some couples think that having sex every day will maximize their chances; however, this can result in 'semen exhaustion' with a reduced number of sperm per ejaculation being placed into the vagina. While trying to conceive, it has been found that four ejaculations per week are ideal and give the best sperm quality.

Ideally, sperm should be deposited high in the vagina, close to the cervix, and the missionary position of sex with the man on top favours this. After ejaculation, the man should rest on top of the woman for a while and not withdraw his penis from the vagina until it has become small and flaccid, otherwise sperm may be pulled out with the penis.

After sex, the woman should relax and remain lying down so

that the force of gravity keeps the sperm high in the vagina. During intercourse, if vaginal lubrication is insufficient, the couple can use saliva from their mouths to moisten the vaginal opening and the penis. Vaseline and other lubricating jellies should be avoided as these may interfere with the mobility of the sperm. It is not necessary for the woman to have an orgasm in order for conception to occur.

What is the role of age in fertility?

A woman is at her most fertile at around twenty-four years of age. After the age of twenty-five there is a slight decline and after the age of thirty there is a more rapid decline, which stays at a steady rate up until the age of forty years, when there is a significant drop in fertility. For women wanting to conceive after the age of forty-five, the chances are quite low; however, if menstruation is still occurring regularly, conception is possible, even beyond the age of fifty.

Men are biologically designed to remain fertile for much longer than women and this could be because the resulting pregnancy carries no risk or strain to their health. After the age of forty-five, there is often a slight reduction in male fertility; however, many men continue to produce large numbers of healthy sperm beyond their seventies.

Overall the optimal age for a woman to conceive and have healthy babies is in the early to mid twenties. This is because some common causes of infertility such as endometriosis, fibroids and tubal blockage become more common in the late twenties and thirties and the risk of congenital abnormalities due to genetic problems increases in the late thirties.

Basic causes of infertility

Many people are surprised to learn that the cause of infertility lies equally with the male and with the female, the ratio being an even 50:50.

What are the causes of infertility in women?

1 Disorders of ovulation (20 per cent).

2 Disorders of the Fallopian tubes (30 per cent).

3 Endometriosis (15 per cent).

4 Disorders of the cervical mucus (10 per cent).

5 Other mechanical causes such as uterine fibroids (5 per cent).

6 Unknown causes (20 per cent).

What are the causes of infertility in men?

1 Inadequate sperm production and/or quality (50 per cent).

2 Disorders of sexual intercourse which may have a physical or psychosomatic basis (30 per cent).

3 Unknown causes (20 per cent).

Of all causes of infertility, infection-related causes are certainly the most *preventable* ones, and the increasing incidence of sexually transmitted infections over the past twenty years should give rise to major concern. The increasing incidence of herpes and AIDS has somewhat put a premature end to the promiscuous society and many prospective lovers are now asked for a past medical history before a chance is taken. This should begin to curb the increasing risk of sexually transmitted diseases, pelvic infection and infertility.

In Third World countries, pelvic infections *after childbirth* are a major cause of tubal blockage and infertility. However, this is no longer a significant factor in developed countries.

Another twentieth-century social phenomenon which has influenced the causes of infertility is the increasing infatuation of women with athletic slender bodies as the epitome of desirability. There is no doubt that inadequate body weight and/or excessive athletic exercise can prevent normal ovulation, menstruation and fertility.

The infertile female

Let us now take a closer look at the specific causes of infertility in the woman.

Disorders of ovulation

Normally an egg is released from one ovary (ovulation) twelve to sixteen days before the onset of the next menstrual bleeding.

A woman may become aware of an absence of ovulation because of:

1 A complete lack of menstrual periods (amenorrhoea).

2 Infrequent periods occurring, for example, every six weeks to every six months (oligomenorrhoea). However, 10 per cent of patients with lack of ovulation may still keep on menstruating regularly on a four-week basis.

How can you find out if you are ovulating regularly?

1 Blood progesterone

After ovulation, the ovary normally produces the female hormone progesterone and your doctor can easily measure this in the blood around the twenty-first day of your menstrual cycle. If he finds no progesterone in the blood, this will confirm a lack of ovulation. See Figure 7 on page 23 which shows a normal ovulation cycle with production of progesterone.

2 Temperature chart

A useful sign of ovulation is the old-fashioned temperature chart. See Figure 35. The temperature should be measured with a special 'basal body temperature thermometer' and taken immediately upon awakening every morning while still in bed. The thermometer must remain in place for at least five minutes and it is best to place it in the vagina. Alternatively you can use one of the new digital thermometers which takes only one minute to give an accurate reading.

If ovulation occurs, the basal body temperature rises by 0.3 to 0.5°C during the one or two days *after ovulation* and stays elevated until the next menstrual bleed begins.

Conversely, with a lack of ovulation, there is no post-ovulatory increase in basal body temperature. A temperature chart must be measured over three cycles to obtain an accurate idea of your ovulation time.

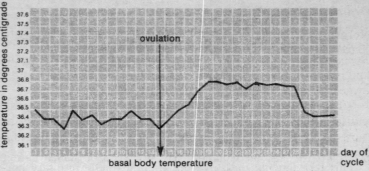

Figure 35

3 Cervical mucus

Just before ovulation, there is an increase in the amount of cervical mucus which appears in the vagina, and this mucus is clear and slippery. On the day of ovulation, there is a peak or maximum amount of this clear slippery cervical mucus. After ovulation the mucus becomes thick and opaque under the influence of progesterone.

4 Endometrial biopsy

Your doctor can also determine ovulation by taking a small piece of the inner lining of your uterus (endometrium) with a special biopsy instrument and looking for the changes induced by progesterone on this endometrial lining. Progesterone causes the endometrial lining to become secretory in preparation for the implanting egg. Without ovulation, no progesterone is produced and these secretory changes do not occur in the endometrium. This is a simple test that does not require hospitalization or an anaesthetic and it can be done at the same time as measurement of the blood progesterone.

5 Symptoms of ovulation pain

Many women who ovulate notice a short-lived sharp pain on one side of the lower abdomen which is due to the egg bursting through the ovarian capsule at ovulation. It may be associated with a small amount of blood loss from the vagina and an increase in libido, and some women find it a very reliable sign of ovulation.

6 A chemical test for predicting ovulation

Recently a brand new urine test has become available which can be done by yourself at home to predict ovulation. It is called 'First Response' and consists of a test stick that is dipped into the urine and mixed with various chemicals to indicate a blue colour in the urine which can then be matched with a graded scale.

When you notice a significant increase in the blue colour, this indicates the most fertile day of the cycle and pregnancy will be most likely to occur if intercourse occurs within twenty-four hours after seeing this significant increase.

This test actually measures the amount of the pituitary hormone 'luteinizing hormone' (LH) in the urine, which reaches a peak on the most fertile day of the cycle and triggers ovulation.

'First Response' predicts that ovulation is about to occur and thus is very useful as, once it has occurred, the egg can only be fertilized for twelve to forty-eight hours and these hours may be missed if you are only using a temperature chart.

Although this home test is quite expensive, it is very worthwhile for women with irregular ovulation, and the manufacturing company also provides a 'hot line' for women to discuss readings with a trained nursing sister. 'First Response' is available at chemist shops and comes with a complete instruction booklet.

All these signs of ovulation are extremely valuable because a woman is most likely to conceive if she has intercourse during the three days before and the three days after ovulation. The most effective time to have sexual intercourse is twenty-four to thirty-six hours *before* the moment of ovulation and the 'First Response' predictor test can be very useful in pinpointing this time.

What causes lack of ovulation?

One cause is premature failure of the ovaries (premature menopause). In other cases, the ovaries are just stubborn and resistant to normal stimulation from the pituitary gland. One might call these lazy ovaries.

Another cause of infrequent or irregular ovulation is polycystic disease of the ovaries, in which the ovaries develop multiple cysts and there is excessive production of male hormones. Women with polycystic ovarian disease are often obese and have excess facial hair and acne.

In all the cases so far mentioned, drugs can be given to stimulate ovulation by the ovaries and this treatment is usually very successful.

Abnormalities of the thyroid gland, situated in the neck, can interfere with ovulation, and correction of this thyroid imbalance will result in normal ovulation. This just goes to show how the function of different hormone glands in the body is interdependent upon normal function of other glands, and they must all work together for normal ovulation to occur.

In some women who do not ovulate, the pituitary hormone prolactin is found to be abnormally high. This may be due to a hormone imbalance in the pituitary gland or a tumour of the pituitary gland known as a 'prolactinoma tumour'. In most cases, excessive prolactin can be successfully treated with the drug bromocriptine and ovulation and pregnancy will commonly follow this treatment. Surgery or radiation of the pituitary gland is needed only if the tumour is very large in size.

After all these causes have been excluded, it will be found that there are a large number of women (around 60 per cent) who do not ovulate satisfactorily because of extremes in weight, excessive athletic exercise, stress, anxiety or psychological problems. These factors upset the delicate balance of the pituitary hormones FSH and LH which normally stimulate ovulation. See Chapter Two, Figure 5 on page 21. Correction of these life-style and psychological factors will usually result in a resumption of normal ovulation, and if it does not, fertility drugs can be used to stimulate the ovaries to ovulate. To be a candidate for fertility drugs you must have a healthy uterus, tubes and cervix and a fertile partner.

Overall, and taking into account all disorders of ovulation, effective treatment with ovulation-stimulating drugs (fertility drugs) results in 80 per cent of women conceiving. The incidence of multiple births (twins, triplets and quadruplets) is approximately 12 to 15 per cent after using these drugs.

Disorders of the Fallopian tubes

Now that we have dealt with infertility due to poor ovulation, let us take a look at another major cause of infertility.

Because fertilization of the egg normally occurs in the outer third of the Fallopian tubes, obstruction, twisting or blockage of the tubes can result in infertility. For pregnancy to occur, there must be at least one healthy unobstructed tube.

Blockage of the Fallopian tubes is often a result of previous pelvic infection, surgery on the ovaries and tubes, abortion, use of an intra-uterine contraceptive device or appendicitis. In a high proportion of cases, no past underlying cause can be found and the first suspicion of tubal blockage occurs only when an X-ray or laparoscopy is done.

In laparoscopy, the surgeon passes a special telescope (laparoscope) through a small incision in the abdominal wall to see all the pelvic organs. By this method, it can be seen whether abnormalities such as adhesions (old scar tissue), cysts, fibroids or endometriosis are blocking the tubes. The surgeon will also try to pass a blue dye through the cervix, uterus and tubes into the abdomen; if the tubes are blocked, the surgeon will not see the dye spilling out of the tubal ends as he looks down the laparoscope. See Figure 36.

The surgical division of adhesions around the tubal openings is quite successful, and pregnancy can be expected in up to 50 per

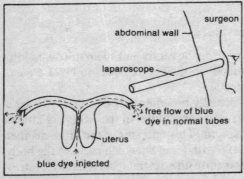

Figure 36

cent of such cases. However, if the tubes are completely blocked internally, plastic reconstructive surgery involving microsurgical techniques may be required but this results in a pregnancy rate of around only 15 to 40 per cent. If the tubes are very dilated and swollen, surgery is usually without much hope and couples should probably choose in vitro fertilization which enables the tubes to be bypassed.

Endometriosis

Another common cause of infertility is endometriosis which causes ovarian cysts and abnormal movement of the Fallopian tubes. Endometriosis is diagnosed by visualization through a laparoscope as, in some cases of quite severe endometriosis, the woman may not complain of any physical symptoms such as pain, swelling, heavy bleeding and so on. Thus the only sure way to diagnose endometriosis is to see it, and that is what the surgeon aims to do. If the endometriosis has produced cysts in the ovaries, their surgical removal may result in ovulation and pregnancy. Small lesions of endometriosis, however, are best treated with hormones instead of surgery. In women with very mild endometriosis, treatment may not be required as the pregnancy rates in such untreated women are similar to those in women who take hormone treatment. Furthermore, the hormone treatment is required for six to nine months and during this time the woman is usually infertile.

Disorders of the cervical mucus

In order for sperm to penetrate the cervix and swim upstream into the uterine tubes, the mucus in the cervix needs to be of a good quality and free from infection.

Occasionally, women actually become allergic to their partner's sperm and produce destructive antibodies in their cervical mucus which react against the sperm. This operates in the same manner as vaccination, for example with tetanus, which induces the body to produce antibodies against the tetanus bacteria to destroy them.

An excellent test for compatibility between a couple's cervical mucus and sperm is the 'post-coital test'. In this test, the woman visits the doctor as soon as possible after sexual intercourse and a small amount of mucus is painlessly removed from the cervix and examined under a microscope. In a normal post-coital test there are sufficient numbers of healthy mobile sperm swimming actively in the mucus. In contrast, an abnormal test will reveal only dead sperm or no sperm at all in the mucus. If the post-coital test is abnormal, the mucus should be checked for infection and anti-bodies against the sperm. If sperm antibodies are found, the woman may have effectively become allergic to her partner's sperm and will need to reduce repeated contact with the sperm by using condoms for at least nine to twelve months. This results in a marked reduction in destructive sperm antibodies in the mucus and an increased pregnancy rate after the condoms are abandoned.

For cervical mucus that is persistently of poor quality, very small doses of oestrogen can be given prior to ovulation, which will stimulate the production of a more favourable type of mucus.

In some cases of very poor cervical mucus, the husband's sperm can be inseminated into the uterine cavity, thus bypassing the hostile cervical mucus, and this will increase the chance of fertilization.

Mechanical causes of infertility

Cases of severe fibroids or an abnormally shaped uterus (as in a congenital abnormality of the uterus) usually require surgical correction before pregnancy can result.

Unexplained infertility

It is surprising to know that in 20 per cent of infertile women no cause or abnormality accounting for their failure to conceive can be found and everything appears just perfect for conception. Experimental treatments with hormones, ovulation stimulating drugs, bromocriptine, antibiotics and so on, do not result in an increase in pregnancy rates. Waiting patiently and optimistically is just as effective as any treatment and should be advocated for at least one year before heroic measures and treatments are attempted.

The infertile male

In many Third World countries, and until recently in many other countries too, infertility in a couple was always blamed on a woman and a man would often seek his luck elsewhere. I found this to be true in India where I was working in a large missionary hospital in the Himalayan foothills. I felt truly sorry for the infertile women there, who were stigmatized as being fruitless and barren failures all their lives. Their husbands would be truly shocked to learn that systematic investigation of the husband in an infertile couple reveals that he is responsible in 50 per cent of cases. Thus, male and female factors are equally responsible in causing infertility, while in a significant percentage, marginal subfertility may exist in both partners. Thus, investigation of both partners should always be done.

So far, we have totally ignored the normal physiology of the male reproductive system and I apologize to any male who may be reading this book; however, do not despair, as we will now describe what happens in a healthy male.

Normally, sperm are continually manufactured in the testicles under the control of the pituitary gland. The sperm leave the testicles via two tubes called the epididymis and the vas deferens and pass to the base of the bladder where they mix with nutritional fluids from the prostate gland and seminal vesicles. See Figure 37.

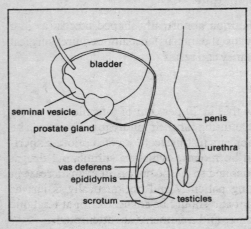

Figure 37

This fluid is now called semen and is stored in the seminal vesicles until it is expelled through the penis at ejaculation. Because a man can perform well sexually, with normal erection and ejaculation, does not mean that he is fertile. He must be able to deliver sufficient numbers of healthy vigorous sperm to enable fertilization of his partner.

Let us now take a closer look at the causes of infertility in the male.

Hormonal disorders

The pituitary gland may produce excessive prolactin, as in the case of the female, and this reduces sperm production by the testicles.

The output of the male hormone, testosterone, from the testicle may be too low, and this will reduce libido and sexual performance. The adequacy of testosterone production can be judged by the rate of growth of the beard and by measuring the level of testosterone in the blood.

Damage to the testicles

This can occur through the use of some drugs, such as cancer drugs or anti-convulsants. It can also be caused by radiation damage, infection with mumps, gonorrhoea or tuberculosis.

Twisting of the testicle on its stalk is a surgical emergency, which if not rapidly operated upon may result in permanent death of the testicle and, therefore, absent sperm production.

Abnormal function of the testicles

If the testicles are underactive, sperm production may be inadequate for conception. Underactivity can be caused by excessive heat (for example frequent saunas, tight underpants or a hot environment in the working place), heavy smoking and heavy drinking of alcohol.

It is thought that in up to six per cent of cases of male infertility, the male actually becomes allergic to his own sperm and makes destructive antibodies against them. This results in a shortened life span for the sperm, reduced sperm mobility and clumping together of the sperm. These sperm antibodies can be tested for by special immunological blood tests.

Testicles which have not descended down into the scrotum are usually underactive and result in infertility. Varicose veins of the testicle, known as varioceles, may cause underactive testicles. In both of these conditions, surgical correction may be effective.

Disorders of the accessory tubes and glands of the testicles

The tubes which carry the sperm from the testicles to the penis are called the epididymis and vas deferens – see Figure 37. These may become blocked or infected and prevent otherwise healthy sperm from being ejaculated into the woman. Microsurgical techniques on these blocked tubes have helped in some cases, but the pregnancy rates still remain low.

The prostate gland and seminal vesicles are responsible for adding valuable ingredients to nourish the sperm and diseases and infections in this area can reduce semen volume and quality. Infection of the prostate gland and seminal vesicles may need prolonged antibiotic therapy.

Genetic disorders

If a male has abnormal chromosomes in his genetic material, he may suffer from infertility. The most common genetic abnormality which occurs in men is 'Kleinefelter's syndrome' and this affects one in 500 men. In this condition, the male has an additional female sex chromosome to that of his normal male counterparts and this results in delayed puberty, infertility and impotence. The only solution is artificial insemination from a donor.

Disorders of sexual intercourse

Abnormal penile erection or ejaculation may prevent sperm from being deposited high in the vagina. Premature ejaculation is a common forerunner of impotence.

The majority of these problems have a psychological cause, but a careful physical examination should be done to exclude medical causes. Such medical causes could be diseases of the nervous system, diabetes, drugs taken against blood pressure and epilepsy, previous surgery on the bladder or prostate gland, fractured pelvic bones, hardening of the arteries, poor circulation and alcoholism.

Unknown causes

After all known causes of male infertility have been tested for and excluded, 20 per cent of cases will still not be able to be explained.

How does one test for male infertility?

In all infertile couples, the male should have a semen analysis and at least three different ejaculation samples should be checked, several weeks apart, to judge an average performance. A diagnosis should not be based on one sample.

Some men find it difficult to accept that they may be the cause of infertility as it undermines their perception of themselves as being virile males and can also wound a sensitive ego. It may take great sensitivity and diplomacy to get your man to agree to a semen analysis.

The semen specimen can be collected by màsturbation or coitus interruptus, after five days of sexual abstinence. The entire ejaculate should be deposited into a clean glass jar, the lid tightly screwed on, and it should be sent to the laboratory within one hour of ejaculation.

The sperm will be analysed for:

1 *Sperm motility:* this is assessed as the percentage of mobile spermatozoa and values of greater than 60 per cent are normal, but less motility does not always indicate infertility.

2 *Sperm count:* sperm concentrations are normally greater than 20 million sperm per millilitre of semen volume, and lesser values mean reduced fertility.

3 *Sperm shape and size:* more than 50 per cent of sperm should have a normal appearance. A high percentage of abnormal-looking sperm is associated with reduced fertility.

It is not uncommon to find that various degrees of abnormality exist in all three of these areas in the same man.

Men with a total lack of sperm (azoospermia) and men with a very low sperm count, less than five million per millilitre (severe oligospermia), have extreme failure of the testicles, and in reality cannot be treated. Artificial insemination by a donor or adoption should be considered, particularly if the couple have tried for more than one year to fall pregnant.

In between sperm values of five to twenty million sperm per millilitre (mild oligospermia) do not necessarily mean infertility, and the chances of pregnancy are good in the long term; it just requires more patience.

What can be done for a man with an in between sperm count?

No specific drugs, hormones or vitamins have been found to increase sperm production dramatically. It is known that sperm counts are very sensitive to life-style and emotional factors, and regular exercise, a healthy diet, rest, avoidance of stress, alcohol and cigarettes can promote a healthy increase in sperm numbers. Some men find a good quality supplement of zinc, vitamin C and vitamin E can cause a worthwhile increase in sperm count.

For some men with low sperm counts, the 'split ejaculate technique' may increase chances. This technique necessitates withdrawal of the penis from the vagina as soon as the first gush of ejaculation arrives, so that the remainder of the ejaculate is placed outside the vagina. The first part of the ejaculate is of premium quality and by depositing the better half of the semen first and leaving it unhampered by the strugglers, the chances of success in fertilization may be increased.

If all these suggestions fail, a worthwhile strategy is to have your partner's semen frozen in a sperm bank, so that three or four separate ejaculations can eventually be pooled together, with a more concentrated specimen being obtained. This concentrated sperm specimen can be inseminated on several occasions around the cervix near ovulation time and the success rates for fertilization are around 50 per cent.

Another useful technique for low sperm counts is that of in vitro fertilization, because only 50,000 to 100,000 sperm are required. If all other factors are normal, in vitro fertilization results in a fertilization rate of 30 to 40 per cent. If the semen is of very poor quality, however, with not only low sperm counts but poor motility and appearance of the sperm, then chances of fertilization drop to 10 per cent using in vitro fertilization. In vitro fertilization is discussed in the following section.

The treatment of infertility

Explanation of modern techniques used in infertility

1 Artificial insemination by a donor (AID)

This almost sounds like AIDS, but thankfully it isn't! Rather, it is the technique of inseminating semen from a sperm bank supplied by male donors into the uterine cavity of a woman. A special injection gun or ordinary syringe is used to inseminate the semen painlessly into the woman around the time of ovulation. The donor semen stored at the sperm bank is frozen and all donors are carefully screened for diseases. Pregnancies have been reported with semen which has been frozen for up to twelve years! Insemination can also be done using fresh semen.

The use of AID is indicated in some cases of male infertility due to poor sperm count, impotence and hereditary diseases which the father may not want to pass on to his offspring. The chances of success are greater using fresh semen as opposed to frozen semen.

Waiting lists for AID vary greatly from one health authority to another. You can obtain specific information by contacting your regional health authority.

In preparation for AID the couple will undergo investigations as to their fertility. If the woman has a normal uterus and one healthy ovary and tube, she will qualify. The couple will also be assessed by a social worker to see if they can cope psychologically with the sperm of a donor.

2 In vitro fertilization (IVF)

This is the technique of bypassing the Fallopian tubes by fertilizing the egg outside the body in a special laboratory dish.

How is an egg collected from the woman?

Firstly, the time of ovulation must be predicted and this is done by measuring the surge of the pituitary hormone LH in the urine that occurs just before ovulation. (Many centres do not rely on natural ovulation and stimulate a strong ovulation with drugs.) Under a general anaesthetic, the surgeon will look into the pelvis with a laparoscope approximately twenty to twenty-one hours *after* the detected LH surge. If the surgeon has chosen the lucky moment, he will see the follicles of the ripe eggs projecting like tiny blisters on the surface of one of the ovaries. These blisters will be aspirated under the guidance of the laparoscope into a small bottle and sent to the laboratory for identification and separation of the eggs. Within a few minutes, the captured eggs will be transferred into a dish containing a fresh preparation of the partner's sperm, along with special nutrients to enable fertilization and growth.

A new technique for collecting eggs, in which a needle is passed through the vagina to the ovary to suck in an egg, under the guidance of an ultrasound video picture, is now enabling some women to have eggs collected without a general anaesthetic.

Of all the eggs fertilized by this method, 80 per cent will advance to a four-cell embryo after forty-eight hours. At this stage, several tiny embryos will be inseminated into the woman's uterine cavity where attachment of at least one of the embryos to the uterine lining will hopefully occur in two to three days.

Surplus embryos produced by this technique are deep frozen for further attempts, although not all survive.

When is IVF indicated?

The main reason for performing IVF is in cases of female infertility due to blocked and damaged tubes. The woman must have a healthy uterus and at least one normal ovary and, ideally, be less than thirty-six years old.

IVF is also used to overcome some cases of unexplained infertility and may be indicated in cases of male infertility due to a low sperm count.

As with AID, waiting lists for IVF vary greatly between regions and access to treatment is often largely determined by ability to pay. In 1987, over 7,000 women were treated using IVF with a resulting 760 live births.

In women who do conceive using this technique, there is no increased risk of congenital abnormality in the child and the chances of having a normal vaginal delivery are as good as any woman's. IVF will not increase the chances of caesarean section or of a difficult birth, unless multiple pregnancy eventuates. In those who do not conceive, the cause is failure of the tiny embryo to implant in the uterus.

3 Gamete intra-Fallopian transfer (GIFT)

GIFT is the technique of collecting eggs and sperm and transferring them to the outer ends of the Fallopian tubes via a laparoscope where, hopefully, fertilization will occur. A fertilization rate of 25 to 35 per cent after each gamete transfer is possible. In 1987, 498 pregnancies resulted out of 2,658 treatment cycles with a live birth rate of about 10 per cent.

The prevention of infertility

There is a direct link between sexually transmitted diseases (STD) and infertility. To prevent STD huge education programmes for pre-sexually active groups need to be started and should stress:

1 Delaying sexual activity.

2 Careful selection and screening of prospective sexual partners.

3 The use of condoms and vaginal diaphragms.

4 Avoiding intra-uterine contraceptive devices in very young women, especially if they have multiple sexual partners.

5 Early attendance to the doctor for symptoms suggestive of STD and compulsory treatment for sexual contacts of patients with STD.

Overall, 30 per cent of infertility is due to pelvic infection and this figure is difficult to reduce as many cases are silent and insidious without obvious symptoms in the early stages. This is all the more reason why prevention should be stressed.

An overall view of treatment

The desperate need for a child makes some infertile couples at risk from exploitation by several groups, but particularly from alternative health quacks who promise magic cures. It is not uncommon for pregnancy to occur independently of any treatment; however, the coincidence is usually interpreted as a consequence of treatments which in reality have done nothing more than let Mother Nature take her course.

Today, all infertile couples, except those with irreversible failure of the gonads (testicles in men and ovaries in women), can now be offered treatment with some hope. The chances of success are dependent on the cause. As can be seen from the graph in Figure 38, women with absent or infrequent periods (known as amenorrhoea or oligomenorrhea respectively) have the best chances of successful treatment. In cases of unexplained infertility, where all tests are normal, there is still a greater than 50 per cent chance of spontaneous pregnancy after twelve months, and therefore, in these cases, a policy of observant expectation should be followed for at least twelve to eighteen months before other measures are instituted.

On the pessimistic side, couples with badly deficient sperm (severe oligospermia) or obstruction of the tubes are most unlikely to conceive without active treatment, and in these cases observant expectation is usually quite useless.

Success in the treatment of severe male infertility (azoospermia or severe oligospermia) is poor, even if artificial insemination or IVF using the husband's semen is attempted. The only option is artificial insemination using donor semen (AID) which is one of the most successful 'treatments' available, albeit that it does not cure the husband of his infertility. Success rates of AID are greater than 60 per cent after twelve cycles of treatment.

In vitro fertilization (IVF) in which the male and female eggs are united in a test tube and then implanted into the uterus, can be used as a treatment in tubal diseases, some cases of male infertility such as low sperm counts, unexplained infertility, endometriosis, immunological cases such as sperm allergy and in cases where AID has failed. IVF is expensive but it is reasonably

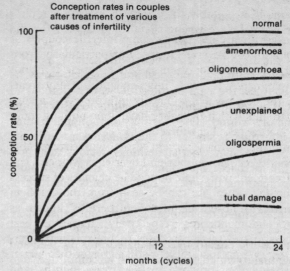

Conception rates in couples after treatment of various causes of infertility

Figure 38

effective with pregnancy rates of around 20 per cent after each cycle of treatment. Approximately 40 per cent of these pregnancies will eventuate in a miscarriage, and thus the 'take home baby' rate is around 10 per cent after each treatment cycle.

The option of inseminating another woman's uterus (surrogacy) is not available in the United Kingdom on a recognized legal basis and has major legal and social implications. It is unlikely that surrogacy will be an option accepted by society in the near future.

Adoption

Couples who have tried to conceive a child for several years will often be inclined to look into adoption. Many hospitals have counselling services for infertile couples which provide up to date information about what is available. Your local social services will also offer help and information about adoption agencies.

In summary

Treatments for infertility have recently improved to the extent that in some conditions it is possible to restore an infertile couple's fertility to near normal. Treatment is more successful for the infertile woman than for the infertile man.

Most couples can be offered treatment with some hope of a child, but the cost – emotional, physical and financial – may be high. To some couples, the pain of infertility is irrevocable and the continual sight of beautiful children belonging to other people reopens the same old wound. The reaction to emotional trauma associated with infertility is similar to the typical reaction of the bereaved. The bereaved have lost something precious they previously knew, but perhaps, for some people, it is even more difficult to lose something they never had, but only dreamed of having.

While society may sometimes bemoan government expenditure on infertility research, and other areas of medicine may seem more pressing in a world already overpopulated, it is the pain and need of the individual to which doctors should be committed, and for this reason, research into more effective treatments will continue.

Infertile couples need a lot of counselling and must be aware that investigations and treatment may worsen the normal feelings of anxiety, frustration, anger, loneliness and despair that infertile couples commonly experience. Infertility places a great strain on any relationship, and many couples find that talking with others who are experiencing the same problem is very helpful. Self-help groups offer support. CHILD is at 367 Wandsworth Bridge Road, London SW8 2JJ, 081-740 6605, and the National Association for the Childless is at 318 Summer Lane, Birmingham B19 3RL. 021-359 4887.

12 The menopause and beyond

The human female is different from other species in that she lives beyond the time of her fertility. During the twentieth century, improved medical technology and public health have resulted in an average life span for women of seventy-five years; this means a woman has on average twenty-five years to live, hopefully a happy and healthy life, beyond her menopause. It is rather startling to compare this to the meagre thirty years of life which was the average life span for women living around AD 1000. Indeed, it was little better during the reign of Elizabeth I when it was forty years, and it wasn't until the turn of the twentieth century that it approximated the menopause (fifty years). It is interesting to surmise what the average age of death will be in women in the year AD 3000, given that medical advances are increasing at a greater rate all the time.

Doctors are now having to cope with new medical diseases related to our ageing population and the menopause is one of these new diseases.

The modern-day fifty-year-old woman is far different psychologically from her fifty-year-old sisters of a hundred years ago. When her family disperses, she no longer needs to feel redundant mentally, physically or sexually, and indeed, often for the first time, she may be really free to pursue a new job, a new career, hobby or latent talent. These desires are reinforced by the current status and prominent role of women in politics and professional life today. To be able to fulfil this capacity for personal satisfaction, she will need to be well informed regarding maintenance of her physical, mental and sexual well-being, which otherwise might be in jeopardy at this time of life. One may have beautiful and passionate desires but, without basic good health, they are likely to be severely suppressed and unrealizable. If a woman takes care of her health, the menopause can be a time of rejuvenation and excitement. Did you know that Nobel Prizes for peace have recently gone to four menopausal women? Alva Myrdal of Sweden for her work on disarmament, Mother Theresa of the Poor in Calcutta and Mairead Corrigan and Betty Williams of Northern Ireland for their efforts to stop terrorism in Ireland. The planet desperately needs more female energy of this mature kind to develop creativity and peace.

What is the definition of the menopause?

The word menopause means the stopping of cyclical menstrual bleeding and this occurs on average at fifty years of age; however, the normal range can vary from forty-five to fifty-five years.

There is a slow downturn in ovarian activity with resultant hormonal imbalance for as long as five years before menstrual bleeding finally stops. During these so-called premenopausal years, one finds abnormalities of ovarian activity, interspersed with some normal cycles. These abnormalities include short and inadequate cycles with deficient production of progesterone, failure of ovulation with very high peaks in oestrogen production and, sometimes, constantly raised oestrogen levels. Later still, periods of absent ovarian activity are frequently observed, interspersed with periods of unbalanced hormone production due to lack of ovulation. The menstrual cycle may become irregular and infrequent, and bleeding may be heavy and prolonged at these times due to the hormonal imbalance. During these premenopausal years, many women require a curettage to exclude cancer of the uterus. Also, during these years of severe hormonal imbalance, a large percentage of women will feel generally unwell, physically and emotionally.

The cause of the menopause is failure of the ovaries. It is predestined that both ovaries have a limited active life span and this is on average thirty-five years. The fact must be accepted as there is no way that the ovary can be brought back to life after its supply of eggs is exhausted.

During their active life span, the ovaries have an amazing potential. Each ovary contains approximately 200,000 eggs at the time of puberty and each month some of these eggs are stimulated to grow. One of these eggs (usually only one) will develop into a small hormone factory called the 'corpus luteum' which makes the two female hormones, oestrogen and progesterone. The function of the ovaries is controlled by the pituitary gland situated at the base of the brain. See Figure 5 on page 21. The pituitary gland sends chemical messengers called FSH and LH to the ovaries in the blood circulation. These chemical messengers stimulate the ovaries to produce mature eggs which produce the two female hormones. After the menopause, there are no eggs left to respond to these chemical messengers (FSH and LH) and develop into hormone producing glands. The pituitary gland tries to compensate by sending increasing amounts of chemical messengers. Alas, the ovaries never respond, but it seems that the pituitary gland cannot 'comprehend' this, as it keeps sending huge amounts of FSH and LH to try to rewaken the dormant ovaries for the remainder of life. This forms the basis of the diagnostic blood tests your doctor can perform to determine if you are really menopausal. The blood tests are simple and if your doctor finds very high levels of the pituitary chemical messenger FSH (greater than eighty units per litre), he can say categorically that you are in the menopause or beyond. In a premenopausal woman, the blood FSH level is usually between five to thirty units per litre. There is no point in measuring the blood levels of the other pituitary messenger (LH), as this tends to change considerably during any twenty-four-hour period.

Thus we can see that the menopause has a physiological or chemical cause, and is not a psychological illness of women in the middle age groups. Doctors are altering their attitudes to the menopause and now regard it as a hormone deficiency disorder rather than, as was often previously the case, merely 'a state of mind'. It can be compared to other hormone deficiency disorders, for example deficiency of thyroid hormones, disorder of the adrenal gland, diabetes and so on, in which hormone replacement therapy is necessary for the maintenance of normal metabolism and, in many cases, the maintenance of life.

The fact that women usually experience problems with the menopause is common knowledge, and indeed way back in 1933, the British Medical Women's Federation Report stated that only 15 per cent of women had a menopause free from symptoms. Effective hormone preparations have been available since this time but it is only in the last decade that the medical profession as a whole has started to use them scientifically.

Immediate symptoms of the menopause

The lack of female hormones causes a disruption in the control of body temperature and this results in hot flushes and sweating, especially at night, which in turn causes disturbed sleep with resultant fatigue the next day. Hot flushes are most intense in the first two years after the menopause and gradually reduce; however, in one third of women they may last up to nine years. Fatter women have fewer hot flushes because their fatty tissues convert male hormones into oestrogen. Hot flushes are usually much worse in very thin women, heavy smokers or women who have had a surgically induced menopause.

The skin often becomes dry, fragile and itchy, particularly in cold weather when a lot of hot water and soap are used.

The female hormones normally exert a slight anti-inflammatory effect and, when they disappear, there is often an increase in rheumatic aches and pains, backache and headaches, and arthritis may flare up for the first time.

The sexual tissues of the pelvis such as the uterus, vagina and bladder become dry and shrink without hormone support. This causes loss of elasticity and lubrication and can result in pain during sexual intercourse, vaginal infections and discharge, urinary frequency and burning and prolapse of the bladder and uterus. Female hormones are also largely responsible for producing a healthy sex drive and, in their absence, there is often a total loss of interest in sexual activities. With all these problems, it is little wonder that marital discord and divorce are rife at this time.

The female hormones also influence the mental state, and indeed it is thought that they may have some controlling influence on the level of the brain's chemical transmitters, and therefore our moods. Thus it is not surprising that the incidence of depression, anxiety, memory loss, confusion, guilt, lack of self-esteem and uncontrollable moods is much higher at this time. These psychological problems may also be precipitated by the physical symptoms previously mentioned and the woman may be caught in a vicious circle.

Long-term complications of the menopause

1 Osteoporosis

This describes the condition in which the bones of the skeleton are weak and prone to easy fracture because of a low level of the mineral calcium. Lack of oestrogen results in an immediate loss of calcium from the bones, averaging about three to five per cent during the first three years, followed by a steady annual loss of one to three per cent for the remainder of life. This results in reduced bone density, and five to ten years after the menopause, a woman may have lost up to 20 per cent of her bone calcium. When a woman has lost more than 25 per cent of her bone calcium, her bones will fracture very easily, in particular the spinal vertebrae, hips and wrists.

At present, osteoporosis is very common and, by the age of sixty, one in four British women is afflicted. By the age of seventy-five one in every four women will have suffered from a fractured hip, wrist or crushed spinal vertebrae. Fractures of these brittle and fragile bones heal slowly and poorly, and often necessitate long and debilitating stays in hospital. If the spine is affected the vertebrae become gradually compressed and narrowed inside, and this results in a curved spine with loss of height, back pain and an ugly dowager's hump just below the neck. Women suffer from bone fractures ten times more frequently than men of the same age and the annual cost of treatment of osteoporosis and its complications is enormous.

In 1985 in the United Kingdom 35,000 women were admitted to hospital with hip fractures, and 20,000 died or became dependent invalids.

2 Degeneration of the circulation (atherosclerosis)

The word atherosclerosis means hardening and narrowing of the blood vessels. Blood vessels can be considered as pipes that carry blood to organs and tissues and, when the pipes become narrowed, the supply of blood to these vital organs is reduced. If the blood vessel is completely blocked, a stroke or heart attack often results. Prior to the menopause, women enjoy a relative freedom from diseases of their circulation compared to men of the same age because of the protective effect of female hormones on their circulation. Before the age of fifty years, the incidence of heart attacks in women is one third of the rate in men. However, by the age of seventy-five, women share an equal risk of death from diseases of the circulation.

How do the female hormones exert their protective effect?

It is thought that they produce a favourable balance in the types of cholesterol fat in the blood. In particular, the amount of the beneficial fat 'high density lipoprotein' (HDL) is promoted by the female hormones and HDL plays a protective role in preventing heart attacks and atherosclerosis. Women have significantly higher levels of HDL than men of the same age group *up to the menopause*. After the menopause, women experience a decrease in HDL fat and an increase in the undesirable low density fats. This results in a large increase in atherosclerosis, especially if other risk factors such as heavy cigarette smoking, obesity and lack of exercise are present.

3 Cancer

The final long-term problem of the post-menopausal years is the increased incidence of cancer of many types. This is probably partly due to an unexplained effect of hormone lack and also because of the gradual reduction in the efficiency of the immune system which occurs in both sexes with age. Without an effective immune system to act as a surveillance and kill cancer cells, the increased risk of cancer is to be expected. Some researchers have found that the risk of cancer can be significantly reduced by maintaining hormone replacement therapy for long periods after the menopause. However this is still slightly controversial and further research is required.

Treatment of the menopause – hormone replacement therapy

If given correctly, hormone replacement therapy (HRT) can maintain the quality of life for many menopausal women, relieve the short-term symptoms and prevent the long-term complications. The operative word here is *correctly* as, when HRT is given haphazardly, it can have disastrous side effects. This was illustrated in the USA in the 1960s, when hormones were considered the elixir of youth and the panacea to cure all ills. The doses of oestrogen used were excessive and prolonged, without progesterone to balance them, and this resulted in a six times greater incidence of uterine cancer. Furthermore, many of these women suffered clots and high blood pressure as a result of excessive doses. Subsequently, in the 1970s, doctors became paranoid about using HRT in all but desperate cases. If they did prescribe hormones, they often used inadequate doses and for too short a time period.

Over the last five years, however, much exciting research has been done using HRT and, now that we know its correct role, we can be confident that in healthy, fit, menopausal women, correctly balanced HRT is very safe.

What are the benefits of hormone replacement therapy (HRT)?

1 The use of oestrogen and progesterone will relieve hot flushes, sweats and vaginal dryness and will improve the muscular tone of the sexual organs. These symptoms will usually be relieved within six weeks of beginning HRT.

The psychological and emotional problems of the menopause are usually improved to a significant degree by the use of HRT and these improvements seem to be long-lasting. Many patients will comment on an improvement in their memory, alertness and concentration while on HRT. The mental improvement often observed in women on HRT may be partially due to the fact that they feel happier simply because the physical and sexual symptoms have been relieved. However, it is also thought that oestrogen has some controlling influence on the brain's chemical transmitters and this alone could result in an improvement in mental and emotional well-being.

2 In general, one can also say that oestrogen given at the menopause, or soon after, will reduce the risk of atherosclerosis. There have been some studies which show that women treated with oestrogen have only half the risk of death from heart attacks, compared to a similar group of women not given oestrogen. A large study involving 7,596 menopausal women at Leisure World, California, revealed that in women taking oestrogen for two to three years, the risk of heart attacks was less than one third that of women not taking oestrogen.

One must be careful not to get carried away, however, as the type and dosage of oestrogen given should be chosen extremely carefully. Some stronger synthetic oestrogens may produce undesirable changes in the composition of the blood, resulting in clots and high blood pressure, especially if the dosage is excessive. They can be particularly dangerous in women who have other risk factors affecting their circulation, for example, obesity, heavy smoking, varicose veins, high blood pressure or a poor family history and, in these cases, the natural oestrogens would be much preferable. In general, the stronger synthetic oestrogens should be given in as small a dose as possible and, if there is any doubt, it is best to use the weaker natural oestrogens.

3 Several studies have shown that oestrogen can stop or even repair the loss of calcium from the bones which results in osteoporosis. It is thought that oestrogen exerts its protection against osteoporosis by stopping absorption of calcium from the bone, thus reducing loss of calcium in the urine and improving calcium absorption from the intestine.

A very well-designed study, reported in the annals of *Internal Medicine* in 1985, involving 245 menopausal women who had been receiving oestrogen for fourteen years, showed a very beneficial effect of HRT in reducing osteoporosis. The incidence of all osteoporotic bone fractures was reduced by half with HRT and it was also shown that oestrogen is particularly good at preserving the calcium content of the spine, thus preventing the ugly dowager's hump.

In summary, it can be seen that oestrogen exerts a protective role against atherosclerosis and osteoporosis, as well as relieving virtually all of the unpleasant immediate symptoms of the menopause. However, there is quite a bit more for you to understand about the various types of hormone available and also their dangers, before you imagine that all your ills can be relieved by HRT.

You should also understand that while hormones may keep your sexual organs younger and more responsive, they will not retard the ageing process of your body. They cannot take away grey hair and wrinkles, although they may improve skin tone and appearance and result in a somewhat thicker skin. In all honesty, it must be said that good nutrition, life-style and naturopathic supplements play an equally big part in retarding the ageing process and we will delve into this later.

Many women have given testimonies as to the value of HRT in relieving their particular menopausal problems and here are some of their remarks:

'I don't get flushes now, I don't feel hot in bed at night and I am sleeping well, also I am less depressed and sexually OK now.'

'Since my oestrogen implant, I can now manage the things I couldn't before. My vagina is not dry and I am getting orgasms as I did before all this menopause trouble started. I do notice I am a bit more hairy and I have put on a bit of weight. My husband tells his friends to send their wives here as it will improve their marital relationship.'

'I had very heavy periods and discharge and used to get hot all the time with headaches and I used to cry all the time, and there was that terrible vaginal odour and discharge and I was dry all the time. Thankfully, all that has now gone.'

'I had oestrogen for my flushes. They were coming every five minutes with rheumatic pains, lack of sleep and headaches. I just couldn't bear it and they have all improved except for the bleeding. I am fantastic.'

'I went to so many people looking for help, many times, telling them I had no sex drive and it was painful with my husband and it had been like this for years. Some people told me to go and see sex films or read pornographic magazines and they didn't realize it was a physical problem. At the Menopause Clinic I was given oestrogen and the flushes went and now I have had an implant, I am back to the woman I was before. We have intercourse twice a week now, and we had not had it for three years while I was so dry. I must remember to get my implant changed as the effect wears off after some months.'

These testimonies come from women who were suffering very much before HRT. Perhaps you can relate to some of their experiences?

Types of hormones available – oestrogen

There are essentially three different chemical types of oestrogen – synthetic, animal and natural.

1 Synthetic oestrogens

Synthetic oestrogens have been used for over forty years and the word synthetic means that the hormone is made in the laboratory and has a different chemical structure from our own naturally produced hormones. Even more importantly, the synthetic oestrogens are *not* metabolized (broken down) in the body in the same way as our own naturally produced hormones. There are several types of synthetic oestrogens:

– mestranol
– ethinyloestradiol
– stilboestrol

2 Animal oestrogens

Of the oestrogens which are extracted from animal sources, 'equine oestrogen', usually known as 'Premarin', is the most commonly used one. Premarin is extracted from pregnant mares' urine and it is metabolized in a similar way to the synthetic oestrogens. Its effects in the body are similar to those of the synthetic oestrogens.

3 Natural oestrogens

The natural oestrogens can be a little difficult to categorize. They are called natural because they are broken down or metabolized in the body in a similar way to our own naturally produced ovarian hormones.

They don't accumulate in the body and are weaker than the synthetic and animal oestrogens, and therefore cause fewer side effects. Some people think that natural oestrogens must come from plants and other human beings' ovaries, but this is not true; indeed, natural oestrogens are fabricated in the laboratory. It is not their source that makes them natural, it is the natural way in which the body can break them down. Yes, physiology can be complicated but it is worth the effort to understand.

There are two commonly used natural oestrogens:

– piperazine oestrogen sulphate (Harmogen)
– oestradiol valerate (Progynova)

These natural oestrogens are a little more expensive than synthetic or animal oestrogens.

What are the risks of oestrogen?
1 Oestrogen stimulates the liver to make more clotting factor proteins and this causes an increased risk of blood clots.

2 Oestrogen stimulates the liver to produce a protein called 'renin substrate' which increases a tendency to high blood pressure.

3 If oestrogen is given continually and without progesterone to balance its effects the risk of cancer of the inner lining of the uterus (endometrium) is much greater. If oestrogen is given in this unbalanced way for more than five years, the risk of uterine cancer is increased by six times.

However, the good news is that if progesterone is given for more than ten days of each monthly oestrogen cycle, there is no longer an increased risk of endometrial cancer.

4 There has been a rumour that oestrogen increases the risk of cancer of the breast and this has frightened many women away from HRT. Unfortunately, this rumour has not been clarified and although some studies have revealed that oestrogen may cause a slight increase in the incidence of cancer of the breast, other studies have suggested that oestrogen reduces this risk. Some research has shown that dietary patterns, life-style and oral contraceptives may equally influence the risk of breast cancer. At this stage more long-term studies are needed before we can be thoroughly sure that hormone therapy is entirely free from risk. The most that can be said now is that hormones probably exert an

influence in both stimulating and protecting against breast cancer. Overall, if any risk does exist, it is very small.

What can modify the risk factors of taking oestrogen?

1 The individual characteristics of the woman
For example, the risk of cancer of the endometrium is greater in women with a delayed menopause (after fifty-two years of age), a low number of children, significant obesity, high blood pressure, diabetes and high oestrogen levels. In this type of woman, oestrogen is probably best avoided, or if it is given, then natural oestrogen should be used and under close supervision.

2 The type of hormones used
Both the synthetic and animal oestrogens are much stronger than the natural oestrogens in their stimulation of:

– breast tissue
– uterine lining (endometrium)
– clotting factors
– proteins that can elevate blood pressure

Therefore, if there is a risk of cancer of the breast or uterus developing, only low doses of natural oestrogen should be used. If there is a risk of high blood pressure, clots or atherosclerosis, particularly in women who smoke heavily, have varicose veins or are very obese, only natural oestrogen should be used.

In summary, in a totally healthy and fit menopausal woman, synthetic and animal oestrogens can be safely used as long as they are in the correct dosage. However, if there are any underlying risk factors, it is much safer to use natural oestrogen.

Types of hormone available – progesterone

The type of progesterone used is also important in determining the safety of HRT. There are essentially two types of progesterone:

1 Androgenic (masculine) progesterone
For example, levonorgestrel and norethisterone.

2 Non-androgenic (non-masculine) progesterone

For example, medroxyprogesterone acetate, desogestrel and dydrogesterone.

The androgenic progesterones can have a detrimental effect on the blood fats, in particular by reducing the beneficial, protective high density lipoprotein fats (HDL fats). This can result in an increased risk of atherosclerosis. Fortunately, the non-androgenic progesterones do not appear to affect the blood fats in this undesirable way, and women with poor circulation or a tendency to atherosclerosis should use these.

Conversely, the androgenic progesterones exert a stronger balancing effect against the stimulation of the uterus caused by oestrogen. One could compare the lining of the uterus to a field of grass – oestrogen acts like a fertilizer and makes it grow. If the growth is excessive, uterine cancer can result. Progesterone acts like a lawn mower, controlling this growth, and the androgenic progesterones are best at this. Thus women at risk for cancer of the uterus should be on an androgenic progesterone.

The reality is that we are still looking for the perfect progesterone and it is best for every menopausal woman to be treated individually, taking all factors into account.

How should hormone replacement therapy be prescribed?

For all menopausal women *with a uterus*, oestrogen should be given *cyclically* to reduce the risk of inducing uterine cancer. This means that there must be seven days in each month during which no hormones are taken. During this seven-day break there will usually be a withdrawal bleed similar to a light menstrual blood loss. Some women don't like this vaginal bleeding, whereas others find it a reminder that they are still women. The very sexy Mae West was said to have menstruated until the age of eighty!

After hysterectomy, where there is no risk of uterine cancer, oestrogen may be taken continually every day and no breaks are necessary.

It is very important that progesterone be added to oestrogen for ten to fourteen days in each cycle, especially when the uterus is still present, to reduce the risk of uterine cancer.

Even in women who have had a hysterectomy, progesterone is generally recommended for at least ten to fourteen days in each month to balance the effect of oestrogen on the breast. If breast tenderness is still a problem, relief may be obtained by giving progesterone every day.

During the seven-day break from the hormone pills, some women complain of a return of aches and pains and hot flushes. If this is a real problem, half to a quarter of the usual daily dose of oestrogen can be continued during the seven-day break to prevent it.

Possible methods of giving the oestrogen and progesterone are shown in Figure 39. In Graph A of Figure 39, the oestrogen is given for 21 days out of 28, and the progesterone is added from day 10 to day 21. Withdrawal bleeding occurs sometime between day 21 and day 28.

In Graph B, the oestrogen is given for 25 days every 31 days and the progesterone is added from day 12 to day 25 of the cycle. Withdrawal bleeding will occur sometime between day 25 and day 31.

In Graph C, oestrogen is given every day as the woman does not have a uterus, and progesterone is added for the first fourteen days of the cycle.

There are various ways of giving oestrogen and your own doctor will work out the best method for you, but remember that progesterone should always be given along with the oestrogen.

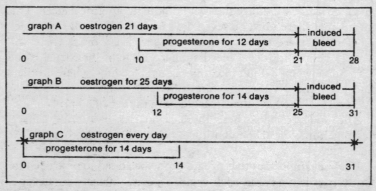

Figure 39

*Is there any other way that oestrogen
can be given besides taking tablets?*

1 Oestrogen implants

If a menopausal woman does not wish to take tablets, oestrogen can be given by implanting surgically, under the skin, a small amount of crystalline hormones. This provides a slow release of oestrogen into the blood which lasts on average thirty weeks, after which time the implant will need to be replaced. Implants are an excellent alternative for women who find hormone tablets induce nausea.

2 Adhesive patch

A very new technique which I feel is superior to the implant is that of supplying oestrogen by applying an adhesive patch impregnated with oestrogen twice weekly to the skin of the buttock or pelvis. One could call this 'band-aid oestrogen'. The oestrogen is absorbed from these patches through the skin and into the blood and appears to control menopausal symptoms very well. Furthermore, the adhesive patches do not induce unwanted metabolic changes in the liver or blood, and thus this seems to be a very safe method.

It is still necessary to take progesterone tablets for ten days of every cycle along with the oestrogen implants or adhesive patches.

3 Hormone injections

Some doctors use injections containing not only oestrogen but also a small dose of the male hormone, testosterone. These combination injections last for approximately six weeks and are effective against hot flushes, vaginal dryness, depression and osteoporosis. They are said to be very good for bringing back sex drive and libido but in some women they can also cause signs of masculinization such as deepening of the voice, increase of facial hair and acne.

4 Vaginal cream

Oestrogen is available as a vaginal cream. This is particularly suitable for women whose only symptom is vaginal dryness and soreness. Dosage is one applicatorful every night into the vagina for two weeks until the symptoms are gone, then a small maintenance dose of one applicatorful, once or twice weekly.

For how long should hormone replacement therapy be given?

This depends on the individual woman and the doctor's philosophy. To relieve the short-term symptoms such as hot flushes and vaginal dryness, HRT may only be necessary for several months. However, if symptoms recur after stopping treatment, it can easily be restarted.

In women who have had a premature or surgically induced menopause, HRT is best continued for many years. Similarly, to prevent long-term complications of osteoporosis and atherosclerosis, HRT should be given for many years. If it is decided to stop HRT this should be done by gradually reducing the dosage.

In 1976 the 1st International Congress on the Menopause was held at 'La Grande Motte' in France, and some golden rules concerning HRT were formulated. These are the following:

1 HRT should be individualized according to the needs of each woman.

2 The lowest effective maintenance dose should be used.

3 HRT should be given cyclically, unless a hysterectomy has been performed.

4 A progesterone should be added for half of the cycle.

5 The patient should be well informed regarding the treatment.

6 If irregular or breakthrough bleeding occurs at any time, other than during the seven-day break from the hormone tablets, a curettage should be done.

What are the hormone doses most commonly used?

This is easily seen by looking at Table G.

Table G

Hormone	Average recommended daily dose	
Oestrogens	Against immediate symptoms	Against osteoporosis
ethinyloestradiol	10 to 20 micrograms	20 to 25 micrograms
Premarin	1.25 milligrams	2.5 milligrams
Ogen	1.25 milligrams	2.5 milligrams

Progesterone	Average recommended daily dose
levonorgestrel (Micronor)	30 to 100 micrograms
medroxyprogesterone (Provera)	5 to 20 milligrams
norethisterone	0.5 to 1 milligram

Remember these are only average doses, and your doctor may vary them according to your particular needs. However, it is helpful to know the best types of hormone and the average doses, as this will enable you to discuss your particular characteristics and needs more intelligently with your doctor.

Are there any conditions in which hormone replacement therapy should be avoided?

Yes indeed. Oestrogen and progesterone should not be given to women with:

1 Unexplained vaginal bleeding.

2 Liver disease.

3 Blood clots presently existing or a past history of severe blood clots.

4 Cancer of the breast, ovaries or uterus.

Furthermore, oestrogen and progesterone should only be used with *extreme caution* in women suffering from:

1 High blood pressure.

2 Fibroids of the uterus.

3 High blood fats.

4 Migraine headaches or epilepsy.

5 Gall bladder disease.

6 Diabetes.

7 Cigarette addiction.

8 Multiple sclerosis.

9 Otosclerosis.

10 Porphyria.

What check-ups should a menopausal woman receive?

Going on HRT should not be taken lightly and a woman under-going it should be kept under regular observation by her own doctor or gynaecologist. Some tests are done before going on HRT, while others are done regularly, usually at yearly intervals, during the programme of HRT. The most important check-ups which should be done are:

1 Blood count for anaemia.

2 Blood pressure measurements.

3 Breast examination and breast X-ray if necessary.

4 Pap smear of the cervix and thorough vaginal examination.

5 An endometrial biopsy may be considered necessary in some women taking HRT. In this test, a small plastic spiral is passed through the cervix and twirled around to catch some of the cells of the uterine lining. These endometrial cells are examined under the microscope to check for any abnormal changes that may have been induced by the oestrogen and could potentially lead to cancer. Some doctors will do an endometrial biopsy routinely at least once a year, while other doctors will only do it if irregular vaginal bleeding has occurred.

6 If there is a risk of atherosclerosis or a family history of circula-tory disease, some doctors will measure the blood fats (cholesterol and triglycerides) and protective HDL fats. If there is a past history of blood clots it is also wise to measure the blood clotting factors.

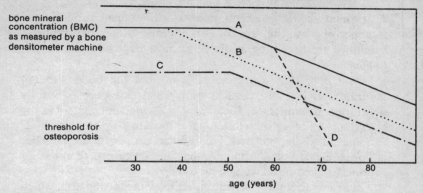

Figure 40

What checks should be done for osteoporosis?

Many menopausal women want to know what check-ups are required to predict their risk of osteoporosis. This is easily answered by saying that, ideally, all women should have a special test called a 'bone densitometer' at the time of the menopause, and another every five years thereafter. This is done with gamma irradiation from a radioactive iodine source and, although it sounds frightening, the radiation involved is very, very small and far less than that of conventional X-rays. It is simply a test to determine the concentration of the bone mineral in various bones, such as the forearm, spine and hip. If the bone mineral concentration (BMC) is high, the chances of osteoporosis are low. Figure 40 shows the average rate of loss of bone mineral concentration, as influenced by specified conditions.

Line A – Normal rate of loss of bone after the menopause (without treatment)

Line B – Premature menopause causing a prolonged period of bone loss

Line C – Reduced premenopausal bone mineral concentration due to genetic and life-style factors

Line D – Accelerated sudden bone loss due to cortisone type drugs.

Note the rapid fall-off in BMC *after fifty years of age* (see Line

A), which is why one in every four women suffers from osteoporosis by the age of sixty years. Bone densitometer machines are becoming available in most large city public hospitals.

Please note that conventional X-rays of the bones are not accurate and pick up changes only when osteoporosis is fully developed. By this stage, 30 per cent of the mineral content of the skeleton has already been lost and it is too late to do anything.

Sometimes computerized X-rays called CAT scans are used but although they are very accurate, they are too expensive to use for routinely screening all women for osteoporosis.

There are other factors, quite apart from the menopause, which put a woman at an increased risk of developing osteoporosis and it is important for you to know if you are in this category.

The following factors can increase the risk of osteoporosis:

1 Being a Caucasian woman with a thin build and fair skin. Negro, Italian, Greek and other Mediterranean races have a lower incidence of osteoporosis.

2 Heavy smoking.

3 Excess alcohol intake.

4 Low calcium diet.

5 Late onset of menstruation (menarche).

6 Lack of exercise.

7 Heavy ingestion of caffeine or aluminium-containing antacids.

8 Lack of childbearing or breastfeeding.

9 Family history of osteoporosis.

10 Surgical removal of ovaries, particularly at an early age.

11 Problems with digestion or absorption of food, for example chronic diarrhoea or operations on the stomach and intestines.

12 Vitamin D deficiency secondary to poor food absorption or lack of sunlight.

13 Crash diets. These can disturb ovarian function and hormone output, particularly in severe cases of anorexia nervosa.

Women with one or more of these risk factors should be sure to have the special test to measure bone mineral concentration at the first sign of the menopause. They should definitely take active steps to reduce their risk factors before osteoporosis rears its ugly head with a wrist, spinal or hip fracture. It is often a slow insidious process, occurring over twenty to thirty years, and a bone fracture can be the first sign. Osteoporosis can begin in the thirties, when the maximum bone mass is reached, and therefore prevention should be started early, ideally in the late thirties or early forties, by making sure that the diet is high in calcium.

With osteoporosis, prevention is much better than cure, because there is no cure once a fully developed case of the disease is present. It is a very salutary experience to sit and chat with the old ladies in any nursing home; they always far outnumber the men and the majority bear some stigma of osteoporosis. One can recognize the short stature, humped spine or limp due to a broken hip. Most of them first heard of osteoporosis when they had their first fracture, and thus they had lived in blissful ignorance for twenty to thirty years while their bones were slowly deteriorating away to thin shells. Many such women have said to me, 'If only I had known about osteoporosis, my life could have been so different.'

You now know that HRT can reduce osteoporotic fractures by half; however, you are still only half-enlightened. If you want to have a complete approach to combating osteoporosis, it will be necessary to read on further about nutritional and naturopathic guidelines for coping with the menopause and ageing.

Treatment of the menopause –
the naturopathic approach

A truly democratic doctor sees every patient as an individual and will modify, if necessary, the standard approach to suit that patient. If a doctor has an open mind, he or she will continually learn, not only from books and ivory towers, but also from the pearls of wisdom that come out of their patients' mouths.

I say these things because I have communicated with thousands of menopausal women and they have taught me a few secrets about naturopathic medicine and its use in relieving their symptoms. I have also learnt that not all women want to take hormone replacement therapy for years, and indeed, that in a significant percentage of those who try it, it does not improve well-being, but rather it produces unwanted side effects.

Up until now, women who were unable to take HRT at the menopause often felt as if they had no choice but to cope with an inevitable decline in the quality of life. This is indeed unnecessary as good nutrition, life-style factors and naturopathic supplementation are in many cases more important than HRT. You might say that they provide the cake and HRT is the icing on that cake. It is rather dull to give a long list of all the vitamins, minerals, herbs and foods that are of specific benefit to menopausal women so I have chosen to present you with this information in a practical reference table. See Table H.

If you look closely at the Table, you will notice that, for osteoporosis, not only the mineral calcium is recommended, but also the added minerals silica, zinc and manganese. These are important in maintaining the strength and fabric of the bone and cartilage. Dosage of calcium should be 1000 to 2000 milligrams per day, but one should be careful not to take more than 3000 milligrams a day as this may result in kidney stones. The best type of calcium to take is calcium carbonate as it has the highest concentration of calcium ions.

If one is not really an outdoor person, it is also advantageous to take vitamin D (see Table H) as this ensures better absorption of calcium from the intestine and is also necessary for the laying down of calcium into the bones.

As far as protecting the ageing circulation from atherosclerosis goes, it is truly amazing to see what Nature's garden has to offer.

Atherosclerosis – what do naturopathic remedies actually do?

1 *Regulate blood fats such as cholesterol and low density lipids:*
The combination of vitamins C and E and lecithin is beneficial in reducing cholesterol and dangerous low density fats.

Garlic is even more powerful in its ability to reduce cholesterol and low density fats and it also increases beneficial HDL fats. In animals on high cholesterol diets, garlic has been shown to reduce fatty blockage of the blood vessels.

Table H

Menopausal problem	Vitamins Daily dose	Minerals Daily dose	Herbals Daily dose	Life-style and diet
Osteoporosis	Vitamin D 20 micrograms – this is a safe dosage	Calcium carbonate 1000 to 2000 milligrams		Do: Regular weight-bearing exercises and obtain 10 minutes' sunlight daily.
	Vitamin C 1000 milligrams			
		Silica 100 milligrams		**Avoid:** Smoking, heavy alcohol, salt, caffeine, excess red meats, aluminium-containing antacids and taking calcium with high fibre foods.
		Zinc 20 milligrams		
		Manganese 800 micrograms		
				Include: High calcium foods in diet, for example, canned sardines and salmon (with bones), sesame seeds, green vegetables, - almonds and dairy products (preferably low fat variety). Dieters concerned with weight gain and

Menopausal problem	Vitamins Daily dose	Minerals Daily dose	Herbals Daily dose	Life-style and diet
				high blood fats can still consume low fat dairy products which contain as much calcium as whole milk.
Atherosclerosis	Vitamin E 100 to 200 inter-national units Vitamin C, as above Lecithin 500 milligrams		Ruscus aculeatus 100 milligrams Hamamelis 40 milligrams Bio-flavonoids Aesculus 40 milligrams Beta rutosides 200 milligrams Arizona odourless garlic 120 milligrams	**Avoid:** Smoking, fatty meats, white flour and white sugar products, high cholesterol foods and alcohol. **Include:** Fish, garlic, green leafy salads, cold pressed vegetable oils, sunflower and sesame seeds, soya beans, fresh fruit, raw vegetable and fruit juices, brown rice and whole grains.
Irritation and dryness of skin and vagina	Vitamin A 8000 inter-national units	Zinc as above	Smilax 400 milligrams	**Include:** Sardines, carrot juice, cold pressed vegetable oils and liver (occasionally).

Menopausal problem	Vitamins Daily dose	Minerals Daily dose	Herbals Daily dose	Life-style and diet
Hot flushes	Vitamin E as above		Cimicifuga 40 milligrams	**Avoid:** Coffee, tea, alcohol and hot spicy foods.
			Crampbark 40 milligrams	**Include:** Primrose oil.
			Smilax as above	
Psychological and emotional problems	Vitamin B1 and B6 40 milligrams each	Zinc as above	Passiflora 40 milligrams	**Do:** Pursue intellectual pursuits and outside hobbies. Try regular exercise, yoga, relaxation therapy and massage. **Avoid:** Excess alcohol.

In women who have real problems with their circulation, the dosage of garlic will need to be high and the tablets must be taken regularly. Any type of odourless garlic capsules can be taken.

Polyunsaturated fats should be included in the diet regularly as they tend to lower cholesterol. Such desirable polyunsaturated fats are obtained from eating cold pressed vegetable oils, primrose oil, sunflower and sesame seeds and their cold pressed oils, corn, soya beans, walnuts and fish (unfried). In general, the diet should contain twice as many polyunsaturated fats as saturated fats to maintain cholesterol at a desirable level.

Ideally, all menopausal women should have their blood cholesterol level checked. The average 'normal' value is five to six millimoles per litre, and if your value is above this, you are at an increased risk for atherosclerosis. Ideal values would be less than 5 millimoles per litre.

2 Reduce tendency to form blood clots:

Once again, that precious little garlic bulb can exert a beneficial influence here because of its effect on platelets. You may have heard of platelets, which are tiny particles normally circulating in the blood, along with the red and white cells. When platelets stick together, they can initiate the formation of a blood clot. Some people have excessively sticky platelets which clump together too easily, forming small clots in the blood vessels, and if this process gets out of hand it can result in the blood vessel becoming blocked. This may cause a stroke or heart attack.

In the *Scientific American Journal*, it was stated that the allicin content of garlic is decomposed to a substance called ajoene, and ajoene can reduce the tendency to form blood clots. Indeed, it has been shown that ajoene is as strong as aspirin in stopping platelets from sticking together.

Not only does garlic reduce platelet stickiness, it also improves the breakdown of blood clots already formed. Please note that this beneficial action of garlic is dose-dependent and the patient must take at least two capsules three or four times daily with food for a real effect.

Diet is also very important when it comes to clot formation. If the diet is high in saturated animal and dairy fats, this leads to the formation of a substance called 'thromboxone A2' which increases platelet stickiness. Conversely, the polyunsaturated fat found in fish and seed oils reduces platelet stickiness and clot formation. This is thought to be the reason why Eskimos have a much lower rate of heart attacks. Some studies have shown that people who eat fish regularly have a 40 to 60 per cent lower chance of heart attacks.

3 Strengthen blood vessel walls and reduce inflammation in the blood vessel lining:

Vitamins C and E are beneficial in promoting strength and elasticity of the blood vessel walls. The bioflavonoids are vitamin C helpers that are always found in nature along with vitamin C and improve its efficiency. The bioflavonoids also reduce the fragility and permeability of the walls of the small blood vessels and this stops fluid leaking out of the blood vessels into the tissues. Thus, in women with swollen limbs and fluid retention in the tissues, the bioflavonoids are excellent.

The bioflavonoids can be combined with several European herbs, namely ruscus aculeatus, aesculus, hamamelis and ranunculaceae, to improve the walls of the veins. These European herbs exert an anti-inflammatory and astringent effect on the walls of the veins and also increase their tone. Therefore, women with varicose veins, varicose ulcers, haemorrhoids and clots in the superficial veins (thrombophlebitis) will gain great benefit from these herbs. They can either be taken individually as shown in Table H, or together with the bioflavonoids.

What can naturopathy do for the psychological and emotional problems of the menopause?

The vitamins B1 (thiamine) and B6 (pyridoxine) are essential for normal metabolism of the nervous system and are also essential enzymes for the manufacture of chemical transmitters in the brain. If they are deficient, one can suffer from depression, anxiety and fatigue, and thus it is wise to take a supplement containing these two vitamins (see Table H).

I would like, however, to warn menopausal women against taking high doses of vitamin B3 (nicotinamide), as it can produce hot flushes, even in young women. Indeed, I once had a very distressed thirty-six-year-old woman rushing into my surgery, horrified to find herself having hot flushes and believing she was going through a premature menopause; the culprit was vitamin B3.

You may find the gentle effect of various sedative herbs very helpful, particularly at night, if insomnia and agitation are a problem. I recommend passiflora, chamomile, valerian and humulus, all of which can be placed in boiling water to make an infusion and sweetened with honey if desired.

Tryptophan is helpful when trying to overcome anxiety, depression and insomnia. Dosage is 500 to 1000 mg on an empty stomach, on retiring to bed.

We have said previously that a calcium supplement is required daily to reduce the risk of osteoporosis. This calcium supplement will also be of benefit for anxiety, especially if muscular spasm or deep sighing respirations accompany the anxiety.

Alcohol should be avoided on a regular basis. A few social drinks once or twice a week are not detrimental but the consumption of alcohol on a regular basis will increase psychological and emotional problems, as well as causing losses of the B vitamins and calcium, zinc and magnesium from the body.

Of course, attitude is crucial in overcoming many of the psychological difficulties experienced at this time. If one realizes that the disorder has a hormonal basis and is not a psychological or personality weakness, then there should be no need for obsessive self-analysis. One can be optimistic as, when the hormonal and nutritional state is improved, the symptoms will gradually lift. For many women, the menopause occurs at a stage in their life which is ideal to cultivate new intellectual and physical interests. So get out of the house, join clubs, learn a new skill or language and take time to find yourself as an individual. It is often beneficial to have an activity that you do entirely separately from your husband and children, and I have known several women who took on new jobs or began international travel at this time. There is only one thing in this life that can really restrict your activities – and that is poor health.

Some menopausal women become tortured by their fading looks. Unfortunately the wrinkles are inevitable and the only solution is to spend less time looking in the mirror! A fading beauty once said to me that as she aged, she stood further and further away from the mirror and tried not to be obsessive. 'Anyway', she said, 'I always appear more beautiful to others than to myself and I am much better than I think I am, especially if I am happy.' This is very true, and don't forget that subtle make-up and tailored clothes to conceal the occasional defect can often work wonders.

Plastic surgeons can also work miracles for those who need it, especially in improving baggy eyes, double chins and saggy jowls, but it should only be done when absolutely necessary, as premature plastic surgery will increase ageing of the skin. When used properly, however, it can take up to fifteen years off a woman's appearance, and off the age of her soul.

Exercise

Exercise should be done regularly and, ideally, every day, or at least four times a week. Exercise will increase blood flow, reduce blood fats and tone the heart muscle; overall it will reduce your risk of serious vascular disease such as heart attacks and strokes. It will also decrease weight. This is important because weight gain will otherwise occur, as lack of oestrogen results in a lowering of the metabolic rate. We now know that many of the changes previously attributable to ageing are simply due to physical inactivity. Middle-aged people who exercise can prevent or reverse degenerative changes in the heart, lungs, bones, muscles and maintain a normal body fat content.

We also know that osteoporosis is far more common in women who do not exercise. It seems that weight-bearing exercises stimulate the laying down of calcium in the bones and even as little as half an hour per day of walking is effective in reducing osteoporosis.

Posture is important too, and the tendency to hunch forward should be avoided. One should do exercises to bring the head and arms back behind the spine.

Any exercise programme should be started gently, especially if there is a tendency to osteoporosis, but if you are in good health, you can gradually work up from walking to aerobics or tennis. Some women with knee, hip or back pain will find swimming and hydrotherapy an excellent form of exercise for them, as it doesn't put any stressful weight on the joints. Yoga also keeps joints flexible and supple and is to be recommended.

If you are unsure of the status of your cardiovascular system, a stress electrocardiograph ('heart stress test') can be arranged by your doctor to detect any latent heart weakness *before* you start your exercise programme.

On a final note, exercise will also improve your state of mind and reduce pain secondary to muscle and skeletal problems. This is because exercise increases production of the brain's endorphins which are naturally occurring pain relievers and mood elevators.

Life-style factors

Avoid things which trigger hot flushes such as hot drinks, caffeine, hot meals, alcohol, emotional upset and hot weather. Ideal body weight is better than too thin, as thin women have excessive hot flushes. Remember to keep cool and keep the house cool, and to eat small frequent meals and drink cool iced juices. These simple points can help to reduce the frequency of hot flushes.

In summary

During my several visits to the retirement havens of middle-class America and Europe, I was saddened by the lack of vitality and mobility in many of the middle-aged and elderly females. These women had the curved stature of weakened calcium-deficient spines and lack-lustre skin and hair. Why do these ironies exist in some of the richest countries of the world?

Over the years it has become obvious to me; many of these women had lived a sedentary life and had smoked and drunk heavily, avoided vitamin and calcium supplementation and consumed excessive amounts of rich artificial devitalized foods. Their menopause was equivalent to old age because they had built their health upon a sandy foundation.

Not only are doctors becoming more interested in the effects of the menopause but also governments and sociologists. The ageing population of developed Westernized societies is dominated by women, and on average 60 per cent of the population over seventy years and 70 per cent of the population over eighty years are female. The cost and social burden of healthcare for elderly women is presently excessive, especially when one realizes that they make up only eight per cent of the total population and yet consume over 25 per cent of total government health costs. Nearly half of the NHS hospital beds are filled with elderly women, and unless something is done to curb the tide of premature old age and disability, huge problems in healthcare planning will occur. One hopes that in twenty years' time, this enormous drain on financial resources will no longer be necessary, and that elderly women will in general be fit and healthy enough to enjoy their longer life span.

13 A little basic psychiatry to help with emotional disorders

The human mind is the most complicated computer in existence, and it is also the most difficult to fathom, as 90 per cent of its programming is subconscious and not available to the average observer. Mental illness may be considered as a derangement in the programming of the brain which leads to behaviour outside of normal limits. This may present itself as abnormalities of emotional behaviour or intellectual behaviour.

The causes of mental illness

Basically, there are three groups of causes, which may operate separately or interact together. They are:

1 Constitutional

2 Physical

3 Psychological

Let us take a look at each individually.

Constitutional

This is the 'physical type' of a person which is inherited genetically and seems to be associated to some extent with a corresponding 'personality type'

The first type is the 'asthenic type' who has a narrow build, well-defined bones and a lean hungry look. These people lack muscle, appear taller than they are, have a long narrow flat chest, pale skin and poor circulation. The associated personality tends to be shy, reclusive, aloof, and is drawn to intellectual and philosophical interests rather than active pursuits. These people tire easily and have a tendency to depression and schizophrenia.

The second type is the so-called 'pyknic type', who resembles 'Humpty Dumpty' in having a wide and deep chest and abdomen, short neck and small but graceful extremities. Pyknics often look shorter than they are, have good musculature if they have not run to fat, a good circulation and ruddy complexion. The associated personality type tends to be emotionally warm and responsive, extroverted and drawn towards activity rather than thought. These people have high energy reserves. There is a tendency to manic depressive illness in the pyknic types.

The third type is the 'athletic type' who is characterized by broad shoulders, narrow hips, good proportions of trunk and limbs, large bones and well-developed musculature. The personality type is less well defined compared to the asthenics and pyknics. However, this athletic physique is disproportionately common in young criminal delinquents.

These basic physical types are necessarily broad generalizations and therefore cannot be held to be true in all cases. However, you may notice that some of your friends fit into these physical and corresponding personality types.

Hereditary factors not only determine our limitations of physique and intelligence, but also make an enormous contribution to our personality and psychological make-up. Inevitably, environmental factors will interact with constitutional factors and may result in unhealthy acquired attitudes of mind and habitual reactions which become so ingrained that they can be considered constitutional.

Physical

The second main cause of mental illness is that of physical factors and a good psychiatrist will always do a thorough physical examination and certain tests to rule out physical causes.

Physical conditions which impair the function of the brain may result in mental illness. Such physical conditions include intoxication with drugs and alcohol, infections of the brain as caused by syphilis, disorders of nutrition, low blood sugar (hypoglycaemia) and hardening of the arteries, and disorders of the hormonal glands, such as the thyroid gland, the adrenal gland and the ovaries. The sex glands (ovaries and testicles) influence the mind and there is an especially high incidence of mental illness in adolescence and at the menopause, these being the early and late stages of activity of the sex glands.

Disorders which involve degeneration of the brain cells, such as Parkinson's disease or senile dementia, may result in depression, anxiety or delusions.

Poisoning with carbon monoxide or heavy metals such as mercury and lead may produce brain damage and a type of dementia.

A brain tumour may first show its presence by personality change, emotional problems and impairment of intellect.

Alcohol is a toxin to brain cells and acute intoxication with alcohol may result in a delirious state with hallucinations and paranoid delusions. Delirium tremens, or the D.T.s, which results from sudden withdrawal of alcohol after a long binge, can cause drowsiness, restlessness, tremor, epileptic fits, hallucinations and terror.

In the chronic alcoholic, dementia will often set in after many years of sustained drinking. This dementia shows itself by disorientation in time and place and reduced judgement and intellect. The patient may wander around the home or hospital getting lost continually. The most striking damage caused by alcohol is severe loss of memory for recent events, and in very advanced cases the memory span may be not greater than ninety seconds. The victim may be aware of a memory loss and in conversation will often invent stories and events to try to cover up this embarrassing loss of memory. These made-up stories can be quite incredible and will often change every five minutes.

Massive doses of B vitamins and total abstinence from alcohol may significantly improve brain damage caused by alcohol.

Psychological

The third main cause of mental illness is psychological factors operating in the individual.

I will be a little traditional here and work from the theories put forward by that well-known scientist of the mind, Sigmund Freud. Freud was the first to see the mind as it really is, an iceberg with 90 per cent of its content hidden in the subconscious and, therefore, inaccessible to the average individual. This is why the average person is surprisingly deficient in introspective analysis; self-knowledge is often limited to only a vague awareness that the individual finds difficult to express in words. In fact, it is very difficult to make a just self-estimate. This difficulty is increased by the normal tendency to attend to those aspects of ourselves which give us satisfaction, with a relative disregard for our weaknesses.

Freud divided the mind into three hypothetical parts: the id, the ego and the superego. See Figure 41.

The id, which is our subconscious mind, contains all our primitive and innate desires for love, sex, security, power, food and so on. These desires are very strong and are not conditioned by society or religious ethics.

The superego is the opposite to our id, and contains our moral code. It is very much the result of our conditioning by society, religion and our parents and dictates to us what is right and wrong.

The ego is the 'meat in the sandwich' between the id and the superego, and must deal with the conflicts between our desires

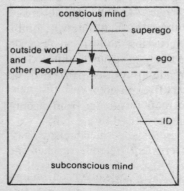

Figure 41

and moral limitations. The ego must also relate to the outside world and other people in an acceptable way, by balancing the conflicts between the id and the superego. The ego makes a compromise to do this and in most people manages to present primitive desires to the outside world acceptably, tempered by the moral scruples of the superego. For example, a homosexual man may be unable to present his desires to young men in society overtly, so his ego chooses a socially respectable means of being with young men, and he becomes a frustrated headmaster.

If the conflict between the id and the superego becomes too great for the ego to cope with, excessive anxiety will result, and it will be necessary for the ego to use 'special psychological mechanisms' to resolve the conflict, or at least make the conflict able to be lived with without unpleasant feelings. These special psychological mechanisms of the ego are called 'defence mechanisms' because they defend us from unpleasant feelings and anxiety.

The most common defence mechanism is that of 'repression' or 'suppression', meaning simply that the ego forgets an unpleasant experience by burying it in our subconscious mind.

Another useful defence mechanism which the ego uses to create mental ease, is that of 'rationalizing' away a conflict. It provides a reason for what one does, not the true one, but one which is more palatable and sufficiently plausible to deceive oneself.

Another very efficient defence mechanism is that of 'sublimation', in which the ego finds a socially acceptable channel for the expression of primitive urges, whose naked appearance would otherwise conflict with personal or social standards. It is often sublimation which causes sexually frustrated women to divert all their sexual energies into a highly ambitious and hard-driving career, especially when that career is in competition with the male sex. Sublimation may influence not only daily events but whole careers and life choices.

If the ego is unable to utilize these defence mechanisms successfully, it may revert to a less efficient defence mechanism known as 'conversion', in which conflict anxiety shows itself as physical symptoms. These physical symptoms can be very varied and affect many parts of the body, but they are only the expression in physical terms of some psychic disturbance.

In such cases, the patient is often completely unaware of the psychological conflict and complains to the doctor only of physical symptoms, such as headaches, cough, stomach pains, diarrhoea, palpitations or tremor. Sometimes this is due to ignorance, but more often the patient is not so much unable as unwilling to see the connection between mind and body. Physical illness is often considered more respectable than mental illness, and it is pleasanter to attribute personal limitation to a physical illness rather than to a personality disorder.

This defence mechanism often operates in chronic hypochondriacs in whom the doctor cannot find anything wrong. The fact is that these people have subconsciously found a socially acceptable reason for not coping with the demands and stresses of life – their poor health is not their fault!

In extreme cases of conversion, hysterical illness occurs, in which the patient develops a loss of function, for example paralysis, loss of memory, deafness or muteness, without there being a physical cause for the condition. The ego has simply converted an extremely stressful and anxiety-provoking conflict into a physical disorder. An example would be the terrified soldier at the front who develops a hysterical paralysis and is unable to fight.

If all these defence mechanisms fail, the patient will develop feelings of anxiety, depression or confusion and may have to seek help in order to maintain his or her ability to relate to the outside world.

A psychiatrist or psychologist can help the patient to explore and understand the contents of the id and superego and aid in developing a new interaction in the ego which is less anxiety-provoking and can be dealt with more productively. This exploration of the subconscious mind and past conditioning can be a lengthy process, but the results are often more than worth it.

A general look at modern psychiatry

In general, women under stress delay seeking help from psychiatrists or psychologists, and this is unfortunate as much needless suffering could be prevented and suicide rates be decreased if timely help were sought. If you were suffering from asthma or heart disease, you would not delay seeking professional help, and the same should apply to mental disorders. The main reason for this resistance in many people, at all levels of society, is that there is a shameful stigma surrounding mental disorders. This stigma is the result of sheer ignorance, especially when one realizes that the brain is a physical organ which can be deranged by physical causes, and that many of these causes are amenable to scientific and objective treatments. Psychiatry is not 'hocus-pocus' and its principles are based on scientific research using sophisticated technology and logical analysis.

In the first instance, if you are aware of a mental or emotional problem, you should ask your doctor to refer you to a psychiatrist. A psychiatrist is a medical doctor who has spent at least seven postgraduate years specializing in disorders of mental function. Thus a psychiatrist is eminently qualified to diagnose both physical and emotional disorders of the brain and, most importantly, can exclude serious physical causes of mental illness such as a brain tumour or dementia. Furthermore, a psychiatrist can prescribe medication specifically for your problem and will be able to view your situation within a broad context, meaning that he or she will have a wide range of possible therapies to offer you.

A psychologist is not a medical doctor and is therefore not trained in the medical diseases of the brain and is unable to prescribe medications. A psychologist spends three years at university, with some optional postgraduate time, being trained in the psychological aspects of the mind. Psychologists use analytical techniques to explore the mind and are proficient in behavioural therapies, hypnosis and relaxation therapy.

A psychiatrist will often refer patients to a psychologist for behavioural therapy after the initial psychiatric assessment, especially for disorders such as panic attacks, phobias, eating disorders, smoking or personality problems.

In general it is safer to see a psychiatrist first if you are suffering from a mental or nervous disorder as he or she is the best qualified person to judge whether you will be helped by a psychologist, or some other type of therapy.

Psychiatrists broadly divide mental illness into three groups, although there is some overlap.

1 Psychotic illnesses

These include schizophrenia, manic depressive illness and some severe types of depression. Patients suffering from these conditions are severely ill. They are often totally out of touch with reality and may be confused by hallucinations and delusions. Their thinking may become disjointed and hard to follow, meaning that they are unable to communicate mentally and emotionally with people who have no understanding of their condition. These illnesses must be taken seriously as they have a 5 to 15 per cent risk of suicide.

Psychotic illnesses are not rare – they affect three to four per cent of the population and often commence in young adulthood.

Until the 1950s most psychotic patients were permanently confined in mental hospitals as they were unable to function safely in society. The introduction of anti-psychotic tranquillizing drugs in the 1950s revolutionized the quality of life for psychotic patients as their symptoms could now be controlled while they were integrated back into society.

Nowadays, the use of anti-psychotic drugs is combined with a programme to educate and counsel the families of these patients, as the importance of the family as 'care givers' and therapists is crucial. All psychotic patients should see a psychiatrist regularly, especially to help prevent an untimely suicide.

2 Neurotic illnesses

These include anxiety, depression, obsessional illness, phobias such as agoraphobia (fear of open spaces), some types of sexual dysfunction and panic attacks. Panic attacks are not uncommon in middle-aged women and consist of a sudden onset of extreme fear or terror accompanied by the physical signs of adrenalin release, namely a racing heart beat, sweating, shortness of breath, diarrhoea and a feeling of imminent collapse.

Neurotic illnesses are very common, afflicting around 20 per cent of the population, with 5 per cent of sufferers being severely disabled by the symptoms.

These days psychiatrists take a holistic approach to treating neurotic illness, meaning that many different treatments may be called upon.

For example, psychotherapy is commonly used – this is an ongoing process in which the psychiatrist explores the thoughts and feelings of the patient. A very close relationship must develop between the psychiatrist and the patient as trust and confidence are essential before the patient will disclose deep and intimate fears. The psychiatrist will analyse the patient's thoughts and feelings, and then explain them to the patient. Patients have described psychotherapy as being like a mirror which the psychiatrist holds before them, thus enabling them to see themselves objectively for the very first time.

Once understanding has been achieved, supportive counselling and suggestions to overcome the problem can be given.

If the psychotherapy is very intense and delves deeply into the subconscious mind, it becomes a more dynamic form of therapy, known as psychoanalysis. During psychoanalysis the patient transfers intense feelings to the psychiatrist and treatment sessions are often required daily as more support is needed.

Medication may be prescribed for neurotic illnesses, but where possible, psychiatrists belonging to modern schools of thought will only use sedative or tranquillizing drugs for as long as is strictly necessary, and only to cope with crisis situations. Thus, the old image of the 'shrink' dishing out upper and downer pills is now quite outdated.

In general, psychiatrists are turning more and more to behavioural therapy to overcome neurotic illness. This encompasses stress management programmes, relaxation therapy, hypnosis, meditation and assertiveness and postive-thinking training. In other words, they are using techniques to change a person who thinks negatively into a person who thinks and feels positively – it is called reprogramming the mind and it works for many people.

3 Personality disorders

At times we all think ourselves to be a little strange or eccentric, and yet we manage to cope, and most of us fit into the curve of 'normality'. It is only when certain personality traits make us unable to cope with daily living and human relationships that we may realize that we really have a personality disorder.

Take, for example, the passive-dependent individual who lacks confidence and relies excessively on others to make decisions. As a result, this person does not handle a crisis well and becomes easily depressed and guilt-ridden.

Another common personality disorder is that of the obsessional person who is pedantic in the extreme and double or triple checks everything. There is nothing wrong in being a perfectionist; however, when it applies to tedious and sometimes irrelevant details it can lead to anxiety and tension. Obsessional types cannot relax as they can never trust anyone enough to delegate responsibility to them. They also seem to have lost faith in themselves. Obsessionals often try to keep everything rigidly tidy and organized, so as to create a feeling of sameness and security. They are also often introverted as they are preoccupied with their own thoughts and fantasies.

Personality disorders can be greatly helped by psychotherapy and behavioural therapy. The passive-dependent type can be taught coping and communication skills and put through assertiveness training. The therapist will find the patient's strengths and build on these, working out realistic goals.

Obsessionals can be trained in relaxation skills and thought control, so as to avoid becoming distracted by internal preoccupations and frustrating insignificant details.

The power of such thought modification therapy is enormous and previously negative people can become towers of strength. Remember, you can do anything in this life – all you need is inspiration, motivation and a little bit of adventurous spirit!

Let us now take a look at three neurotic illnesses commonly suffered by the twentieth-century woman, namely anxiety, depression and insomnia.

Anxiety

The condition of anxiety, which is commonly known as stress or tension, is usually accompanied by a feeling of apprehension or fear.

Not all anxiety is abnormal, indeed a certain amount of useful anxiety is experienced by most people under stress such as when sitting exams, learning a new skill or public speaking. This so-called healthy anxiety keeps you on your toes, increases concentration and rapidity of reaction and prepares for the task ahead.

Conversely, abnormal or neurotic anxiety serves no useful purpose and tends to be *present all the time*, even when there is no definite external stressful situation. If you suffer from neurotic anxiety, you may be aware that your fears are irrational and without cause and yet you will tend to magnify and brood on your anxiety, often making it worse.

What are the symptoms of anxiety?

The mental symptoms are tension, fear, difficulty in concentrating, difficulty in falling asleep and broken sleep throughout the night. The patient may lie awake worrying about exaggerated fears. Sex drive and appetite may decrease and feelings of unhappiness and depression may add to the underlying anxiety.

Anxiety causes excessive excitement of the automatic nervous system which results in the release of adrenalin in the body. Adrenalin is a very powerful chemical which prepares our body for flight or battle in the face of danger. The problem is, however, that there is no battle to fight and therefore we find ourselves continually stimulated for a non-existent stressful experience. This constant stimulation of our automatic nervous system results in typical physical symptoms of anxiety. These are:

1 Fast pulse rate, fast or irregular heart beat and raised blood pressure.

2 Dry mouth.

3 Diarrhoea, stomach cramps or nausea.

4 Dilated pupils, excessive sweating.

5 A frequent desire to pass urine.

6 Excessive contraction of the muscles in the scalp, which may result in a 'tension headache'.

7 Deep sighing breathing with a feeling that you cannot get enough air into your lungs. If this is not recognized, you may

continue to overbreathe and this results in a very alkaline state in the blood which causes blood calcium to become low. This may result in spasm of the muscles in the hands, feet and face, so that you feel as though you were having an epileptic convulsion or fit. These unpleasant muscle spasms due to overbreathing can be quickly relieved by breathing slowly into a paper bag.

Now you can understand why the strong and unpleasant physical symptoms of emotional anxiety may cause you to visit your doctor because you think you have a physical disease. The astute doctor will recognize that your physical symptoms will be alleviated if your anxiety neurosis is relieved.

Common therapies to relieve anxiety are analytic psychotherapy, hypnotherapy, behavioural modification and tranquillizing drugs. A cure may take from many months to several years.

A closer look at tranquillizing drugs

Tranquillizing drugs are amongst the most commonly prescribed drugs, with millions of prescriptions written every year, the vast majority being for women, as it is still true that 'men swill and women pill' to escape stress. The prescriptions are often written in haste with inadequate thought being given to the value of alternative treatments such as psychotherapy, hypnosis, meditation, and nutritional or hormonal programmes, which may be far more effective and better for the well-being of the patient in the long term. The doctor may be under pressure with a full waiting room and the patient may be ignorant as to the value of alternative psychiatry – so it is easy to see why this unfortunate event occurs.

The most commonly prescribed sedative drugs are benzodiazepines, of which Valium is the best known. Until recently, few reports on the serious side effects of sedatives were ever published. Doctors were encouraged to rely on the 'efficient and safe' effect of sedatives because of high-powered pharmaceutical advertising in which the risks of dependence and more rarely, drug-related personality changes and suicidal thinking, were swept under the carpet and called 'paradoxical reactions'. However, they occur too frequently to be considered merely as idiosyncrasies of the patient. The truth of the matter is that sedative drugs should only be used for the minimum time possible, say to overcome a short-term severe life crisis; they should not be prescribed for the long-term treatment of chronic anxiety or personality disorders. In general, benzodiazepine sedatives should not be prescribed for more than four months.

There are many similarities between the use of sedative drugs and alcohol, as both relieve anxiety quickly, albeit temporarily; however, in both cases the anxiety is really only being suppressed and it is the symptoms which are being relieved. The underlying cause remains and will recreate the anxiety as soon as the drug effect wears off.

Both alcohol and sedative drugs can produce psychological dependence and physical addiction. Long-term use of either, especially if combined with other drugs, may also produce gradual intellectual deterioration and personality changes.

How do you know if you are hooked on tranquillizers?

This is easy to find out, as if you stop taking the drugs you will develop unpleasant physical and psychological symptoms, which are known as a 'withdrawal syndrome'. The withdrawal syndrome is far more likely to develop if you have been taking a high dosage, in which case physical dependence can develop after only two or three weeks and certainly within four months. In one study of women taking sedatives, a withdrawal syndrome occurred in between one third to one half of them.

What can the withdrawal syndrome experience be like?

1 *Recurrence* of the original anxiety, with tension and insomnia. However, there will be no new symptoms.

2 *A worsening* of the original anxiety, called a 'rebound phenomenon', with tension and insomnia. There will be no new symptoms.

3 *Onset of new symptoms* that were not present before tranquillizing drugs were started. These can constitute a new type of anxiety, with poor concentration, irritability and insomnia. Other new symptoms may be physical problems such as palpitations, tremor, sweating, nausea, abdominal pain and loss of appetite and

weight. There may be changes in perception of the environment and sounds may seem very loud or lights excessively bright. Some people have complained of a crawling sensation under the skin and new pains in the head and face during withdrawal from sedatives.

All these symptoms can occur after stopping normal or high dose sedatives. If very high doses have been taken, withdrawal may result in muscular twitching, epileptic convulsions and psychotic illness with paranoid delusions and hallucinations.

The withdrawal syndrome usually lasts from seven to twenty-one days, although some lingering anxiety and depression may persist for several months.

How should you stop taking tranquillizing drugs?

When you feel ready to try, you should only do so under the supervision of a sympathetic doctor or psychiatrist. Remember that other support methods should be used during withdrawal to substitute for the drugs, such as hypnotherapy and vitamin and mineral supplementation. Your doctor or psychiatrist should give you constant explanation and encouragement. And try to keep the company of positive optimistic people and to avoid criticism.

The withdrawal should occur slowly over a six- to twelve-week period, with a gradual reduction in dosage, and there should be no need to introduce new sedative drugs or tranquillizers. A withdrawal period of longer than twelve weeks will be counter-productive.

The natural tranquillizers

These provide a natural alternative to the use of chemical sedatives and tranquillizers and, although they may take more time to work, they are free from side effects and improve well-being. Dependence and withdrawal syndromes do not develop while taking natural tranquillizers.

What natural tranquillizers are available?

1 Magnesium
This is an essential mineral for normal function of the central nervous system and in large doses can act as a relaxant and

anti-convulsant in animals and humans. Magnesium deficiency is not uncommon in people eating a lot of red meat without vegetables and fruit, or in people drinking a lot of fizzy soft drinks. It is also not uncommon in women on the oral contraceptive pill.

Magnesium should be taken in a dosage of 200 to 400 milligrams daily by those suffering from anxiety, tension, insomnia, muscular twitching and tics.

2 Vitamin B1 (thiamine)

An excellent nerve supplement is vitamin B1 or thiamine, which tends to be deficient in alcohol drinkers and lovers of junk foods which are full of sugar and white flour. Thiamine helps reduce the toxic effect of alcohol on the nerves, and it is also necessary for the body to metabolize carbohydrates, especially junk foods, because without sufficient thiamine they are converted into pyruvic acid and lactic acid which lower blood calcium and may result in anxiety and panic attacks. For anxiety-prone individuals, it is beneficial to take thiamine, 50 to 100 milligrams daily, and also to reduce consumption of refined carbohydrates and sugar. Along with the thiamine, take a daily calcium supplement of 1000 milligrams elemental calcium in effervescent tablet form, for example, Sandocal 1000.

3 Vitamin B6 (pyridoxine)

The faithful old vitamin B6 can be a useful tranquillizer as well as a fighter against depression. Vitamin B6 is required for the production of the brain chemical 'gamma amino butyric acid' (GABA), which is a naturally occurring brain tranquillizer. The dosage of B6 is 50 to 100 milligrams daily.

4 Vitamin B3 (niacinamide)

This form of vitamin B3 has been shown to have a useful tranquillizing effect in cases of schizophrenia by noted Nobel Prize winner Linus Pauling. To obtain a significant tranquillizing effect, large doses are needed to enable niacinamide to pass the normal barrier existing between blood and brain. Doses of niacinamide required are between 500 and 3000 milligrams daily.

Please note that the nicotinic acid form of vitamin B3 does not have such a powerful tranquillizing effect as niacinamide.

5 Zinc

The mineral zinc is well known for its beneficial effect on the immune system, yet not many people realize that supplements of zinc can also have a calming effect on the central nervous system. We think zinc achieves this by antagonizing the excitatory effect of copper on the nerves. Many people on the oral contraceptive pill or who have copper plumbing in their homes have excess copper in their cells which can irritate the nervous system. Dosages of zinc are 50 to 100 milligrams daily.

6 Vitamin C

The world's most prominent orthomolecular psychiatrist, Dr Abram Hoffer, has successfully used vitamin C as a tranquillizer and claims that, in large doses, it can be as active as some powerful major tranquillizing drugs which are commonly used to sedate schizophrenic patients. It seems that vitamin C is found in very high concentration in the brain and adrenal glands and, thus, is obviously needed for the body to fight stress. Dosage required is 2000 to 10,000 milligrams daily, higher doses being required in heavy smokers. Smoking is particularly harmful for sufferers of anxiety as it reduces the blood oxygen level which in turn increases production of lactic acid and, thus, tension and fatigue.

7 L-Glutamine

This substance is an amino acid of great nutritional importance, especially for the treatment of alcohol addiction and low blood sugar (hypoglycaemia). It exerts a gentle and lasting tranquillizing effect if taken in a dosage of 100 milligrams, three times daily.

8 DL phenylalanine

This essential dietary amino acid has the unique property of reducing the breakdown of the brain's naturally occurring painkillers known as endorphins. The endorphins also have a mood elevating effect and are produced in higher amounts during times of stress. Phenylalanine is known as the 'endorphin shield' and if taken for a two- to three-week period, it will lead to an increase in brain endorphin levels which is particularly good for patients suffering from pain and depression, as well as anxiety. Dosage of

DL phenylalanine is 600 to 1200 milligrams daily until a response is achieved, when the dosage can be reduced to 300 milligrams daily. DL phenylalanine should not be taken by pregnant women or people suffering from the rare metabolic disease, phenyl-ketonuria.

9 Sedative herbs

In preference to caffeine-containing beverages which are stimulating, you should drink herbal teas with a calming effect, especially at night. Suitable calming herbs are camomile, passi-flora, humulus, angelica and valerian. They can be obtained from a health food store.

Depression

Let us try to understand the experience of depression, commonly known as unhappiness or melancholy. Such miserable states of mind are often associated with feelings of inadequacy, guilt and pessimistic gloom. The patient may become obsessed by worrying thoughts which seem to haunt the mind, and this situation could lead to suicide.

Depression causes the automatic nervous system to become under-active and this may result in typical physical symptoms, such as:

1 Lack of sleep with early morning awakening.

2 Tiredness.

3 Loss of appetite and weight loss.

4 Constipation.

5 Reduced sex drive.

6 Irregularity or absence of menstruation.

7 Slowing down of movement, thought and speech.

8 The patient may become a hypochondriac, imagining, for example, that his or her constipation is causing the bowels to rot away. There may be exaggerated delusions concerning many different parts of the body.

In manic depression, the patient alternates between extreme highs and lows in mood, and may develop paranoid ideas of persecution and punishment.

The greatest risk of depression is *suicide* and anyone who talks about the possibility is at risk. Factors which make a person more likely to commit suicide are:

1 Severe sleep disturbance.

2 Previous suicide attempts.

3 Family history of suicide.

4 Suicidal talk and preoccupation.

5 Social isolation with persistent feelings of guilt and unworthiness.

The causes of depression

Common causes of depression are loss of a precious thing or person, a family history of depressive illness (constitutional), certain drugs such as the oral contraceptive pill, blood pressure drugs or sedatives, and hormonal imbalances such as premenstrual syndrome, menopause and post-natal depression. Depression and anxiety may be very much worsened by nutritional deficiencies of the B vitamins.

The treatment of depression

If suicide is a risk, urgent admission to a psychiatric hospital should be arranged. Supportive psychotherapy, occupational and social rehabilitation may be necessary and are available through a community health centre, utilizing a team approach of psychiatrists, occupational therapists and social workers.

In extremely severe cases of depression, in which the patient becomes totally lethargic and vegetable-like, electroconvulsive therapy (ECT), popularly known as 'shock treatment', may be the only effective treatment. It is given two to three times a week and an average of ten treatments should take away the depression.

For moderately severe cases, anti-depressant drugs are some

times effective. These are different from the sedative and tranquillizing drugs commonly used in anxiety states.

Stimulant drugs such as amphetamines (speed) should be avoided, as when they are stopped a severe rebound depression will occur.

The most common type of anti-depressant drugs are the 'tricyclic anti-depressants' and examples of these are imipramine, amitriptyline and doxepin. They are effective in relieving depression in about 70 per cent of cases, and early improvement, particularly a reduction in anxiety, may occur by the end of the first week. However, the depression may take six to eight weeks to be fully relieved, and thus patience is needed.

Side effects of the tricyclic drugs are dry mouth, sweating, faintness, a fine tremor and, occasionally, low blood pressure and sexual impotence. These side effects gradually wear off as the patient becomes adjusted to the drug.

Another range of very powerful anti-depressant drugs are the 'monoamine oxidase inhibitors' (MAOI) and patients who fail to respond to the tricyclic drugs frequently do better with these. However, the MAOI drugs can result in life-threatening side effects if the patient does not stick to a diet which is free from tyramine-containing foods such as mature cheese, yeast, meat extracts, alcohol and various others.

For manic depressive illness, the drug lithium is usually given and can effectively stop the roller coaster highs and lows. However, it must only be given under careful supervision as it can cause damage to the kidneys and thyroid gland.

All patients suffering from depression, especially if associated with sleep or eating disorders, should take the following natural supplements:

1 A high dose vitamin B complex tablet, containing B1, B2, B3, B6 and B12. Dosage is one to two tablets daily, with food.

2 Tryptophan, one to four grams daily, on an empty stomach, with fruit juice, before retiring. This is usually well tolerated, although the occasional patient may experience nausea.

3 Other amino acids, in particular tyrosine and phenylalanine,

can be effective in overcoming depressive moods if they are taken three times daily, on an empty stomach, with a sweetened beverage.

Insomnia

An inability to sleep normally is surprisingly common, and up to one quarter of the adult population is affected by sleep problems. There are no universal criteria for the minimum amount of sleep required per night in order to function normally and there is tremendous variation between individuals. Some people seem to need ten hours, while others can be amazingly productive on only four hours' sleep a night. Habit and mental discipline play a big role.

In general, the amount of sleep required decreases with advancing age. A baby needs approximately sixteen hours, but by forty years of age, seven and a half hours is usually sufficient, and by seventy, this is further reduced to six hours.

As a general rule of thumb, we can say that the ideal maximum amount of sleep needed by an adult is seven and a half hours, as this can accommodate, very neatly, our ninety-minute sleep cycles. If you sleep even a few minutes longer than this, you will be into the next cycle and may find it difficult to wake up.

The nature and function of sleep

When a person sleeps normally, he or she is totally unconscious and unaware of the external world, and enters an inner world where the problems and pressures of daily life are no longer troubling. Ideally, this inner world of sleep should be like a state of deep meditation in which peace and total escape are found and in which fantasies have no limits to their ability to create perfection. Daily life will always have its upheavals whereas sleep can provide a domain of total release. When life becomes too much, sleep can be seen as a safety valve which stops excessive tension from causing damage to the psyche.

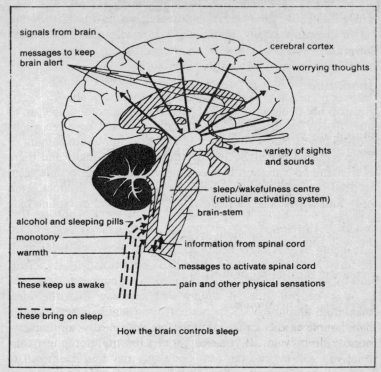

Figure 42

Which part of the brain puts us to sleep?

Deep inside the brain stem lies the centre which controls our cycles of sleep and wakefulness. This centre is called the 'reticular activating system' (RAS). See Figure 42.

The RAS is like a railway station, receiving impulses from all over the body and also from the higher brain (cerebral cortex). If the ingoing impulses to the RAS reach a low level, such as during a monotonous concert in a warm room, the RAS will become underactive and fail to stimulate the higher brain, and the person will fall asleep. In Figure 42 you can also see how worrying thoughts coming from the higher brain will stimulate the RAS and so keep us awake.

What are the two stages of sleep?

1 Orthodox sleep

During this phase of sleep the activity of the brain is very quiet and it has entered a state of true rest during which the body can restore itself. This type of sleep occurs at the beginning of a sleeping period and makes these first hours very valuable.

2 Paradoxical or rapid eye movement sleep (REM)

During this phase of sleep the brain becomes very active and its blood supply is much greater than during normal wakefulness. REM sleep occurs in bursts throughout the night, lasting for about twenty minutes every two hours of sleep. During REM sleep a person has vivid dreams and fantasies which he or she is usually unable to remember unless forcibly awoken during the dream. If a person is woken repeatedly during REM sleep, he or she will become increasingly irritable and when sleep is again allowed to progress, there will be a compensatory rebound increase in the time spent in REM sleep.

The causes of insomnia

Most people who complain of insomnia do not have any serious mental illness and are unable to explain the cause of their problem.

However, that aside, probably the most common causes of insomnia are *anxiety and stress*. Because the mind is preoccupied, it keeps reactivating itself, and thus the more primitive part of the brain, the RAS, cannot gain dominance. Anxious people have particular trouble falling asleep and often lie awake for hours worrying or counting sheep. They may have an underlying fear of sleep because of regularly occurring nightmares or an unconscious fear of death. Some people have unrealistic fears of the consequence of lack of sleep, believing that it will result in poor physical and mental health, brain damage or insanity. These misbeliefs create anxiety and an overinterest in sleep which, in itself, can prevent sleep.

Depressive illness can often cause a sleep disturbance. The depressed, unhappy individual typically wakes in the early hours of the morning (three to five) and is unable to go back to sleep because of obsessive and morbid thoughts. The early morning waker can be so anxious to return to sleep and blot out those hours of waiting that he or she becomes increasingly wide awake.

Physical diseases such as breathing problems, heart disease, cough, fever, pain, itchy skin or frequency of passing urine can all easily disrupt the sleeping pattern. In particular, menopausal women are often awoken from sleep by drenching hot flushes and have to throw off the blankets and change their clothes.

The external environment of sleep is extremely important and noise, bright lights, a restless, snoring bed companion or a crying child can be the last straw.

Old age and retirement are a common cause, as the brain is no longer fatigued by a normal day's physical and mental work.

Alcohol, if used as a nightcap in small quantities, may assist sleep for some people but in others it can disturb sleep. Heavy and sustained alcohol use will grossly disorganize sleep patterns as it reduces REM sleep and causes frequent awakening.

The treatment of insomnia

There are many effective possibilities and it is usually necessary to experiment with a few to find the ones that work for you. A combination of several different treatments may be required, so let us go through them one by one.

1 Hypnotic drugs (sleeping tablets)

These are a mixed blessing, yet despite this their use is widespread and it is estimated that in the Western World one night in ten of sleep is induced by drugs. Some sleeping tablets are highly addictive (for example, barbiturates and methaqualone or mandrax), while others such as the benzodiazepines, of which Valium is one, are only slightly addictive. The benzodiazepines have a quick action and produce sleep lasting between six and eight hours and the sleeper usually awakes free from a hangover.

Unfortunately, with most hypnotic drugs, resistance to their sleep-producing effect develops over a period of four to twenty-four weeks and thus they do not provide a permanent cure for insomnia.

If a depressive mental illness is the cause of insomnia, sleeping tablets should be avoided and instead, a specific anti-depressant tablet should be taken, if necessary, to correct the insomnia.

Why is it often difficult to stop taking sleeping pills?

Sleeping pills not only induce sleep but they change the quality and type of sleep, so that the REM phase of sleep with all its vivid fantasies and dreams is drastically reduced.

When the drugs are stopped, there is a rebound increase in REM sleep, with vivid dreams and nightmares, often resulting in insomnia which is worse than it was before the sleeping tablets were commenced. It is incredible to think that it takes a whole two months after cessation of these sleeping drugs before REM sleep settles down to normal, and thus coming off sleeping pills is not just mind over matter.

Ideally, sleeping pills should only be used temporarily to cope with a crisis situation until more natural methods to induce sleep can be found. However, this can be a bit academic for the thousands of older people who are petrified to face life without their certain nightly drug-induced sleep. In these cases, it may be best to let sleeping dogs lie.

2 Life-style modification

It is important to retire to bed at the same hour each night. However, it may be necessary to change the 'same old rut' of your sleeping environment. For example, you could move your bed to a new position, sleep alone or with someone! Glamorize the bed and its decor – some people swear by waterbeds which enable them to flow off into oblivion. Soft music and lighting, or a beautiful view may help to induce a sleepful state.

Research has shown that 'white noise' (the humming of a fan or the ticking of a clock, for example) is much more effective in inducing sleep than ordinary music. People who listen to white noise fall asleep more quickly and sleep more deeply. This is because white noise has a predictable nature, whereas music tends to distract a person's attention.

Don't forget that sex can be a powerful relaxant and stepping-stone to sleep, so it is important to try to overcome any sexual frustration.

Avoid eating a large heavy meal at night or snacks late at night.

Physical exercise is beneficial for sleep and can be done before retiring – it may be vigorous or take the form of yoga and muscular relaxation. It is often helpful to take a hot bath, followed by a warm milky drink such as Horlicks just before retiring.

A particularly difficult time can occur after childbirth when a woman may find that she not only has to cope with post-natal depression, engorged breasts and a painful vaginal scar, but the broken sleep that comes with demand feeding. This may interrupt the essential REM sleep and the woman may become too irritable and anxious to fall asleep again in between feeds.

It is necessary to fall into the swing and sleeping pattern of the baby and a good idea could be to snatch smaller intervals of sleep with the baby, even during the day. Give your sleep priority, get it when you can, forsake the housework, your social obligations and marital demands and relax when and how the baby wants.

I have a patient who is a prime example of natural mothering. She would never think of keeping the baby in a separate room or getting up from bed to heat bottles. Rather, she makes a bed within the marital bed for the new-born child, and thus does not have to get up to breastfeed. Her new-born's bed is fashioned from soft pillows and blankets so that the child is protected from smothering or falling out, and yet is still able to feel the warmth of the maternal body and breath.

This is not absolutely necessary and a crib or cot adjacent to the marital bed can be just as good. Having the child so close helps to overcome the fear of the 'sudden infant death syndrome' which can be a potent parental worry preventing restful sleep.

3 A change of attitude

For all insomniacs, it can be very beneficial to change one's attitude and reaction to the hours of sleeplessness. If all other measures fail, try to be positive about it. For example, think 'I have three extra hours of conscious life in which to do all those things I need and want to do and yet never have time for'. Think of all those books you want to read, the new skills you want to acquire, the poetry you want to write, the dreams to plan – and do it while you have those peaceful nocturnal hours with no one to distract you. Don't waste your time becoming anxious about it – this will only set up a vicious cycle of anxiety – insomnia – anxiety – insomnia.

Many famous and rich people tell how they need those lonely late hours or early hours of the morning to set out their dreams and plans. If you use your energy productively while awake, this will bring a natural fatigue which will eventually lead to sleep. Tomorrow or the day after, you will need to sleep more and natural compensation will occur – relax and go with the flow and in the meantime, nothing dreadful or serious will happen.

It is wise to avoid taking sleeping pills after 4.00 a.m., as you will awake with a pill hangover and find yourself too drowsy to face another day. If you don't feel like sleep after 4.00 a.m., get up and do something and catch a short nap in the afternoon or evening – sleep when you feel like it, as a one-hour nap can freshen you up for many hours ahead.

4 Naturopathic sleeping aids
(a) Homoeopathy
These gentle drops seem to help some insomniacs and are free from side effects or addiction. They can be taken in a dose of ten to twenty drops in a teaspoon of water and repeated every ten minutes until sleep comes.

For those who wake soon after midnight with a sense of anxiety and physical restlessness, the homoeopathic remedy 'arsenicum album' may be taken. If there is a feeling of fright and tension in the stomach, it may be combined with the remedy 'camomile'.

For those who wake at dawn after a deep sleep and have one or two hours of insomnia and then want to fall asleep just when they should be getting up, the remedy is 'nux vomica'. These people often have nausea or a repulsion to food on awakening and nux vomica will also aid this digestive problem.

For those who develop a fear of not sleeping, just as they are about to go to bed, associated with feelings of being shattered or in emotional turmoil, the remedy is 'gelsemium'.

For those who have fatigue following a bout of insomnia or late nights, the remedy is 'cocculus'.

(b) *Nutritional supplements*

The brain chemical 'serotonin' has a powerful influence on our moods and sleep pattern and, if it becomes depleted, this can result in insomnia and depression. Serotonin is made in the brain from a small protein known as tryptophan and its manufacture is also helped along by vitamin B6 (pyridoxine). The reason why some insomniacs find a glass of warm milk useful in inducing sleep is because milk contains a large amount of tryptophan which can be converted to serotonin in the brain. Thus logically, supplements of tryptophan and vitamin B6 should help to maintain normal serotonin levels which will aid in promoting sleep. The addition of a zinc supplement has also been found to aid the sleep-enhancing properties of tryptophan and B6.

Trytophan will not work effectively unless it is taken on a completely empty stomach (at least two hours before or after a meal) and with some readily absorbed form of carbohydrate such as honey, bananas or fruit juice.

(c) *Sedative herbs*

Insomniacs should avoid drinking caffeine-containing beverages after 6.00 p.m. and, in preference, should drink herbal teas which have a gentle tranquillizing effect. Useful sedative herbs are valerian, hops, passiflora, camomile and angelica, and these can be made into an infusion, just like ordinary tea, and sweetened with honey or brown sugar as desired.

5 *Hypnosis for insomniacs*

This can be very useful, especially in mild cases before dependence on sleeping pills develops. Nevertheless, if a patient is really motivated, dependence on drugs can also often be gradually broken down by using hypnosis.

It is interesting to note that, of all patients, insomniacs are the most difficult to hypnotize, especially if the word sleep is used by the hypnotist, as this sets up the old chain reaction which causes them to become more awake. The hypnotist should use words like drowsy, relaxed, groggy, tired and so on, rather than the word sleep, and try to create tranquil images and scenes in the subject's mind within which total relaxation is possible.

I myself practised hypnotherapy for some months on my own

patients and found that my deep melodious voice made me very good at hypnotizing insomniacs – there was one little problem, however, in that I became so involved in the sound of my own suggestions that I wanted to fall asleep before the patient! I also discovered that hypnosis will not have a very deep effect unless the patient is fully reassured that lack of sleep does not ruin physical or mental abilities.

Let us go through a typical hypnotizing routine together, similar to the standard routine used by many hypnotherapists in clinical practice. This is the voice of the hypnotherapist talking to you:

'Lie back in the chair and stretch out your legs,

Make yourself comfortable,

Fix your eyes on the centre of my watch,

Concentrate deeply on this and don't let your eyes wander,

While doing this, begin to count slowly backwards from 400, silently to yourself,

Continue counting until I tell you to stop,

Breathe in and out slowly, in and out, in and out, in and out,

I am going to talk to you while you are counting, but try not to listen to me, just concentrate on my watch and your counting,

Your eyes are becoming heavier and heavier and very tired,

Your vision is a little hazy and you are beginning to feel drowsier and drowsier,

You can sense a heavy feeling in your legs, arms and head,

Your eyelids are feeling heavier and heavier and you are wanting to blink,

Let your eyelids blink as much as they want and as they do so, they are beginning to feel very, very heavy and want to close,

Let them close, closing, closing, tighter, let them close completely.'

By this stage you will be feeling extremely relaxed, if not totally hypnotized. The hypnotherapist could then give you further suggestions of relaxation and reassurance such as that sleeplessness will not harm you and that worry will cause more harm than insomnia. Further suggestions may be given to reduce tension and build up your self-confidence – this is called 'ego strengthening'. The suggestion can also be given that you will now be able to cope with a smaller dose of sleeping tablets.

Auto-hypnosis or self-hypnosis can also be practised by you at home and is very easy and natural. For example, sit back in a reclining chair and relax completely, close your eyes and stare into the darkness and concentrate on the darkness. Some people see a light 'inside' when they close their eyes; if you see this light inside, concentrate on it. Now begin to breathe in and out slowly and deeply and *stop thinking*; instead, direct all your concentration on to your breathing. Let your mind flow with the in and out of your breath and, with every breath, you will be more relaxed and more sleepy. Let your muscles relax, sink deeply back into the chair and with every breath – in and out – your muscles will become looser and floppier and you will become drowsier.

You may prefer to practise this technique of self-hypnosis in bed so that you are not disrupted after becoming drowsy. The key to success is concentration; do not allow your thoughts to wander – concentrate intently on your slow rhythmic breathing.

As a closing note, I would like to say that many cases of insomnia are due to our exaggerated preoccupation with the future, and thus we lose the ability to relax in the present moment. Try to be still within yourself and feel the beauty and strength of your inner being – let go a little and be like Scarlett O'Hara in the epic film *Gone With the Wind* – she always said, 'I'll think of that tomorrow'.

Alternative psychiatry

These days women are really looking for alternatives to chemical drugs and always having to suppress their fears. They are searching to express their deepest desires, ambitions, intellect and creativity in an individual way, free from the imposition and obligation that men and often a chauvinistic medical fraternity have hitherto placed upon them.

Thankfully, the stereotype of the neurotic young or middle-aged woman is no longer acceptable and now many women will not tolerate a condescending diagnosis that puts them in a box with a lid tightly shut by tranquillizers and cynicism.

Let us take a look at some of the more daring and fruitful methods of self-exploration that, with practice and persistence, may open profound realms of emotion, understanding and tranquillity within an individual.

Meditation

The word meditation has many religious and Eastern philosophical connotations; however, in reality it simply means concentration. The important thing is not meditation itself, but the experience upon which one meditates. You can meditate on a horror movie, an unhappy news event or a painful memory of a broken love affair, the result being an increase in anxiety and depression. You can meditate on an inanimate object outside yourself, such as a candle flame or a beautiful painting and this may bring a temporary experience of peace, but it is confined to the time during which you concentrate upon the object. Some people meditate on music or a sentence known as 'a mantra' which they repeat over and over again and this also brings an experience of tranquillity, but usually only for so long as one is actually meditating.

The most effective techniques of meditation allow one to concentrate on an energy which exists within oneself, so that one remains independent of the environment, and the experience can then be transported and not confined in time and space. Furthermore, the experience is natural and does not require fabrication.

To do this type of meditation it is necessary to seek instruction from a professional meditation teacher on the techniques which enable one to concentrate on inner energy in its various forms.

If one can concentrate effectively on inner energy, an experience of tranquillity, pleasure and self-understanding can result. This can be very beneficial to individuals who are usually preoccupied with unpleasant thoughts and feelings in their conscious mind. As one meditates on the inner energy, or inner self as it is sometimes called, the unpleasant thoughts and feelings in the mind become more distant and eventually cease until total concentration on the inner self is obtained. With this experience comes an increase in understanding of the mind as meditation is often able to show an individual that she is tormented by thoughts which exaggerate and create problems. It is as though one is taken to a quiet seat, deep inside, from which one can objectively examine the ranting and raving of the mind. Some people have described the meditation experience to me as if it seemed like their crazy thoughts and feelings had been locked up in a cage from where they could no longer be hurt by them and, instead, they found a lovely peaceful experience of deep concentration on their inner self. They found that the inner self was like an ocean, enormous, tranquil and profound, while their thoughts were like the waves upon its surface.

This type of meditation gives the choice to an individual of staying with the experience of troubled thoughts and emotions or leaving them behind to dive deeper into more tranquil experiences. During meditation it should not be necessary to change the state of consciousness and one can remain completely awake, active and involved in the outside world, while still being aware of the inner meditation.

There are many different methods of meditation around, some of them promising levitation, instant paradise or improved intellect and sex life. These things are really marketing techniques to get your money and, although I feel it is important to get some sort of instruction initially, you should be very cautious of such promises. It is usually true in this life that anything worthwhile does not come without sincerity and commitment, and 'fast food take-away' expensive meditation techniques are likely to disappoint you. It is you that must take the plunge of discovery inside yourself and, with time and practice, you will understand the benefits. You cannot buy this experience, as your time, effort and sincerity are priceless, and in any case, no one can tell you exactly how it will be for you, as every person is unique.

Hypnosis

The use of the hypnotic state as a healing tool dates back into the mists of antiquity. It was used during the days of ancient Greece and the early Egyptian and Babylonian empires.

Dr James Braid, a Scottish doctor, first used the term hypnosis in 1843 and he initially thought it was a special form of sleep – that is why he derived the name from the Greek word for sleep, *hypnos*. He later discovered that hypnosis is really nothing to do with sleep, although the word has become popularized and so survived.

It was the scientific brilliance of Sigmund Freud which revealed, fifty years ago, that the state of hypnosis can give a great insight into the workings of the subconscious mind in determining behaviour. Freud proved beyond doubt that, if the subconscious mind could be reached and given a voice through hypnosis, many emotional and psychosomatic illnesses could be cured, especially if guilt and fear were removed.

Many incorrect ideas exist about hypnosis; let us first clarify what hypnosis is *not*:

1 It is not a form of sleep.

2 The hypnotized person cannot be made to do anything she does not want to do and she does not lose control.

What is a realistic definition of the hypnotic state?

It is a state of 'heightened suggestibility', in which the suggestions act on the subconscious mind rather than the conscious mind. It is not a natural state and must be induced by oneself or another person using special induction techniques.

During the hypnotic state, electrical recording of the brain (an electroencephalogram) will show alpha waves, typical of a high level of concentration such as during study, but there is no low voltage pattern seen as during sleep. The subject allows herself to go into the hypnotic state, under the guidance of the hypnotist, and usually experiences tranquillity and relaxation but is able to hear everything and respond normally. The subject will also be able to open her eyes and talk normally.

Why does hypnotherapy work so effectively?

In the normal everyday state of mind there is a sharp division between the conscious and subconscious mind. We are aware only

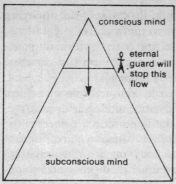

Figure 43

of what our conscious mind is doing, and yet, it is the sub-conscious mind which has the greatest determining effect on our behaviour. It is best explained symbolically and one could say that there is an eternal watchman on guard who maintains the division between the conscious and subconscious minds by stopping new suggestions and ideas from penetrating into the sub-conscious mind – see Figure 43.

In the normal conscious state the guard is very active and, if someone suggests something to your conscious mind that you do not believe, the guard will reject it and prevent it from entering the subconscious mind.

The problem of neurosis often arises because the subconscious mind is full of negative and detracting ideas about, for example, our personality, appearance, ability to love and form lasting rela-tionships, and so on. Thus, deep down, we don't believe in ourselves and this causes our conscious mind to act with less conviction, confidence and success. It may be very nice for some kind person to tell you that you are not hopeless, that you are indeed very gifted, but unfortunately the guard will stop these suggestions from penetrating your subconscious mind and chang-ing the subconscious self-image – so alas, the ego boosting effect is only temporary. Nevertheless, it is still preferable to live with positive people who reinforce your belief in your abilities and encourage you, rather than to be always surrounded by negative suggestions.

The great advantage of hypnosis is that it gets the annoying paranoid little guard out of the way, so that positive suggestions, whether from the hypnotist, yourself or others can easily penetrate the subconscious mind, where they can begin to change a negative self-image for the better. See Figure 44.

For example, for people who have a poor self-image and feel that they are boring, stupid, below average intelligence, unattractive or terrible lovers, and so on, the hypnotic state enables the hypnotist to give opposite suggestions to these negative impressions. The hypnotist will tell you that you are now exciting, clever, attractive and have above average intelligence and so on, and because the unbelieving little guard is no longer there, these wonderful new ideas can travel straight to the subconscious mind where they can gradually overcome your negative self-image.

The effect of hypnosis is gradual and several sessions will be required. You will find that with time, however, the negative subconscious mind will gradually grow a new positive self-image and, as a result, your conscious mind will work more efficiently, more freely and without so much anxiety. This newfound confidence engendered by the hypnotic suggestions will often also decrease your need for social crutches such as food, alcohol, smoking or nail biting, and eventually such negative needs will fade away.

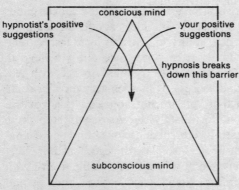

Figure 44

For what conditions can hypnotherapy be useful?

If you suffer from anxiety or a poor self-image, you may be just the candidate for hypnosis. The following is a list of the many conditions which may respond beautifully to hypnosis, and all without the use of drugs.

1 Anxiety.

2 Phobias for school exams, open spaces or closed spaces.

3 Chronic pain such as migraine, tension headaches or back pain.

4 Smoking, alcohol and drug addiction.

5 Obesity.

6 Preparation for childbirth.

7 Insomnia.

8 Sexual dysfunction including frigidity and impotence.

9 Nail biting and tics.

10 Speech problems such as stuttering.

11 Bed wetting.

12 Irritable colon and ulcerative colitis.

13 Obsessions.

14 Loss of confidence.

15 Personality problems.

16 Anorexia nervosa.

17 High blood pressure.

18 Asthma.

19 Some cases of dermatitis and chronic itchy skin.

Indeed, this long list of problems for which hypnosis can be of benefit is very surprising and, yet, the value of hypnosis in such cases has been proved beyond doubt.

How does the hypnotist hypnotize you?

Hypnosis is not magic, it is just a tool that can be mastered by any doctor or the patient can do it herself (auto-hypnosis) and control her own treatment. (See page 365 in the section 'Hypnosis for insomniacs' for more guidance on auto-hypnosis.) There are various techniques to induce the hypnotic state, most of which depend on getting the patient to fix her attention upon a definite object such as a pencil top or swinging pendulum, while ignoring the rest of the environment. Meanwhile, the hypnotist gives strong and soothing suggestions, telling the patient that she is becoming relaxed and drowsy. Often suggestions are given to the effect that the patient is in the midst of a beautiful scene, where peace, love and tranquil sleep are all-pervading. Eventually, the patient enters the hypnotic state and the therapist can begin positive suggestions to strengthen the ego and overcome negativity in the subsconscious mind. The hypnotist may try to learn more about the hidden contents and fears of the subconscious mind by getting the patient to talk under hypnosis and disclose dreams or perform automatic writing. Such valuable material would otherwise remain inaccessible.

After all necessary positive suggestions have been given, the hypnotist then suggests to the patient to wake up, move the muscles and by the count of ten, find herself fully awake and in a normal state of mind. The patient comes out of the hypnotic state easily, and wakes up feeling very alert. A hypnotic session usually lasts thirty to forty-five minutes at the beginning of a course of treatment. However, with practice, the hypnotic sessions become shorter and shorter.

If you want to know more about hypnosis, contact the British Society of Medical and Dental Hypnosis at 42 Links Road, Ashstead, Surrey KT21 2HJ, tel. 0372 273522 but, please, avoid unqualified persons. A helpful publication on hypnosis is the book, *Relief without Drugs*, by the famous Melbourne psychiatrist, Dr Ainsley Meares.

14 Chronic painful conditions

I have given this chapter a broad title as I want to deal with the alleviation of pain arising from various conditions. I receive numerous letters from women suffering from pain of many different origins, who are dissatisfied with the prospect of taking painkilling drugs (analgesics) for many years. This chapter describes nutritional programmes and special naturopathic supplements that can reduce pain and inflammation. With their use, the patient may be able gradually to wean herself off drugs, or at least drastically reduce the dose of drug required.

Of course, there will always be a need for drugs, especially for quick relief of severe pain, but for chronic nagging pains, there are other effective, more natural therapies.

Unfortunately, thousands of patients abuse analgesics and many of them are unaware of their dangers. Health authorities in several European countries and Australia are hoping that recent attempts to control analgesic drug abuse will help to overcome the epidemic of kidney failure and, in some cases, cancer of the urinary tract, that has emerged in the last two decades. In Sweden and Australia, where the analgesic abuse problem and associated kidney damage is severe, legislation that regulates advertising and sales of various analgesics seems to be making an impact. The analgesic abuse problem is now being felt very strongly in the older age groups, especially amongst women; for example, it is known that analgesic-induced kidney damage causes over 40 per cent of kidney failure in older females in some parts of Europe. Other studies in Europe have shown that cancers of the urinary tract are six to twelve times higher in analgesic drug abusers.

The painkilling drug 'phenacetin' has been shown to be a culprit, but other drugs such as aspirin, caffeine and paracetamol can also be dangerous if abused. Kidney damage can result from a daily intake of three tablets of an 'aspirin-phenacetin-caffeine' mixture taken over a five-year period, or from as little as one tablet a day taken for fifteen years. These analgesics also increase the risk of high blood pressure, kidney stones, pus in the urine and gastric and duodenal ulcers.

There are various times when a woman is more vulnerable to physical pain, especially premenstrually, post-natally, during the menopause and when under psychological stress. This is because of a reduction in the female hormones which in turn causes a reduction in the brain endorphins. The endorphins are natural painkilling hormones produced by the brain, and they act like the opiate drugs (for example, heroin and morphine), in reducing pain and depression. During these vulnerable times they are thought to be inadequate in amount and the pain threshold is therefore lower.

During pregnancy, many women who have previously suffered from headaches or arthritis will tell their doctor that they don't need their painkilling drugs. This is because of the extremely high levels of female hormones and endorphins during pregnancy. There is no doubt that the female hormones and endorphins exert a protective role against pain and depression. In fact, tests have proved the endorphins to be mighty painkillers and mood elevators. One of the endorphins, called beta endorphin, is around thirty times more powerful than the drug morphine. Unfortunately, endorphin pills are not able to be effective as they are destroyed by the digestive juices, so the only way of taking endorphins as a supplement is to inject them directly into the brain, a dangerous procedure.

What causes pain?

Irritation and inflammation of the ends of nerve fibres in any part of the body can result in pain. When a tissue is inflamed, there are often redness, heat and swelling caused by the release of irritating chemicals. These chemicals are such things as 'enzymes' which are released by the white blood cells, 'prostaglandins' and 'leuko-trienes'.

The importance of the prostaglandins and leukotrienes in the genesis of pain is illustrated by the fact that doctors write pre-scriptions for anti-prostaglandin drugs more commonly than any other drug, after the oral contraceptive pill. These anti-prostaglandin drugs block the synthesis and action of prostaglandins in the body. Anti-inflammatory steroid drugs such as cortisone also reduce leukotriene and prostaglandin production in the body.

What are prostaglandins?

Prostaglandins are a group of chemicals which are produced in almost every tissue of the body and are made from essential fatty acids in the diet. Prostaglandins have critical involvement in practically every aspect of life's physiology; for example, they are involved in controlling inflammation, the circulation and platelet stickiness, and in regulating body temperature and the automatic nervous system.

When researchers discovered how prostaglandins were made, the century-old mystery of how aspirin worked was unravelled. Aspirin relieves pain and inflammation by blocking the enzyme which is necessary for the body to manufacture prostaglandins.

Basically, there are three families or types of prostaglandins made in the body, and we shall call them the families prostaglandin 1, prostaglandin 2 and prostaglandin 3.

To simplify a rather complicated issue, it can be said that there are desirable and undesirable families of prostaglandins. The family that increases inflammation and therefore pain, is the undesirable prostaglandin 2 family. The good families are prosta-glandin 1 and prostaglandin 3 and these families reduce inflam-mation and pain.

Thus, the obvious solution is to increase the amount of families prostaglandin 1 and 3 and reduce the amount of the family prostaglandin 2 in the body. Thankfully, Mother Nature allows us to do this by changing the types of fats in our diet. You will remember that prostaglandins are made from dietary fatty acids, and each prostaglandin family is made from a specific fatty acid which comes from specific foods. See Table I to find the foods which give the specific fatty acids required to form the correct prostaglandin families.

Many people think that the fats contained in vegetable shortening and margarines are beneficial to health. This is very doubtful as they contain 'trans-fatty acid' which exerts an unfavourable effect on the balance of the prostaglandin families.

Now that we understand the basic cause of chronic pain in the muscles, tendons, bones, joints and blood vessels, it will be more interesting to look at some of the painful conditions which commonly occur in women. These conditions may not be life-threatening, but they can severely affect the quality of daily life and, more importantly, they can lead to the destructive abuse of painkilling drugs.

Table I

Foods	Essential fatty acid	Prostaglandin family	Effect in body
Sunflower seeds and oil, cold pressed vegetable oils (polyunsaturated), blackcurrant seeds and their oil, oil of evening primrose	Linolenic acid, dihomogamma linolenic acid	Prostaglandin 1 (desirable)	Reduces pain and inflammation
Saturated animal fats in animal meats (especially red meat), dairy products, preserved meats	Arachidonic acid	Prostaglandin 2 (undesirable)	Increases pain and inflammation, can result in sticky platelets and poor circulation
Linseed oil, blackcurrant seeds and their oil, cod liver oil, mackerel and fresh fish from cold deep oceans (must not be fried)	Alpha linolenic acid, eicosapent-aenoic acid (EPA)	Prostaglandin 3 (desirable)	Reduces pain and inflammation

Headaches

The vast majority of headaches, indeed 97 per cent of them, are called 'functional headaches', which means that they are caused by abnormal function in muscles, fibrous tissue, blood vessels or nerves, and not by serious diseases such as brain tumours. In a patient who suffers from functional headaches, the physical examination, special tests and X-rays will all be completely normal.

What type of headache may have a serious underlying cause?

If your headaches are constant in severity and do not fluctuate from day to day, or if the pain is particularly severe for long periods of time, then this could be the sign of an underlying serious physical cause such as a brain tumour. Another sinister sign is the patient who suffers from headaches which are particularly bad on awakening in the morning and are associated with vomiting and weight loss – these headaches are often the first sign of a brain tumour. If the headaches are associated with symptoms from the nervous system such as trouble with vision, pins and needles in the legs, weakness of a limb, clumsiness, or an epileptic fit, then there is much more chance that a serious underlying cause is present.

If your headache has these features, then your doctor will do a complete physical examination, skull X-ray, CAT scan of the brain – and a recording of the brain's electrical waves (electroencephalogram). He will be looking for such serious causes as cancer of the brain, haemorrhage into the brain, brain abscess, very high blood pressure and so on.

In only 3 per cent of headaches will a serious cause requiring hospitalization be found. The remaining 97 per cent of headaches are labelled functional headaches, and in this group there are various types.

What are the types of functional headaches?

1 Migraine
Migraine is due to the contraction and dilatation of blood vessels in the head which stretches various nerve endings, causing pain.

The pain is often preceded by visual changes (such as blind spots and flashing lights) and numbness and tingling in the hands. It is throbbing and pulsating and may be associated with vomiting and a dislike for bright lights.

2 Cluster headaches

A cluster headache is a severe pain, usually localized over one area of the head, typically the forehead and face, and is associated with the running of the eyes and nose with clear fluid. These headaches have a tendency to occur several times a day during a six- to eight-week period and then to disappear completely for months. Cluster headaches come on suddenly and generally disappear after one to two hours of intense pain.

3 Headaches due to spasm and inflammation of the scalp and neck muscles

In this type of headache there is often chronic anxiety, producing increased contraction in the muscles which causes the so-called 'tension' headache. Sometimes arthritis or misalignment in the bones of the neck ('cervical vertebrae') causes pain which is referred to the head area. The scalp muscles may be very tender and the pain is usually a constant dull ache which may last for days.

4 Headaches secondary to toxins

These toxins may be such things as heavy smoking, drug taking or excessive alcohol consumption.

5 Hormonal headaches

Hormonal headaches are very common and occur around period time when the female hormones are at a low level in the blood. They may also occur at other times when the female hormones are especially low, such as during the menopause or post-natally. They may take the form of a migraine headache or a constant dull ache, and there may also be an element of muscle pain, inflammation and spasm. These headaches may last for several days and will typically be relieved by the onset of the menstrual blood flow. However, they may persist during menstrual bleeding and for a few days after. It can be very demoralizing for a woman to face the prospect of suffering from these chronic premenstrual headaches every month of her reproductive life, knowing that analgesic drugs will only relieve the pain temporarily, while she waits for the onset of the menstrual blood flow.

Conventional drugs prescribed to prevent or treat functional headaches

1 Prevention

(a) *Drugs which antagonize various brain chemicals*. Certain brain chemicals are important in determining our moods, sleep, appetite and basic drives. The most important brain chemicals are 'serotonin', 'histamine', 'tryptamine' and 'acetylcholine'.

If drugs are given to antagonize or block these brain chemicals, the frequency of headache attacks will be decreased. These drugs will not alleviate a headache once it has appeared, but they can prevent them from occurring in the first place. They can have side effects such as depression, drowsiness and weight gain, and certain ones may be dangerous if used for long periods as they can cause fibrosis of various parts of the body and kidney damage. Thus although these drugs may sometimes be necessary and are very good at headache prevention, the side effects may be unacceptable to some women.

(b) *Sedatives and muscle relaxing drugs* such as Valium (diazepam) and phenobarbitone can be useful if anxiety and muscle spasm are present. There is a potential, however, for drug abuse and dependency and they should not be taken for a long period. Drowsiness and impairment of mental function are common side effects. If a woman is suffering from associated depression she may be given anti-depressant drugs which may also reduce the frequency of headaches.

(c) *Female hormone tablets* may be necessary for sufferers of hormonal headaches occurring premenstrually, post-natally or during the menopause. Many menopausal women find that hormone replacement therapy cures their headaches and, similarly, women with premenstrual or post-natal headaches may find that a low dose contraceptive pill will bring a cure because it prevents the hormonal fluctuations and deficiencies that typically cause these headaches. Your doctor can make a tailor-made pill especially for you to try and overcome the hormonal fluctuations which produce the headaches. Some women notice that their headaches return during the standard seven-day break from the contraceptive pill and, if this is a real problem, it may be overcome by using a very small dose of oestrogen during the seven-day break.

2 Treatment of the acute headache attack

(a) *Migraine*. Ergotamine drugs can be very effective in relieving acute attacks if they are taken very early, at the first sign of the headache. They are much less efficient when the migraine is fully developed. The ergotamine preparations are prescribed by your doctor in the form of tablets to be swallowed, or dissolved under the tongue (sublingual). If vomiting has set in, ergotamine can be given in the form of an inhaler just like asthmatics use, or in the form of suppositories or injections. The maximum safe dose must not be exceeded as otherwise reduction of blood circulation to the limbs can result. Ergotamine should *always* be given with one or two painkilling tablets (analgesics) such as aspirin, codeine or panadol. These analgesics may be repeated every three or four hours. There are many effective analgesics and you can try a few different ones as some people respond differently to the same drug. In general, analgesics are safe if used infrequently, but please avoid phenacetin-containing preparations.

If the migraine progresses despite the ergotamine and analgesics into a severe pounding headache, an injection of a narcotic preparation along with a drug to prevent vomiting may be necessary. However, narcotic drugs are highly addictive, and I have seen many women who have become addicted to their euphoric effect and later found it very difficult to live without these injections again.

(b) *Cluster headaches*. These may prove very difficult to eradicate and treatment is still a little experimental. Some doctors have had success in relieving a bout of cluster headaches using cortisone drugs and major tranquillizing drugs. However, these drugs should be used only as a last resort, as unpleasant and dangerous side effects can develop.

The naturopathic treatment of headaches

Many women come to me suffering from chronic functional headaches, seeking a natural alternative to relieve their pain. They find that the analgesic drugs cause such side effects as pain in the kidneys, constipation, drowsiness and skin problems.

There is no doubt that natural medicines can help alleviate headaches, but in a woman who is used to taking analgesics regularly, it will require great patience, courage and will-power to resist the temptation to pop a pill, as the battle may take years. Let us take a look at the many natural ways you can try to alleviate headaches:

1 Regular exercise is crucial and this may take several forms. Swimming and yoga are particularly beneficial, but during headache-free times more vigorous exercise such as aerobics and jogging can be tried.

Exercise definitely increases the pain threshold as it stimulates the production of the brain's natural endorphin hormones which are powerful painkilling and mood elevating substances.

2 A series of treatments from a physiotherapist or a good chiropractor can help, especially if neck problems and tender contracted scalp muscles are contributing to the headaches.

3 In patients with a lot of muscular pain in the shoulders, neck and scalp, a series of deep massage treatments from a trained masseur is invaluable.

4 Acupuncture can help, especially if there are painful localized areas to touch, 'trigger points' in the neck, scalp and face.

5 Diet is very important, especially if the patient has a toxic lymphatic system and unhealthy life-style. I usually suggest to the patient that they try a diet to stimulate the body's elimination process, called a 'cleansing diet'.

This can be achieved by:

Drinking six glasses of water daily.

Drinking raw vegetable juices, sweetened with raw fruit juice, three to four glasses daily.

The diet should include plenty of salads with fresh vegetables and fruit. Avoid white sugar, sweets, fast foods, white flour and processed, canned or salty foods. Avoid constipation and maintain a regular bowel movement by eating three to four tablespoons of raw bran daily.

6 If you suspect that 'food allergies' could be playing a part in furthering your headaches, it would be wise to see your doctor for allergy testing of skin and blood to try to pinpoint the foods in question. Some people can pick the culprit food simply by the after-effect and in these cases it is best to eliminate all suspect foods for six to eight weeks. You can then introduce the suspect foods or drinks, one at a time, and observe the after-effect. If the food brings on pain or other unpleasant symptoms, it should be avoided indefinitely.

Food allergies don't always show up in the conventional blood, skin and urine tests and this elimination diet may be the only way to diagnose food allergies.

7 All headache sufferers should modify their diets to reduce the production of the inflammatory prostaglandin 2 family and to increase the production of the desirable prostaglandin families 1 and 3. Please refer back to Table I, page 376, to see the necessary foods that should be included regularly in the diet to maintain an adequate balance of the prostaglandins.

8 All migraine sufferers should eliminate 'tyramine'-containing foods from their diet – these include red wine, beer, chocolate, lima and Italian beans, cheddar cheese, chicken livers, raisins, nuts, avocados, plums, salty foods and monosodium glutamate.

9 Herbal medicines: instead of drinking caffeine-containing beverages, headache sufferers should drink herbal teas which can be sweetened with honey. These teas have a calming action on the nervous system and the best ones are valerian, chamomile, echinacea, angelica, passiflora, sarsparilla and humulus.

One European herb called 'gelsemium' has a good reputation for alleviating neuralgic, deep, stabbing-type headaches. The dosage of gelsemium should not exceed six milligrams of the dry extract in any one dose, and should not be repeated more than four times a day. In general, herbal medicines should not be taken by pregnant women.

10 Homoeopathic medicine is extremely popular in Europe as a means of treating headaches, and beneficial homoeopathic medicines are iris versicolor, viola oderata and sanguinaria. The dosage is ten drops of each in water and this may be repeated as often as required. They are very safe and free from side effects.

11 Pure vitamin C, in the form of pure calcium ascorbate powder, should be taken, a quarter of a teaspoon, four times daily, dissolved in fruit or vegetable juices.

12 The amino acid 'phenylalanine' can act as a natural painkiller, and this has been revealed by studies done at the Chicago Medical School. Phenylalanine is an essential small protein (amino acid) that must be taken in the diet, as the body cannot manufacture it. Studies have shown that if phenylalanine is given as a supplement to the diet in the form of 'DL phenylalanine', in a dosage of 600 to 1200 milligrams daily, more than 60 per cent of chronic and musculo-skeletal problems are significantly alleviated. It does not work immediately like a conventional painkilling drug, and indeed it may take four to six weeks to bring 'maximum' relief. Thus, it should be taken daily as a preventative. Tests have shown that after eight weeks, the dosage can usually be reduced to 400 milligrams a day to maintain the effect.

Phenylalanine acts as a natural painkiller because it protects the brain's endorphins from being broken down by enzymes, and indeed, it has been called the 'endorphin shield' because the brain's natural endorphins have a longer life and are increased in amount. This is an entirely natural way to increase the body's threshold to pain and phenylalanine is very safe in all but a few circumstances. It should not be taken by people suffering from the rare metabolic disease known as phenylketonuria, nor should it be taken by pregnant women during lactation or by children under the age of twelve years. DL phenylalanine can be obtained from your chemist or naturopath.

In summary

Many headache sufferers have an abnormal degree of anxiety and frustration in their lives. One of my patients once said to me that she frequently suffered from dull throbbing headaches but that she had immediate relief after sexual orgasm. I prescribed a few herbal and vitamin preparations along with sexual intercourse twice daily! It is very important that the headache sufferer lead a relaxed life-style and, if you are trying to achieve a thousand goals at once, it may be necessary to drop a few. Migraine sufferers, especially, tend to be very self-demanding and obsessional perfectionists, worrying about every little detail. It is important not to set yourself unrealistic goals and to be patient in waiting for the right time and place to present themselves.

The very bohemian terms of 'stay cool' and 'be more laid back' are perhaps very illustrative of the desirable state of mind that headache sufferers need to acquire in order to be able to surrender gracefully to life's many sudden surprises.

I vividly remember my grandmother who was a small thin-lipped and anxious woman. She was a perfect cook, housewife and business woman – when she didn't have a migraine headache. By contrast, my mother was very 'laid back', and the dishes would often lie in the sink until the next day, while she took time to relax or talk with her friends and students – and I have never seen her with a headache to this day.

Arthritis

Arthritis is one of the epidemics of the twentieth century and is responsible for much chronic pain and loss of social and economic status. This is particularly so in the older age groups, where it is almost universal. However, the destructive process begins in the third and fourth decades of life. Modern-day pharmacology has produced several powerful drugs to suppress pain and inflammation but, unfortunately, they do nothing to arrest the underlying destructive cause. This is not to decry the use of these drugs, as they may be necessary, but sufferers should be aware that naturopathic therapies are powerful in their own way, and although relief may be slower in coming, such remedies are free from side effects and improve well-being. After using naturopathic medicines in my practice for many years, I have observed that, in many arthritic cases, they will also actually stimulate the healing process and arrest destructive changes.

Basically there are three types of arthritis:

1 Degenerative

The most classic example is osteoarthritis in which the bone and cartilage of the joints wear out and large lumps and roughenings develop on their surface. The joint space becomes narrow and the rough hardened surfaces of the bones rub on each other. Sufferers often complain of cracking noises in their joints. Factors which increase your chances of osteoarthritis are increasing age, obesity and previous injury to the joints.

The joints most commonly affected are the base of the thumb and big toe, the last joint in the fingers, the hip and knee and the spinal column in the neck and lower back.

2 Inflammatory

The most classic example of this is rheumatoid arthritis (RA) which affects about three per cent of the population and is much more common in women. This presents itself as pain, swelling, stiffness and heat in many different joints, and is due to a destructive inflammation in the bones, cartilage and fibrous tissues.

Other types of inflammatory arthritis are rheumatic fever, infection of the joints with bacteria or viruses, auto-immune disease, such as systemic lupus erythematosis (SLE) and collagen diseases.

Rheumatoid arthritis is thought by many researchers to be an auto-immune disease. The auto-immune diseases are very interesting and result because the immune system seems to go 'haywire' and, instead of attacking outside bacteria and toxins, it turns in on itself and attacks various tissues of the body.

There is much speculation in research as to what sets the immune system against its own body, but the most accepted theory is that the nucleus of the cell, which contains all the genetic programmes, becomes damaged, and thus the programme is damaged, causing loss of regulatory control. The immune cells can no longer recognize some tissues of the body as being different from outside toxins, and it attacks these tissues in the same way. There are several things which can cause damage to the nucleus of cells, namely cigarettes, air pollution, excessive amounts of processed and saturated fats, some drugs, nuclear radiation, some viruses and excess alcohol.

3. *Arthritis due to acidic crystals*

In these cases, crystals of acid are deposited in the joints where they produce irritation and inflammation. The most classic example is gout, in which crystals of the waste product, uric acid, are deposited in the joints. The typical gouty patient is a middle-aged man, very fond of alcohol and rich foods, who comes to the doctor several days after a festive period with a very red, swollen and excruciatingly painful big toe, although other joints may also be affected.

Other acid crystals which may cause arthritis are calcium pyrophosphate dihydrate and calcium hydroxyapatite.

Apart from these three physical categories of arthritis, the philosophy that arthritic sufferers are born and not made has many advocates. This is partly true as many arthritic patients are people who suppress their anger and frustrations, never losing their 'calm, complacent composure'. It appears that, somehow, this suppression of intense emotion produces an accumulation of acid in the tissues of the body. A naturopathic doctor will look into the eyes of such a sufferer and note the yellow staining of 'acidity' over the natural colouring of the iris, and immediately diagnose excess acidity. Arthritic sufferers who are aware of such an inability to express their emotions and feelings should seek help in finding a more natural release for these things.

The naturopathic treatment of arthritis

All arthritic sufferers should try the following:

1 Remain as active as possible, except during acute flare-ups of

arthritis when temporary rest is required and indeed very painful swollen joints may need total rest in a padded splint until things have settled down.

2 Receive regular treatments from a physiotherapist who will also give you instruction in specific muscle building and stretching exercises. Hydrotherapy and yoga are often excellent. Other physical therapies such as acupuncture, ultrasound and massage can provide pain relief.

3 Try to use the minimum amount of painkilling anti-inflammatory drugs and avoid synthetic steroids such as cortisone, if at all possible.

The following are some long-term naturopathic treatments for arthritis:

1 Manipulation of prostaglandins

Several researchers have shown that the pain of rheumatoid arthritis can be decreased by a diet high in polyunsaturated fats and eicosapentaenoic acid (EPA) and low in saturated animal fats, as this causes a decrease in the production of the inflammatory prostaglandin 2 family. Please refer back to Table I (page 376) to see which foods you should eat regularly in order to maintain the production of the desirable prostaglandin 1 and 3 families, and reduce the production of the undesirable prostaglandin 2 family.

There is no doubt that prostaglandins are important in the genesis of pain and inflammation, because one of the most common prescriptions written by doctors is for anti-prostaglandin drugs which block the synthesis and action of prostaglandins. The anti-prostaglandin drugs are also the most commonly prescribed drugs for arthritis and they can be very effective; however, they are not entirely free from side effects on the stomach, intestines and kidneys.

Would it not then be preferable to balance the prostaglandins naturally by diet? I think it is worthwhile for anyone suffering from a chronic painful inflammatory disorder such as arthritis, headaches, rheumatic pains and so on, to try a diet high in polyunsaturated vegetable oils, sunflower seeds, linseed oil and fresh fish and low in saturated animal fats.

2 Reducing acidity

Some doctors would laugh at such a vague and unscientific term as 'acidity' and they would also be incredulous to hear of the many cases of arthritis I have seen cured by juice fasting. However, there is no doubt that some foods are toxic for arthritis sufferers and I have even seen a case of 'ice-cream arthritis' which was completely cured by measures aimed at reducing acidity.

To reduce acidity:

(a) Drink four to six glasses of water daily.
(b) With a juice extractor make fresh vegetable juices, for example, cucumber, celery, green pepper (not chilli), fennel, parsley, carrot, beetroot, apple, lettuce or watermelon, and drink four glasses daily.
(c) Avoid white flour, white sugar, salt and artificial processed foods.
(d) Reduce alcohol.
(e) Eat plenty of salads and fresh fruit. A good salad dressing is cold pressed vegetable oil with lemon or pure apple cider vinegar.

3 Herbal medicine

It has not been proved in any large trials, but I have heard several anecdotal reports that the following anti-inflammatory herbs have reduced pain and swelling. These herbs are safe and non-toxic but should be avoided by pregnant women. Useful herbs are:

(a) Chinese rhubarb (diacerhein) – this has the ability to reduce destructive enzymes which break down cartilage and damage the joints.
(b) Yucca (sounds ghastly!).
(c) White willow bark.
(d) Devil's claw.

Homoeopathics may be added, especially arnica, rhus tox and apis mel. Enzymes may also be added. These include bromelain, papain and trypsin.

4 Vitamins and minerals

I feel specific vitamins can be very important in strengthening bone, cartilage and fibrous ligaments, as well as in reducing cellular and nuclear damage.

(a) Pure calcium ascorbate powder, a quarter of a teaspoon four times daily in juices.

(b) Vitamin B1 (thiamine), 100 milligrams, and B6 (pyridoxine), 50 milligrams daily.

(c) Minerals: calcium 1000 milligrams, manganese chelate 10 milligrams, silica 100 milligrams, zinc chelate 50 milligrams, daily.

(d) Vitamin D in a dosage of 20 micrograms daily is very beneficial for those arthritic patients who do not get sufficient sunlight, or who suffer from problems of food absorption, or kidney or liver problems.

5 Amino acid proteins

Just as in the case of headaches, the amino acid DL phenylalanine may be an effective preventative against chronic pain. The dosage of DL phenylalanine should be initially 600 to 1200 milligrams daily, and it may need to be taken for up to eight weeks before the full effect is obtained. However, once reduction in pain is obtained, the patient may be able to reduce the dose to 400 milligrams daily to maintain the analgesic effect.

6 Homoeopathic medicines

The best homoeopathic medicines to try for arthritis are rhus tox, arnica and hypericum. You may need to see your naturopath to get these remedies and you can try different potencies to find the one that is most effective for you, but in general, in the chronic sufferer, the very high potencies will be necessary.

The efficiency of homoeopathic treatment for the condition of chronic rheumatoid arthritis has been proved by trials which were published in the *British Journal of Clinical Pharmacology* in 1978 and 1980. In these trials, it was shown that patients who received homoeopathic medicines did better than those who received aspirin. A further trial compared patients suffering from rheumatoid arthritis who were being treated with conventional drugs plus homoeopathic medicines, to patients being treated with conventional drugs alone. In the cases where homoeopathic medicines were added, a significant improvement in pain, movement, stiffness and grip strength was noticed after three months, compared to those patients who were receiving conventional treatment alone. In all trials there were no side effects observed in the homoeopathically treated patients.

It is not known at present how homoeopathic remedies work in the body, but the proved efficacy of homoeopathic therapy in reducing pain suggests that at least part of the effect may be produced through brain endorphins, and further research to investigate this possibility would be of value.

In summary

Arthritis may affect the spine, from the neck to the tail bone (coccyx), and, if severe, it may pinch the nerves which go to the extremities, causing symptoms of weakness, pain and pins and needles in the spine or limbs. Furthermore, any joint in the body may be afflicted with arthritis. Little wonder that there are new 'magic bullet' drugs coming out every day for this increasingly common affliction. Many patients think that just because a drug is new, colourful and high powered, it will be a wonderful panacea. Please be careful and remember that Mother Nature's remedies may be simple and sound insignificant, but they are not – they act at the grass roots level. They may take a few weeks or even months longer than the magic bullets to bring relief, but the effects will be longer lasting, free from side effects and accompanied by an increase in suppleness, energy and general wellbeing.

15 Skin disorders

Your skin is one of your greatest assets, so is it not worth it to invest time, care and understanding in keeping it an asset that will withstand the ravages of time? The most common problems that beset feminine skin are acne, scarring, eczema, dryness, cancer, damage caused by exposure to the sun, superfluous hair and ageing.

This chapter contains many pearls of wisdom to prevent and reduce these problems. These pearls are drawn from the art of natural healing, as well as from modern drugs and surgery – read on and you will be infinitely the wiser!

Structure and function of the skin

The skin is made up of two main parts. The outer part is called the 'epidermis' and consists of several layers of cells, the lowest of which are called the mother cells, because they are continually regenerating. The mother cells then move up to the surface where they flatten, die and are transformed into a material called keratin which is shed as tiny scales. Underneath the epidermis, one finds a much thicker layer, called the 'dermis', which contains bundles of collagen and elastin, and this is what gives the skin its elasticity and prevents wrinkling – see Figure 45.

Embedded in the dermis are sweat, sebaceous and apocrine glands, and also hair follicles, blood vessels and nerves. The sebaceous glands open into the hair follicles and produce grease or sebum and their secretion is controlled by sex hormones. These glands, along with the sweat glands, serve to keep the skin moist and oily.

The apocrine glands develop at puberty and are found in the

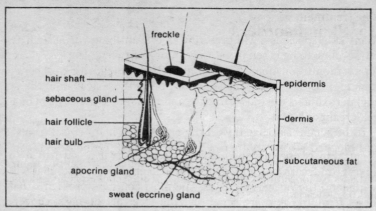

Figure 45

skin of the armpits, breasts and surrounding the genitals. They are odour-producing and are stimulated by sexual activity. When they begin to function, they produce a thick milky substance.

Acne

Acne can have a devastating effect on the psyche of the adolescent and may even result in personality disorders and depression. An adolescent girl often tends to be obsessed with every little pimple and to exaggerate in her own mind the severity of the acne. In her fervent desire to make the spots disappear, she may pick and squeeze continually, with the long-term result of scarring and premature ageing of the skin. She will look back when she reaches a mature age and wish very much that she had left her skin alone.

If a young woman is psychologically disturbed by the presence of even mild acne, she should be taken very seriously and active physical and mental treatment should be instituted. This applies at any age, because although acne usually gets better with advancing age, many people with acne major still have large pimples in their twenties and thirties and become severely depressed by the fact that their teenage acne has lingered on.

The treatment of acne

Many skin specialists will prescribe an oral antibiotic drug such as tetracycline to be taken in a dosage of one or two tablets every day for six months or more. This should be combined with a preparation applied directly to the skin and, of all those available, 'benzoyl peroxide' is the most effective and is available in the form of a gel, cream or lotion.

If the acne is associated with the presence of many 'blackheads' and blocked pores, another preparation called 'retinoic acid' can be applied to the skin. Retinoic acid is available in gel or cream and acts by loosening the keratin plug of the blocked acne lesions and blackheads.

What about hormone therapy in relieving acne?

In patients who respond poorly to the above conventional treatments, a trial of hormone therapy is well worth the effort.

The various possibilities are:

1 An oral oestrogen such as 'ethinyloestradiol', 50 micrograms daily, can be taken in an oral contraceptive pill or by itself from days 5 to 25 of the menstrual cycle. A low dose contraceptive pill containing only 30 micrograms of oestrogen will not relieve acne, as this amount is not sufficient to reduce sebum production from the sebaceous glands.

2 The oestrogen can be combined with a small dose of synthetic cortisone (for example, prednisolone, 5 milligrams daily) from days 5 to 25 of the menstrual cycle. This combination must be given for six months and is very effective as it reduces sebum production by 50 per cent.

3 An 'anti-male hormone' in the form of 'cyproterone acetate' 100 to 200 milligrams daily, may be given in combination with the oestrogen, 50 micrograms daily. The cyproterone is given from days 5 to 14 of the menstrual cycle and the oestrogen from days 5 to 25 of the menstrual cycle. Cyproterone is an excellent drug, especially in women with raised levels of male hormones, and is available on prescription. Cyproterone does not appear so far to have any adverse effect on future fertility. In any case such a risk

would be very small, but further studies are needed. The side effects of cyproterone can include nausea, weight gain, breakthrough bleeding, breast tenderness, headaches, reduced libido and mild depression, and are thus similar to those of the oral contraceptive pill.

The results of hormone treatment can be striking; however, side effects may occur and if you want to have this type of treatment, I advise you to see a specialist endocrinologist as well as a dermatologist.

Have there been any new breakthroughs in the management of acne?

In the last few years, a revolutionary new drug has become available to sufferers of severe acne. This drug is a synthetic complex form of vitamin A called '13-cis-retinoic acid' and has a unique action of converting the oily sebaceous glands into nongreasy epidermal buds. After six weeks on this drug there is a dramatic improvement and the severest acne cases can be cured. The drug can only be given by a skin specialist (dermatologist) as side effects can occur. It must not be taken by women who are not using effective contraception as it causes birth defects if taken during pregnancy.

Can naturopathy offer help to the acne sufferer?

The answer is definitely yes, and the following supplements are to be recommended:

1 A zinc supplement containing zinc chelate, 50 milligrams, in a dosage of one tablet twice daily with food. This supplement should also contain the helper factors for zinc, namely magnesium, manganese, pyridoxine and vitamin A.

2 Garlic capsules (odourless), 300 milligrams, in a dosage of two capsules, three times daily with food, are excellent for acne sufferers.

3 'Blood purifying' herbal teas, namely sarsparilla, burdock, echinacea and golden seal.

4 Pure calcium ascorbate powder (vitamin C), in a dosage of a

quarter of a teaspoon, four times daily, in raw fruit and vegetable juices.

5 If scarring is a problem, vitamin E with pectin, 250 milligrams daily.

What about diet for acne sufferers?

Avoid: foods high in fat, oils and sugar, for example, high fat dairy products, snack foods, chocolate, fried foods, lollies and soft drinks.
Eat regularly: fresh fruit and vegetables, lean meats, fish, steamed vegetables, whole grain cereals, fresh fruit and vegetable juices and fresh herbs, such as garlic, parsley, basil and chives.

What can be done for permanent scarring caused by acne?

Acne may result in large depressions, ridges and creases in the skin which give a generally lumpy and rough appearance. This can often be corrected by the technique of injecting purified bovine 'collagen' into the scars, which fills out and smooths the depressed and lumpy areas. The collagen is injected with a fine needle and several sessions may be required for optimal results. This can be combined with dermabrasion, which is the technique used by plastic surgeons to 'sandpaper' away lumpy protrusions.

Eczema and dry skin

In these conditions, the skin becomes dehydrated and fragile, and develops areas of redness, roughness and scaliness associated with chronic itchiness. If scratching is persistent, the eczema may develop cracks and hard crusts and the lesions may be aggravated to the point of bleeding.

In these conditions, steroid cortisone creams are often prescribed to be rubbed in liberally on a long-term basis. However, this is not a satisfactory treatment by itself, because the only thing these steroid creams achieve is suppression of the inflammation, and they do nothing for the cause. Furthermore, after years of use, the sufferer becomes dependent on these creams and finds that the skin has become thinner and more fragile as a result of their use.

It is no use treating the skin from the outside only – this stubborn skin condition needs to be treated from the inside. This means that you must 'feed your skin' to bring back its natural oils and suppleness and to reduce swelling and exudation of inflammatory irritants into the skin. To achieve these vital things you should take:

1 Cold pressed vegetable oils, cod liver oil or primrose oil daily.

2 Raw vegetable juices, three to four glasses daily (especially carrot juice).

3 Zinc chelate, 50 milligrams daily.

4 Calcium, 1000 milligrams twice daily, preferably as an effervescent drink. Calcium reduces exudation of fluid into the skin and exerts anti-inflammatory and anti-allergic activity.

5 Vitamin C, in the form of pure calcium ascorbate powder, a quarter of a teaspoon three times daily in juices, to reduce inflammation and promote healing.

Women with dry itchy skin should avoid hot soap and water on the affected areas and instead cleanse the skin with aqueous creams which have rehydrating action. These creams should be bland and free from perfumes and preservatives. Vaseline, although cheap, is pure and natural and when rubbed into the skin is effective in preventing dehydration, especially in hot climates.

Superfluous hair

This means excessive hair growth on areas such as the face, chest or abdomen. The medical term for such superfluous hair is 'hirsutism' and a hairy woman is called a 'hirsute woman'. Mild hirsutism is a common complaint of women and about one third of women in the reproductive age group have some noticeable hair on the upper lip and sides of the face.

What are the underlying causes of severe hirsutism?

Many women with this problem have an excessive production of the male hormones (androgens) from their ovaries and adrenal glands. See Figure 46 for location of the adrenal glands. These male hormones stimulate hair growth in a male pattern.

1 In five per cent of cases this will be due to a physical disease of the ovaries and/or adrenal glands and the hirsutism will be very severe. The excess male hormones in these cases often produce other masculine effects such as absence of menstrual bleeding, enlargement of the clitoris, deepening of the voice and balding over the temples.

The physical diseases are such things as tumours of the ovaries and adrenal glands which secrete excess male hormones or excess cortisone, and polycystic disease of the ovaries. Women with polycystic disease of the ovaries are often overweight and infertile, as well as being hirsute, and have large multiple cysts of both ovaries.

2 In 95 per cent of hirsute women, there is no physical disease to be found. For some unknown reason, the ovaries and/or adrenal glands overproduce male hormones or the hair follicles are excessively sensitive to normal levels of male hormones. In a significant percentage of hirsute women the production of male hormones is not excessive, and in these cases the problem is often caused by genetic and racial factors. This applies especially to Mediterranean and dark-skinned races.

Should a woman worried by hirsutism have any special tests?

I feel that all hirsute women should visit a specialist of the hormone glands (endocrinologist) to have the amount of male hormones measured in the blood and urine. The most important male hormones to measure are testosterone, androstenedione, 17-hydroxyprogesterone and dehydroepiandrosterone sulphate. These tests are very reliable and, if you are one of the five per cent of hirsute women who have an underlying physical disease of the glands, your blood level of these male hormones will be extremely high. In the remainder of hirsute women, more subtle elevations of the male hormones may be found.

Are there any hormonal treatments
that really work for the hirsute woman?

Quite definitely yes, and that is why you should always seek the

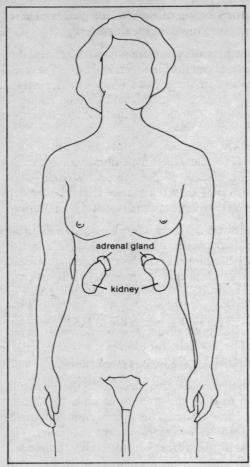

Figure 46

help of a good endocrinologist. In the small number of cases where a tumour of the glands is found, surgical removal is necessary. In the majority of cases where simple overactivity of the glands is found, there are various hormonal treatments that can safely and effectively suppress this overactivity.

Commonly used hormonal treatments are:

1 Small doses of a cortisone-like substance called 'dexamethasone'. This is taken at night to suppress the adrenal gland.

2 A combined oral contraceptive pill containing a high dose of oestrogen and a feminine progesterone.

3 A remarkable new drug called 'cyproterone acetate'. This is an anti-androgen and blocks the action of the male hormones in the body. In order to obtain regular menstrual bleeding, cyproterone must be given with an oestrogen from days 5 to 25 of the cycle. This treatment yields excellent results in over 70 per cent of patients treated for nine months or longer. Cyproterone is available only through a specialist endocrinologist.

4 Aldactone, 100 to 200 milligrams daily, is an effective treatment.

Can physical treatments be combined with hormone therapy?

Yes indeed, and in some women physical treatment alone can bring sufficient control of hair growth. If there are relatively few hairs, electrolysis is quite successful; however, this is a somewhat long and expensive process. Bleaching a moustache with hydrogen peroxide is an effective camouflage. For women who have developed a large area of excess hair (for example, a true beard), hot wax removal is effective, reasonably priced and does not damage the skin. A good beautician can be of invaluable help in these matters.

Skin cancer and damage caused by exposure to the sun

In the vast majority of cases, this is due to solar damage in fair-skinned people. Prolonged exposure to the sun's rays, in particular to the ultra violet-B (UVB) range, will cause not only skin cancer but degeneration of the collagen and elastin fibres in the dermis. The young girl who persists with a beautiful tan will later regret this when she develops premature wrinkling, crow's feet around the eyes and discoloration of the skin as an older woman.

The most typical lesions caused by the sun are 'solar keratoses', which are scaly, reddish or brownish patches of irregular shape and size on the face, hands and other sun-exposed areas. The lesions may be firm with a rough surface, from which sticky scales can be scraped. Some 1 to 10 per cent of solar keratoses will turn into skin cancers. The sun may also produce large pigmented freckles known as 'Hutchinson's melanotic freckles' of a blue, black, brown, grey or red colour, and these may also undergo invasive cancerous changes. Other lesions caused by chronic exposure to the sun are broken capillaries, loss of pigment in the skin or a yellowish thickening of the skin.

Given that the sun can produce such hideous and disfiguring skin damage, it seems very strange that young women do not take preventative measures against it. The best prevention is avoidance of strong sunlight and the use of protective clothing, large hats and sunscreens. The best sunscreens contain zinc oxide or titanium dioxide, but these may be cosmetically unsuitable for women who like to look glamorous in the sun. The invisible sunscreens which block out UVB range rays contain para-aminobenzoic acid or methoxycinnamate, but broader spectrum creams are more effective because they also block out ultra violet-A (UVA) rays.

The treatment of solar keratoses and melanotic freckles is by freezing them with liquid nitrogen which produces blistering and healing, usually with no scarring. If the freckles are large or suspicious looking, surgical excision is required and this inevitably leaves a scar.

For those women who have run into trouble with sun-damaged skin and notice brownish scaly areas on their face and hands, there is a remarkable little cactus called 'aloe vera' which may help to reverse these changes. I personally have seen one case of a rosette cancer of the lower eyelid and several cases of solar keratoses which totally reversed after several weeks of treatment with aloe vera, much to the amazement of the respective specialists. It is best to obtain the aloe vera plant fresh, or grow it yourself in your garden, and apply the juice fresh from the plant, directly on to the skin, six to eight times daily. It definitely seems to have an anti-cancer property, although at this time we cannot explain how it works.

Old-age spots

One of the first signs of ageing of the skin is the appearance of flat brown marks which progressively darken and affect the back, hands, face, neck and upper chest. Their development is accelerated by prolonged sun exposure. They are due to skin cells called melanocytes which group together and overproduce the dark pigment melanin. See Figure 45 on page 392.

There is a new lotion available in France from Ethnodex Laboratories called Ethnoderm, which consists of a vegetable and herbal extract high in the enzyme melanolysine. If this lotion is massaged into the spots twice daily, they will often gradually fade over a period of months as the melanolysine breaks down the high content of melanin pigment. This lotion is not abrasive to the skin and is free from side effects.

The fresh gel from the cut leaf of the 'aloe vera' plant also seems to have an ability to reduce old-age spots. Grow a plant in the garden and apply the gel four to six times daily.

Malignant melanoma

The most malignant and dangerous skin cancer of all is the 'malignant melanoma', which is much commoner in fair-skinned people living in sunny climates. The first signs of a malignant melanoma are new changes occurring in a pre-existing mole, such as enlargement, itching, darkening in colour, bleeding or pain. Any *one* of these changes should demand urgent removal of the mole.

If a malignant melanoma is ignored and allowed to become thick, the natural course of events will be rapid spread of cancer throughout the body and death but, with early surgical removal, the outlook is now very good.

Cosmetic surgery for the face

The twentieth century offers to women and men the possibility of appearing physically younger for a price which is now within the reach of many. Thousands of years ago, humans dreamed of magic potions which would guard the beauty of youth and now, thanks to the clever surgeon's knife, these dreams have partially come true. Of course, not everyone is in agreement intellectually or spiritually with cosmetic surgery – it is a truly personal matter.

Then there are the purists and health fanatics who believe that, with good diet, exercise and a healthy life-style, one need never look old. They are partially correct, as indeed such things as alcohol, smoking, poor diet, lack of exercise and stress can all make us age twice as fast. This is because these habits produce 'free radicals' in our bodies which damage our vulnerable cells by excessive oxidation – a process which has been proved to cause rapid ageing.

But what are the issues for those women who do feel a deep need to tighten those excessive bags and wrinkles, whether they be public figures, executives, famous stars or just ordinary people? The desire for surgery translates into a desire to improve one's self-image and the perception that others have of us. With it comes greater self-esteem and self-confidence in all spheres of life.

What issues need careful consideration by a woman planning to have cosmetic surgery?

The first issue is to realize that, although the results can be fantastic and revolutionary, it is necessary to *search*, ask many questions and then, once decided, to plan carefully, as the field is mined with traps.

The search for a plastic surgeon should be arduous, as they are not only technicians, but artists too. Not every artist is capable of producing a *chef-d'oeuvre* and some people have come out looking worse than before. Always get recommendations, go only to the best and, preferably, to a surgeon who specializes in the particular procedure you want done. For example, there are surgeons who do mainly noses, faces or chins, and so on. If you are still not sure after talking to your first choice, then go to a second surgeon, or a third or a fourth and so on, until you find the one with whom your ideas click.

Then ask the questions and make sure the surgeon really understands what you want and exactly how you want your face to look. This is a very subtle subjective thing, and a stereotyped look from a textbook of photos simply won't do. If you can't find a capacity within the surgeon you have chosen to empathize with and conceptualize your idea of your desired change, look for another surgeon. Remember, Picasso may have been a superb artist and painted technically excellent portraits, but they could be of a face that you did not ask for, or do not like. *Communication and planning* is the name of the game – in the consulting room; it is too late on the operating table. And it is quite all right to be demanding and to make sure all your minutest concerns will be catered for – this is not the time for being polite or shy.

Another cardinal rule is never to have plastic surgery done because someone else thinks you should – only ever have it for yourself.

So you have found a surgeon, one could say an artist and technician, on your 'wavelength', and you have decided yes – what next?

It is most beneficial to follow a dietary and nutritional supplement programme for two weeks pre-operatively and six weeks post-operatively. I speak as a medical practitioner with a long clinical experience in the therapeutic value of nutritional substances. Furthermore, I have recently been in France and spoken with an eminent plastic surgeon who is recommending similar programmes to his patients.

Let's take a look at the supplements you should take for two weeks pre- and post-operatively. After this you should continue the same supplements at a reduced dosage until the sixth week post-operatively. These supplements are harmless and the only side effect you will notice is an increase in physical and mental well-being.

1 A high dose multivitamin twice daily with food.

2 Pure vitamin C in the form of pure calcium ascorbate powder – half a teaspoon, four times daily, in fruit juices. If this produces any diarrhoea, reduce the dosage gradually until the diarrhoea disappears and maintain that dosage.

3 A zinc supplement, 50 milligrams, three times daily with food or juices.

4 Vitamin E with pectin, 250 milligrams twice daily.

These minerals and vitamins have been proved to be invaluable in the healing process. Not only will your wounds heal more rapidly, but scars will be strong and sure, and therefore your face lift, eyelid lift, chin tuck or whatever will last longer.

It is also necessary to take something to aid your circulation during these eight weeks. This will reduce the bruising and swelling and also often reduce bleeding. I recommend a combination of the European herbs ruscus aculeatus 50 milligrams, aesculus 50 milligrams, hamamelis 50 milligrams, ranunculaceae 10 milligrams along with bioflavonoids 500 milligrams and beta-hydroxy-rutosides 400 milligrams. These are daily dosages of these natural circulatory tonics. It is also important that people preparing for any type of plastic surgery avoid taking aspirin tablets two weeks before and two weeks after the operation, as this can increase the incidence of bleeding.

So if all that sounds too complicated I am sorry, but I am going to demand even more of you! First, stop or reduce smoking drastically during these eight weeks and, second, treat the bottle with respect.

After a facial operation, and particularly a face lift, you will usually find it painful to chew or open your mouth widely. In any case, I feel it is best to avoid chewing hard or large pieces of food and opening your mouth widely in the first two weeks post-operatively. This will give the scars and swelling a chance to rest while they are healing. Any orthopaedic surgeon will place a patient's leg in plaster until the tendon has healed strongly and firmly – in other words, immobilize it, and the same should apply to your face.

Your diet should be full of fresh fruit and vegetables, and something particularly useful is the inclusion of fresh juices, which means you need to invest in a juice extracting machine. The juices provide a concentrated source of living vitamins and minerals essential to your healing process, are an excellent source of nutrition and will also stop you from losing too much weight or becoming excessively fatigued or depressed. In particular, fresh pineapple juice has an enzyme 'bromelaine' which is excellent in reducing swelling and puffiness.

If you follow this advice you should feel even better two weeks after your operation than you do normally, as well as maximizing and maintaining the results of your surgery.

About 50,000 cosmetic surgical operations are carried out in the United Kingdom each year and this number will probably increase.

Why does some women's skin age faster than others?

A most sensible and practical way to end this section is to discuss the ways in which the factors of daily life age our skin. Ultraviolet radiation from the sun is a big ageing factor. Extremes of temperature and picking and squeezing acne and blackheads will also contribute to ageing of the skin.

Another factor is lack of oxygen, and women who smoke heavily and are sedentary will age their skin much faster than their healthier active sisters.

Genetic factors also play a large part in determining the rate of ageing of the skin. Anglo-Saxon women with fair, fine, thin skin, prone to freckling, will usually find they need to take extremely good care of their skin to prevent early deterioration.

Diet is also very important as are the vitamins A, E, C and riboflavine which are anti-oxidants that protect us from free radicals. Free radicals can irreversibly damage our body's cells including the skin cells. To avoid this it is necessary to eat foods from all five major food groups:

1 Bread and cereals.

2 Vegetables and fruit.

3 Meat and fish.

4 Dairy products.

5 Butter and table margarine.

If this is not possible, supplement the daily diet with the anti-oxidant vitamins A, E, C and riboflavine.

Dehydration is also important and an adequate daily intake of water and fruit juices is essential for a youthful skin.

Another interesting factor affecting the skin is the female hormone oestrogen. After the menopause, most women notice a rapid increase in the rate of skin ageing. This is partly because of oestrogen deficiency and some eminent cosmetic surgeons are recommending the use of oestrogen skin cream containing ethinyl oestradiol. This is a doctor's prescription item.

What are the stages of ageing of the skin?

1 Fine creasing. At this stage a face lift is unnecessary and the recommended treatment is dermabrasion or collagen injection which should be done by a plastic surgeon. The most common cause of this type of skin damage is exposure to the sun.

2 Weakening of the collagen tissue with general slackening of the skin and deep wrinkling. It is as if one is wearing a size 16 skin on a size 12 face! At this stage the only effective solution is the surgeon's knife to lift the face and other sagging structures.

16 Obesity and eating disorders

I am fortunate enough to be one of those congenitally slim people who never has to calculate what passes between their lips. I have always relished my feeling of 'lightness' as it has enabled me to jump and run without straining my knees and to feel like a leaf in the wind. However, it is not all roses, as I have never been able to look voluptuous in a low-cut dress and I envy the rounded feminine contours of my young sister who looks as if she has stepped out of a French Renaissance painting. Oh well, 'c'est la vie', and I could never achieve those delightfully rounded contours no matter how much I stuffed myself.

It has become obvious to me that obesity is a very complex disorder as I usually find myself eating significantly more than several of my obese friends with whom I eat out. It is not just a matter of calories and exercise, but also temperament, metabolic rate, childhood patterns and hereditary factors.

Obesity can become like a prison, restricting an individual physically, emotionally and psychologically and obese individuals always seem to be searching for a new key to unlock the door of that prison. Obesity can be very destructive, creating enormous dents in a person's ego, self-image and confidence, and often stopping people from attempting to realize their ambitions. This in turn creates frustration and anxiety which leads to more overeating and a vicious circle is established. The key lies in escaping from the vicious circle for ever and realizing that you *can* beat it, you *can* be the master of your destiny and overcome the torment of obesity. The power of your own mind is far greater than your destructive eating habits, or thinking habits for that matter, and all that is required is for you to create new habits using your newfound will-power.

If you suffer from obesity, you must learn and practise new

positive thinking patterns which will take your mind away from failure and seeking solace in food, into a new experience of life where your reactions are beneficial and lead to productive use of your body and mind. For example, for the obese person who takes refuge in food when life is a little out of kilter, the decision must be made to find comfort in something completely different; this could be one of a million non-fattening things such as sport, dancing, learning a new skill, making love or meditation upon the fullness of your inner being, even while your stomach remains relatively empty.

You must believe and tell yourself repetitively that you can do it, and you will, much to the surprise and admiration of everyone. The power of the mind when it is inspired and informed can be formidable!

Table J

Desirable Weight
Age 25 years and over

Height		Small frame		Medium frame		Large frame	
cm	ft	kgs	lbs	kgs	lbs	kgs	lbs
142	4'8"	42–44	92–98	44–49	96–107	47–54	104–119
145	4'9"	43–46	94–101	44–50	98–110	48–55	106–122
147	4'10"	44–47	96–104	46–51	101–113	49–57	109–125
150	4'11"	45–49	99–107	47–53	104–116	51–58	112–128
152	5'0"	46–50	102–110	49–54	107–119	52–59	115–131
155	5'1"	48–51	105–113	50–55	110–122	54–60	118–132
157	5'2"	49–53	108–116	51–57	113–126	55–63	121–138
160	5'3"	50–54	111–119	53–59	116–130	57–64	125–142
163	5'4"	52–56	114–123	54–61	120–135	59–66	129–146
165	5'5"	54–58	118–127	56–63	124–139	60–68	133–150
168	5'6"	55–59	121–131	58–65	128–143	63–70	139–154
170	5'7"	57–61	126–135	60–67	132–147	64–72	141–158
173	5'8"	59–64	130–140	62–68	136–151	66–74	145–163
175	5'9"	61–65	134–144	64–70	140–155	68–76	149–168
178	5'10"	63–67	138–148	65–72	144–159	69–78	153–173

Note: For ages between 18 and 25 years, subtract half a kilogram or one pound for each year under 25 years of age.

Now that we have become inspired, let us examine the technicalities and find out if you really are obese or simply flabby. Take a glance at Table J to see if you fall into your desirable or 'normal' weight bracket.

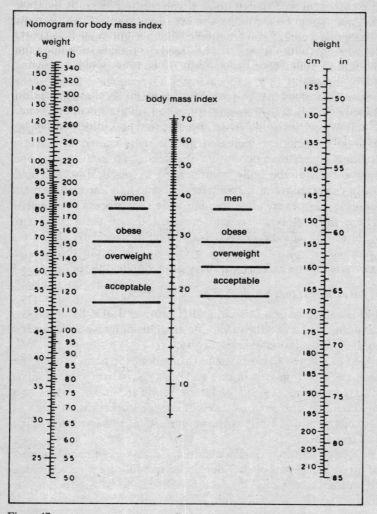

Figure 47

In general, obesity is defined as an increase in weight of greater than 10 per cent above desirable weight; for example, if a five foot tall, small-framed woman weighs more than 121 pounds, she is considered obese, albeit mildly so. See Table J.

Another method to determine if you are overweight is by using the 'nomogram for body mass index' – see Figure 47. To use the nomogram place a ruler between your weight (undressed) and your height (without shoes). Then read the body mass index from the middle scale. The normal limits for body mass index are 19 to 24 for males and 18 to 23 for females. Overweight is between the upper limit of normal body mass index and a body mass index of 29. Obesity is a body mass index greater than 29.

It is important to analyse why you are too heavy – it may be due to fluid retention or increased muscle mass caused by athletic training, rather than deposition of excessive fat in the body. The composition of the body is influenced by physical activity and during physical training, body fat decreases and lean muscle mass increases; however, after training ends this process is reversed. These shifts of body fat into muscle and vice versa can occur without any change in total body weight. Normally, body fat increases between the ages of twenty and fifty, but this can be prevented if you exercise regularly throughout adult life.

What exactly is that horrible yellow fat made of?

Fat is called 'adipose tissue' and is composed of cells which are very elastic and filled with varying amounts of fat which is carried to them in the blood – see Figure 48.

Fat or adipose tissue is found throughout the body – under the skin and covering vital organs and muscles. In overweight individuals, excessive deposits of fat are found in all soft tissues and organs. The degree of overweight depends upon the number of fat cells present as well as the amount of fat that each individual cell contains.

Obesity acquired during childhood is due to an excess *number of fat cells*, whereas obesity developed in adult life is basically due to an increased *size of the fat cells*. During weight reduction the individual fat cells shrink in size, but the number of fat cells remains constant throughout life.

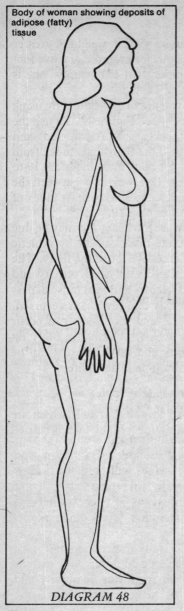

Body of woman showing deposits of adipose (fatty) tissue

DIAGRAM 48

Figure 48

The causes of obesity

There is no doubt that subtle differences in metabolic rate between individuals play a big part in determining the tendency to obesity. For example, we all know people who seem to eat enormous quantities of all the wrong foods, and yet remain disgustingly slim, despite no exercise. These people have a higher metabolic rate, meaning that they burn up calories faster and tend to use more 'nervous energy'; they are often described as 'highly strung'.

Conversely, those individuals who tend to gain pounds at the mere sight of food, have a lower metabolic rate and burn up calories at a lower rate. The best solution to this problem is regular aerobic exercise, as it increases the metabolic rate. Some of these easy weight gainers have told me that the regular consumption of seaweed products seems to speed up weight loss, so that's worth a try too. The very least it can do is act as a valuable nutritional supplement of protein and minerals.

In the vast majority of cases of obesity, the cause is simply that we eat more energy in the form of food than the amount of energy used in maintaining and exercising the body. A certain amount of energy, measured in calories or kilojoules, is needed to maintain internal body functions and this is usually around 1000 to 1500 calories for every twenty-four hours. Kilojoules are a metric measurement and 4.2 kilojoules equal one calorie.

The body seems to regulate its storage of calories, as most adults on a normal diet for their weight fluctuate around the same body weight over many years. For example, if a person consciously overeats for some reason, weight will be gained. However, when overeating stops, the weight will return to its previous level. Likewise, if a person is starved, as in anorexia nervosa, body weight will return to pre-starvation levels when normal eating recommences.

This regulatory mechanism is not fully understood and it can fail in a number of situations, such as a high fat diet, extreme physical inactivity, some rare hereditary forms of obesity and, very occasionally, in some diseases of the hormonal glands (endocrine disorder).

People who tend to gravitate towards obesity will need consciously to control their eating habits. To see how many calories you need to maintain a certain weight, look at Table K on page 421.

Inherited fatness

A susceptibility to develop obesity can be inherited through the genes, whether it be through a dominant or recessive gene or several different genes combined. In ordinary obesity, at least one parent is obese in 65 to 75 per cent of cases, and twin studies show a greater incidence of obesity occurring in both twins when they are identical than when they are non-identical. There is also a very rare group of diseases associated with extreme obesity in which genetic factors are of prime importance. Individuals suffering from these diseases always have other physical abnormalities, besides being obese.

Obese parents tend to provide an excess of food in the environment of their children which exaggerates the genetic tendency to obesity. In obese children, the number of fat cells can be increased two to four fold. The critical periods for the onset of obesity are the first two years of life and between the ages of four and eleven when more serious forms of obesity begin. In patients who have reached 140 kilograms (300 pounds) or more by the age of thirty, their average weight gain will have been 4.5–11 kilograms (10 to 25 pounds) each year. The future prognosis for these cases of obesity is not good and more than 80 per cent of such people will remain overweight throughout life. In general, the more overweight an individual is in childhood, the worse the chances of losing this excessive weight.

Obese families are often physically inactive and this plays an important role in the development of obesity. In affluent societies, the caloric requirement for weight maintenance has declined by 10 per cent in the last decade.

Obesity caused by disorders of the hormonal glands

Many endocrinologists (hormone specialists) are consulted by obese women in the hope that a 'glandular disorder' may be found responsible for their excessive weight. In a patient in whom obesity is the main complaint and who is otherwise generally well, it is rare to find a glandular or hormonal cause for their obesity.

Some of the hormonal disorders that can cause obesity are:

1 Underactive thyroid gland (hypothyroidism)

The thyroid gland situated in the front of the neck controls the metabolic rate of the body via its production of the thyroid hormone, 'thyroxine'. If this gland is underactive and produces insufficient thyroxine, the basal metabolic rate of the body will slow down, meaning that calories will be burnt up at a slower rate. This results in a mild form of obesity (an increase of 10 to 20 per cent above ideal weight), due to fluid retention and the deposition of fat. Patients with this disorder will always have other symptoms in addition to obesity, such as hoarse voice, intolerance to cold temperatures, dry-cold-yellow-puffy skin, thick tongue, slow heart beat and anaemia.

An underactive thyroid gland can be checked for by a simple blood test which measures the amount of thyroxine in the blood. If the thyroid gland is found to be underactive, tablets of the thyroid hormone (thyroxine) will be prescribed, and a significant weight loss will usually result.

Some women who have normal thyroid glands take courses of thyroid hormone and claim that it stimulates their metabolism, so that weight loss results. This may be true; however, if thyroid hormone is taken in excessive amounts for any reason it can produce side effects detrimental to the heart and nervous system, so be cautious about this practice.

2 Overactive adrenal gland (Cushing's disease)

The adrenal glands situated on top of each kidney in the abdomen manufacture the hormone cortisone, which is essential to the normal maintenance of blood sugar control, circulation and the immune system. If, for some reason, the adrenal glands over-produce cortisone, the syndrome of 'Cushing's disease' can develop. This results in a characteristic type of obesity in which excessive fat is deposited on the chest, abdomen and back of the neck with a moon-shaped face developing. The legs and arms, however, remain slender.

In patients with Cushing's disease, the skin becomes thin and develops red stretch marks and there may be diabetes, high blood pressure, osteoporosis and absence of menstruation.

It is simple to test for Cushing's disease. Two blood samples are taken, one at nine in the morning and another at midnight, to measure the levels of blood cortisone. If the level of cortisone is high in both samples, Cushing's disease is diagnosed. It can be treated by drugs or surgery, and after treatment the obesity will gradually go away.

In ordinary obesity, stretch marks are also common; however, they lose their red colour and become white again after several months, and the general texture of the skin is normal.

3 Polycystic ovaries

In this disorder, the ovaries develop multiple cysts and over-produce male hormones which can stimulate the appetite, resulting in obesity. These hormones also cause increased body hair, absence of menstruation and infertility. The disorder is diagnosed by laparoscopy (see page 293) and blood tests. Polycystic ovaries are treated by surgery and anti-male hormone drugs such as cyproterone, to reduce obesity, excess facial hair and acne.

4 Diabetes

In diabetics who are receiving large doses of insulin by injection, a stimulation of the appetite can occur which will lead to increased food intake and fatness.

Obesity caused by medical drugs

Some drugs prescribed for psychiatric and emotional illnesses may stimulate the appetite, leading to weight gain. These drugs are the tricyclic anti-depressants, lithium, and the major tranquillizers used in schizophrenia.

Some analgesics used to prevent headaches, and also cortisone-like drugs, may cause a significant increase in weight over a short period of time.

Some brands of the oral contraceptive pill containing strong masculine progesterones can stimulate appetite and weight gain. Some women gain up to fourteen pounds during the first six months after commencing the oral contraceptive pill. This is best avoided by taking a low dose oral contraceptive pill containing a weak progesterone.

Be sure to check with your doctor when you are prescribed new medications as to whether they are likely to stimulate your appetite. If they are, then you can go on a low calorie diet while taking the drugs.

Smoking marijuana stimulates the appetite centre and, if its use is prolonged, a significant weight gain is likely.

Obesity caused by disorders of the brain

The centre that controls appetite and appetite satisfaction is located in the primitive part of the brain called the hypothalamus – see Figure 5 on page 21. Occasionally, the hypothalamus can be damaged by trauma, cancer or inflammation and this may derange the appetite control centre, resulting in an enormous appetite with lack of satisfaction after eating and resultant obesity. These patients are usually very ill and have other symptoms such as headaches, poor vision, menstrual irregularities, convulsions and an inability to maintain a normal body temperature. Such patients are often very difficult to treat effectively, whether it be with drugs or surgery.

The risks of being obese

In significantly obese people, the life span tends to be shorter and this is revealed by statistics from large insurance companies. The heart must work harder to supply the large body mass with blood and, for this reason, the heart muscle tends to thicken and enlarge to cope with its increased work-load. The blood pressure is often elevated, and as high blood pressure can result in brain haemorrhages and damage to the kidneys and heart, it is essential that obese people with high blood pressure lose weight to bring their blood pressure down.

Obese people have a marked increase in the disease of atherosclerosis in which fatty deposits are laid down on the lining of the blood vessel walls. This results in a reduced diameter of the blood vessels and thus a reduction of blood circulation to many organs.

In a large study in Framingham, Massachusetts, involving 5,000 subjects, those with obesity ran a significantly higher risk of heart pain (angina pectoris) and sudden death from heart disease.

Adult onset diabetes is often precipitated by obesity and an increased carbohydrate intake. Fortunately, this type of diabetes can often be controlled by diet alone.

Very obese people often feel tired and short of breath, as their lungs must work harder to supply oxygen to an increased number of body cells. Furthermore, breathing is often restricted by the presence of large fat deposits in the abdomen which restrict movement of the diaphragm. Asthma and chronic bronchitis often improve remarkably when obese persons lose weight.

The chances of developing gall stones, abdominal hernias and menstrual irregularities are increased in obese persons.

During pregnancy, obesity is not a bonus, as it leads to a higher incidence of prolonged and difficult labour, distress of the foetus and surgical intervention in labour. Obese women also tend to have more complicated pregnancies with a higher incidence of maternal and infant deaths.

In obese persons, the increased weight pushing down on the spine, hips, knees, ankles and feet hastens wear and tear on these joints, which tend to become arthritic at an early age. This arthritic pain discourages physical activity and leads to more obesity, which in turn results in more joint strain; thus the patient becomes trapped in a vicious circle of inactivity.

There is an inexplicable increase in the incidence of various types of cancer, namely of the breast, uterus, gall bladder and colon in obese persons.

Thus, overall, obesity will not only harm your ego and vanity but, over the years, will gnaw away at your vital organs and circulation with the potential to reduce your longevity. Unfortunately, obesity has become a serious epidemic in this indulgent twentieth century, and many people are slowly but surely digging their graves with their teeth.

Eating disorders

Bulimia

A significant proportion of obese people, especially young women, suffer from the eating disorder known as 'bulimia'. Bulimia is the term given to recurrent episodes of engorgement with a large amount of food, each episode lasting up to several hours. The sufferer usually eats in secret and is riddled with guilt and depression regarding this gluttony. The episodes of engorgement result in abdominal bloating, discomfort and sleepiness. As these people are obsessed by their weight, they often resort to severe diets, induced vomiting and the use of drugs which reduce the appetite or stimulate the bowels and passing of urine. As a result, their weight frequently tends to vary by several kilograms due to alternating episodes of engorgement (binge eating) and starvation. The bulimic person lives in fear as she feels she cannot control her sudden urges for food and thus she becomes a victim of these primitive desires.

Bulimic patients are usually very depressed with low self-esteem, and they are in need of professional support and counselling as they often run a high risk of suicide. There is sometimes a need for them to be cared for by several different therapists – a psychiatrist to help with personality problems, a dietician to organize eating habits, and a physician to deal with any medical complications caused by their induced vomiting and abuse of appetite suppressants and laxative drugs. Patients with bulimia are often very hostile to any forceful suggestions to change or control their lives, which means that the therapist will need to be very tolerant until the patient is ready to drop her defences and participate honestly and voluntarily in the treatment programme. Such patients also often display childish thinking and expect magical cures and the counsellor will need to give them great support in the gradual maturing process.

In general, patients with bulimia should avoid appetite suppressant drugs and the aim of therapy should be to help the patient regain self-control over sudden desires to eat enormous quantities of food. If this can be done without the crutch of medications, the patient will gain much more self-confidence.

Anorexia nervosa

Anorexia nervosa is a serious mental illness in which the patient, typically a young woman, stops eating and develops severe malnutrition. The incidence of anorexia nervosa is increasing because of the high prevalence of obesity in Westernized societies and the contemporary obsession that beautiful is thin. There is also an increase in anorexia amongst middle-aged women, perhaps because, for some people, the menopause is associated with weight gain.

What causes anorexia nervosa?

Sufferers often have underlying psychological problems such as an inability to cope with sexual maturity and responsibility. Some feel that by remaining unattractively thin, they will maintain a child-like form with its connotations of being protected. Anorexic illness may start with a severe depression and loss of interest in the pleasures of life. To the anorexic person, food becomes the symbol of the enemy to be avoided at all costs and self-satisfaction and pride is only felt when food is effectively refrained from, despite an often voracious appetite and near starvation. Some young anorexic girls feel terribly guilty and it is as if their enforced starvation is a form of necessary punishment, perhaps to expiate some hidden sin. If these young girls are forced to eat, they become more guilty and anxious, and may resort to drugs which cause vomiting or diarrhoea in order to rid themselves of the food.

What are the symptoms of anorexia nervosa?

An anorexic person will often be very boring company as she will be totally preoccupied with her thoughts of weight, food, calorie counting and self-control.

She will be abnormally thin, although in her own mind she will probably think she is fat and insist to her doctor that she needs to lose more weight. In other words, her body-image will be distorted. The doctor will find signs of severe malnutrition and a slow metabolic rate such as low body temperature, low blood pressure and pulse rate, and cold hands and feet. The metabolic rate becomes slow in order to conserve the body's energy and to stop it feeding upon its own internal organs.

Other common symptoms will be constipation, dry skin and hair, hair loss and absence of menstrual periods. Eventually the anorexic will become weak and tired, although she may continue with a vigorous exercise programme to keep up her weight loss.

How is anorexia nervosa treated?
If you are suffering from anorexia you should seek the help of a psychiatrist and doctor who have a special interest in this area, as it is not an easy illness to recover from.

Doctors are usually worried by anorexic patients as they have a habit of lying about their food consumption, often hide food and do not stick honestly to a prescribed meal programme. If weight loss gets out of hand the only safe thing to do is to try to persuade the anorexic to go to hospital where food intake can be supervised. Anyone dealing with an anorexic person must remember to treat them diplomatically – sometimes it is necessary to bribe them with childish rewards and special privileges in exchange for the attainment of a certain weight. It is necessary to work gently and slowly with the anorexic patient as force-feeding is ineffective, at least outside hospital. If the doctor becomes aggressive the anorexic patient may reject the doctor's help and it may be necessary to search around a bit until a sympathetic doctor is found. If the anorexic patient is severely depressed or suffering from marked disturbance of thoughts, the use of anti-depressant drugs and tranquillizers can be life-saving.

If you are feeling that all this sounds a bit too drastic for a mere eating disorder, you are wrong, as even with treatment 10 per cent of people with anorexia nervosa die from their self-enforced starvation.

Dieting, fasting and exercise

Dieting

To lose weight it is necessary to eat fewer calories than are required to *maintain body weight*. In Table K you can see how many calories are required at certain ages to maintain a given body weight.

Table K

Calories required for maintenance of various body weights

| Weight | | Calorie intake | | |
kg	lbs	25 years	45 years	65 years
40	88	1550	1450	1400
45	99	1700	1600	1550
50	110	1800	1700	1650
55	121	1950	1850	1800
60	132	2050	1950	1900
65	143	2200	2100	2000
70	154	2300	2200	2100
75	165	2400	2300	2200

Small people need fewer calories to maintain their weight than heavyweight people. This is obvious from Table K where it can be seen that at twenty-five years of age, a woman weighing forty kilograms needs only 1,550 calories a day to maintain her weight, whereas a woman weighing seventy-five kilograms needs 2,400 calories a day to maintain her weight.

An intake of 500 calories a day fewer than the amount required to maintain body weight should lead to a weight loss of around half a kilogram (one pound) every week. Thus, from Table K, you can see that a forty-five-year-old woman weighing fifty-five kilograms could lose half a kilogram every week on a 1,350 daily calorie diet. This is a little slow for some people and a safe and more satisfactory weight loss is usually achieved with a daily caloric intake of 800 to 1,200 calories. Some dieters become too impatient with themselves, especially if they have unrealistic expectations, but the key is persistence, as even a small loss of 140 grams (5 ounces) a week adds up to 7.3 kilograms (16 pounds) over a year.

Some dieters prefer to use a calorie counter as this enables them to swap and substitute a wide variety of foods, adding up the individual caloric contents of the foods to keep the total within the specified allowance. You will find the calorie counter provided at the end of this chapter, page 443, a handy guide for this purpose. Foods with a higher caloric content will easily cause obesity if they are eaten in excess.

Other dieters prefer not to add up calories but rather to use ready-made menus with a total caloric value given for each meal. Some sample menus giving 300 calorie value meals are included for your convenience at the end of this chapter. Table L may also be helpful to you. It gives the food servings allowed per day in order to make up daily caloric intakes of 800, 1,000, 1,200 and 1,500 calories.

Planning your meals

This can involve some life-style modification which, in practice, means distracting yourself from food, except at mealtimes. For example, if you tend to snack when arriving home from work before dinner is ready, stop off and do a gym class, see a movie or walk in the park with a friend. Consciously eliminate any thoughts of food from your mind, unless you are actually sitting at the table ready to eat.

In between meals, snacking should be strictly confined to raw vegetables and fruits. Many fruits are fattening so their caloric value should be checked to prevent overshooting your daily caloric allowance.

Table L

Foods to be distributed into regular meals during the day

Amount of calories:	800	1000	1200	1500
Breads, enriched white or whole grain*	½ slice	1 slice	2 slices	3 slices
Fruit, unsugared (1 serving = ½ cup)	3 servings	3 servings	3 servings	3 servings
Eggs, any way but fried	1	1	1	1
Fats and oils, butter, mayonnaise	None	3 teaspoons	5 teaspoons	6 teaspoons
Milk (nonfat, skimmed or buttermilk)	2 cups	2 cups	2 cups	2 cups

Amount of calories:	800	1000	1200	1500
Meat, fish or poultry, any way but fried★★	113 grams	142 grams	170 grams	170 grams
Vegetables, raw or in salads (1 serving = ½ cup)	2 servings	2 servings	2 servings	2 servings
Vegetables, cooked, green, yellow or as soup (1 serving = ½ cup)	2 servings	2 servings	3 servings	3 servings
Starch, potato, and so on (1 serving = ½ cup)	None	None	None	1 serving
Artificial sweeteners	As desired	As desired	As desired	As desired

  ★ You can substitute half a cup of cooked cereal or 1 cup of dry prepared cereal for one slice of bread.

★★ You can substitute half a cup of cottage cheese or 85 grams (3 ounces) of cheddar for 85 grams (3 ounces) of meat.

Always eat your high fibre, high bulk foods first, as such foods, for example, a big green leafy salad, will prevent you overdosing on richer foods during the meal.

Probably the most undisciplined eater of all is the 'nocturnal nibbler' who seems to pick continually at a variety of foods from the time of arrival back home to the time of sleep. Some nocturnal nibblers become so obsessed by food that it awakens them for a night raiding of the refrigerator.

However, a cardinal rule of dieting is three to four small meals a day and, unless illness has occurred, this should be religiously adhered to. Because your meals are calorie restricted, they will be smaller, and your stomach will gradually shrink.

Do not indulge in fad diets as in the long term you may induce severe nutritional imbalances. For good health and well-being it is advisable to eat foods from the five food groups every day, unless you are on a juice fast or other cleansing programme.

The five food groups are:

1 Bread and cereals.

2 Meat and fish.

3 Dairy products.

4 Butter and table margarine.

5 Vegetables and fruit.

Protein should be adequate to maintain muscle mass of the body and normal immune function. In general, for every kilogram that you weigh, one gram of dietary protein is necessary every day. If this proves difficult you can use a protein powder concentrate.

Proteins are body builders and, unlike some animals, human beings cannot manufacture eight of the essential proteins and must obtain them from the diet. These are called the eight essential amino acids. They cannot be stored in the body for very long and must be eaten daily in the form of first class protein. First class protein can be obtained from lean meats, eggs, dairy products, fish, unfatty chicken or by combining three of the following four foods at the same meal – nuts, seeds, grains and legumes.

Carbohydrates are burnt in the body to give energy and are like petrol to a piston engine. Refined carbohydrates are found in foods such as white flour, sugar, bread, cakes and pastry. In general, obese persons should avoid these and eat only complex natural carbohydrates. These are found in vegetables, grains, seeds and cereals. People on a strict diet should only eat fruit in moderation as it contains a high amount of carbohydrates.

Fats are a concentrated source of energy for the body to burn, and they also supply the fat-soluble vitamins A, E. D and K. They should be carefully controlled, whether they are saturated or polyunsaturated, and should always form the smallest part of the diet for the weight watcher.

To reduce calories and improve health, fats must be decreased. After your daily protein requirements have been met, the remaining calories should be divided between fats and carbohydrates in the following proportions:

Protein	20 to 30 per cent
Complex carbohydrates	45 to 60 per cent
Fats	15 to 20 per cent

What are the relative energy values of the following nutrients?

1 gram protein	= 4.1 calories/17 kilojoules
1 gram carbohydrate	= 4 calories/16 kilojoules
1 gram fat	= 9 calories/37 kilojoules
1 gram alcohol	= 7 calories/29 kilojoules

These figures show how easy it is for fat and alcohol to add on the pounds when eaten in excess of your allowed diet. Butter, margarine, oil, cream, peanut butter and salad dressing, for example, must all be avoided.

If you look at Table L on page 422 of this chapter, you will find diets of 800, 1000, 1200 and 1500 calories displayed. You will notice that, on the strictest diet of 800 calories, no fat is permissible at all.

When on a restrictive diet of between 800 and 1000 calories a day, a good high dose multivitamin tablet should be taken with food every day. This tablet should contain the fat-soluble vitamins A, E, D and K, as well as the water-soluble vitamins C and B. Extra minerals can be obtained from raw unsweetened vegetable juices.

Fasting

The process of fasting involves excluding all solid foods and nutritive liquids from the diet. The patient is restricted to low calorie liquids and, in some cases, water only with the addition of multivitamins.

Another drastic measure for losing weight is to eat only very small amounts of food or liquid totalling 500 calories or less per day.

These extreme methods of weight reduction are usually reserved for the very obese and are not without hazards. There are certain situations in which fasting should never be practised, namely diabetes, adolescence, pregnancy and breastfeeding, liver disease and severe gout.

In any case, fasting is best done in hospital under medical supervision as the chances of successful fasting at home where one is exposed to food and advertising are remote.

The fasting patient is confined to water, weak tea, low calorie soft drinks and raw vegetable juices with the addition of multi-vitamins.

Unpleasant side effects may be experienced during the fasting period and these include low blood pressure and dizziness, muscle cramps, fatigue, nausea, hormonal imbalance and bad breath. Fasting will also produce some temporary metabolic disturbances such as the breakdown of body proteins and the appearance of acid waste products in the urine. Very occasionally, prolonged fasting in unsupervised conditions has resulted in liver damage and even death – so always consult your own doctor before attempting any kind of fast.

For the very obese, there is no doubt that fasting in hospital can be extremely effective and losses of nine to fourteen kilograms (twenty to thirty pounds), over a two week period, are usually attained.

For the moderately obese patient in whom the fat seems to stick like stubborn glue, a twenty-four-hour period of fasting once or twice a week can act as a powerful trigger to set in motion the breakdown of body fat. During this twenty-four-hour period, weak tea and unsweetened raw vegetable juices can be taken every hour.

Some golden rules for dieters

1 You must change your mental attitude to dieting and not see it as an unpleasant punitive exercise. Do it positively and re-educate your palate and stomach to enjoy healthy low fat natural foods.

2 Over a long period, you should make sure you eat foods from *all the five different food groups*, see page 423. Just eat less of each group, particularly fats, rather than totally rejecting any one food group.

3 Reduce sugars, as the average Western person eats more than 50 kilograms (110 pounds) of sugar each year, especially in refined and processed foods. Refined sugar, white or brown, is high in calories and devoid of nutritional value.

4 Eat lots of fibre in the form of raw vegetables and fruit, whole

grain cereal and bran. Fibre gives a satisfying feeling of fullness and also slows down the absorption of carbohydrates and fats.

5 Drink more water and raw vegetable juices, especially during the morning, as this will keep your stomach full and reduce acidity and hunger pangs. Reduce salt intake, as a salt-free diet can cause a weight loss of two to three kilograms over several days due to loss of fluid. The weight will be regained, however, if salt is reintroduced into the diet.

6 Eat slowly, chewing your food thoroughly and tasting all the subtle flavours of each small mouthful. Become a gourmet, not a gourmand. While chewing, place your knife and fork on the plate and do not pick them up again until you have swallowed your food.

7 You must *never* exceed the allowed caloric content of any meal and if you feel full or satisfied before the allowed meal is finished, leave whatever remains, get up from the table and immediately begin some other activity.

8 Do not keep high-calorie fast foods in the house; rather, have a selection of fresh raw vegetables for snacking if hunger pangs occur.

9 Do not go shopping when you are hungry as you will be tempted to buy high-calorie tasty snack foods. Attempt to buy foods that will take a reasonable amount of preparation. Only take enough money with you to buy the planned foods on your shopping list and stick to your list of items.

10 Eat only at the dinner table and not while doing other activities such as studying, reading or watching TV.

11 Keep an accurate record of everything you eat and write down its caloric content so that you do not exceed the total daily allowance.

12 When cooking, make enough for only one serving so that you cannot come back for seconds.

13 Eat three regular meals a day at set mealtimes, and do not skip

meals. If breakfast really turns your stomach, delay it until mid or late morning, and then eat a late lunch and late dinner.

14 Involve someone else with the progress of your weight loss – your doctor, your lover or a friend, so that you receive encouragement and support. Some people find that group support is a tremendous help and if you are one of these people, join 'Weight Watchers' or a 'Jenny Craig' centre.

15 Allow yourself only a fixed amount of money each week to spend on food, and save the remainder for a treat for yourself when you have achieved a certain goal in weight reduction. You can spend the extra money on a hobby, new clothes or a holiday.

16 Weigh yourself once a week to get an average perception of your weight loss. But concentrate on your diet, not on the scales. Remember that premenstrually you may retain extra fluid and salt and thus weight loss may slow down at this time. Don't be disappointed as you will catch up once the menstrual period is over.

17 Eating out can be the excuse of many would-be slim people, especially if their job involves a lot of entertaining. You must plan a pattern of defensive eating if this is your plight. For example, before leaving home, drink two glasses of water and eat one piece of fruit, which will take away the pangs for an entrée. Allow yourself only one glass of dry wine and dilute it with water during the meal. Avoid all other alcohol. Do *not* eat the accessories such as bread, rolls and chocolates. Avoid fried food and rich sauces and ask for grilled foods with a large salad and an extra serving of vegetables. You can take along your own low-calorie salad dressing or if you find this embarrassing, ask for a light French dressing. Drink lots of mineral water to reduce stomach capacity.

18 Some foods are positively dangerous and should be treated with red flags. These are cakes, pastries, biscuits, condensed milk, soft drinks, flavoured milk drinks, alcohol, fried foods, snack foods in packets, sweet chutneys and pickles, preserved meats (such as sausages, salami, fritz), lollies, chocolates, sugar, jam and honey, ice-cream, dried fruits, butter and margarine,

cooking fats and oils, mayonnaise, cream and fatty cheeses. You should be on the alert that fats, whether polyunsaturated or saturated, are very high in calories. Learn to feel danger when you see these foods if you are on a diet.

19 To maintain a stable blood sugar level and avoid hypoglycaemia when dieting, it may be useful to take a homoeopathic preparation containing kelp 75 milligrams, natural vitamin E 10 milligrams, zinc chelate 50 milligrams, manganese chelate 5 milligrams, magnesium phosphate 50 milligrams, vitamin B6 50 milligrams, nicotinamide 100 milligrams, vitamin B1 (thiamine) 50 milligrams, chromium chelate 500 micrograms, iron phosphate 50 milligrams, potassium chloride 50 milligrams and the herbs uva ursi, parsley, juniper and crampbark. The dosage is one tablet daily. This seems particularly helpful for women who have uncontrollable desires for chocolate and sweets, as it reduces these sudden cravings.

20 If you have an unbearable empty, gnawing or burning feeling in your stomach in between meals, make yourself a fresh vegetable juice and add to it two to three tablespoons of raw bran which can be obtained from a health food store. This swells in the stomach and suppresses the appetite. It is also a cure for constipation and aids stubborn skin problems.

21 Once you have finished restrictive dieting and, hopefully, have achieved a normal weight, you must remember that your period of dieting will have caused a slowing down of your metabolic rate. This means that you will now be burning up food calories at a slower rate than before dieting and thus, if you resume a normal food intake straightaway, rapid weight gain may result. To maintain your newly found slender figure, it is safer to stick to your diet for six days a week, leaving one day free to indulge in your normally forbidden foods. Once you are confident that you can maintain your weight, you can allow two to three days off the diet a week as your metabolic rate gradually returns to normal.

Exercise

This is an essential part of your weight-losing programme and, without it, you are stacking the odds against yourself. Exercise will speed up your weight loss, distract you from eating, improve the health of your heart and lungs and regulate your desire for food. It will also help you to fight against depression which is one of the enemies of the dieter who can no longer attain emotional solace in food. Exercise will improve your moods, as it stimulates the production of endorphin chemicals in the brain which give a feeling of relaxation and well-being. It will also tone up the flabby parts so that when you look in the mirror and see the gradually evolving new you, a sense of satisfaction and achievement will arise.

Whatever exercise you choose, it must become a disciplined programme so that you do it *every day*, or at least three or four times a week, rain or shine. For some mothers with young children, it may be difficult to get out of the house to go to the gym and, if this is the case, you can perform your own aerobic exercises at home for thirty to forty minutes a day while listening to the radio or a set of programmed exercise cassette tapes. Or go for a long energetic walk – take the children to the park and play tag for a change.

In very overweight individuals, the best exercise to start with is gentle swimming or walking. As weight is lost, more active forms of exercise, such as aerobics or jogging, can be engaged in. If you have time it is preferable to join a local fitness club and attend regularly for your programme of exercise. You should always be on the lookout for opportunities to exercise, such as by leaving your car at home, stopping for a walk in the park, getting off the bus a few stops earlier or taking the stairs instead of the lift. It may seem hard at first, especially if you are a heavyweight, but you must force yourself to overcome laziness and lethargy. Things will get easier as you become lighter and the exercise will eventually become effortless and very enjoyable.

The more you can exercise the better. If you burnt up 250 calories daily with exercise, this would lead to a weekly loss of 230 grams (half a pound). Better still, if you burnt up 500 calories daily with exercise, a weight loss of half a kilogram (one pound) a week would result. Very light activity uses two calories a minute, moderate activity 3.5 to 7 calories a minute and heavy

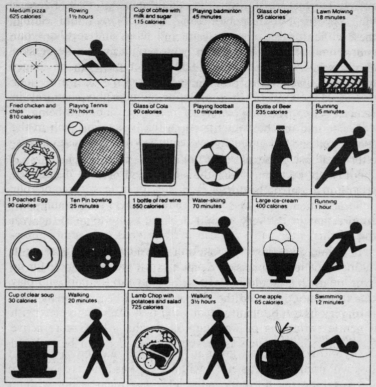

Figure 49

activity more than 7.5 calories a minute. Figure 49 shows how much exercise is required to burn up the caloric content of various types of foods.

The use of drugs to stimulate weight reduction

1 Appetite-reducing drugs

These drugs can be helpful for seriously overweight people who have tried unsuccessfully several times to lose weight by diet and exercise alone. Such people have often developed huge appetites and become habituated to large meals in order to fill their enlarged stretched stomachs. They find that they cannot control their appetite by will-power alone. There is no doubt that, in these difficult cases, appetite-reducing drugs can be the solution and several of them have been demonstrated to be effective in clinical trials. They can be especially useful during the first three months of a weight loss programme or when the patient becomes depressed or is subjected to undue stress which may lead to the return of comfort eating patterns.

A safe and reliable appetite suppressant is found in the drug 'Ponderax' and it is easy to take as only one tablet daily is required after breakfast. Ponderax does not cause dependence; however, it should only be taken under the supervision of your doctor who should also control the dosage.

Some patients may find that they only need to take an appetite suppressant drug every second or third day, rather than every day.

It is still important to follow a calorie-restricted diet while taking appetite-suppressant drugs and, in general, the course of drug treatment should not extend beyond three months. During this three-month period the stomach should become smaller and eating habits can be changed.

2 Hormone tablets

If thyroid hormones are given in large doses, a significant weight loss will occur, but this effect will only last as long as the patient keeps taking the hormone pills. This treatment is not without risk, as thyroid hormone pills also increase the metabolic rate which results in loss of muscle and bone mineral. Furthermore, heart problems may arise such as palpitations and the long-term use of thyroid hormone pills is not advisable.

3 Hormone injections

Not long ago, in some fashionable and expensive weight losing centres, injections of the hormone 'human chorionic gonado-trophin' (HCG) were advocated as a cure for obesity. Normally these injections are used to treat delayed puberty, infertility due to failure of ovulation and severe hormonal imbalances. Unfortunately, injections of HCG have never really been shown to be effective in the achievement of weight loss. They do not cause a more attractive or even distribution of fat and nor do they reduce the appetite. Any claims for the weight reduction properties of these injections must be based on the enforced 600 calories a day diet that is prescribed with them.

Surgical procedures for weight loss

1 Intestinal bypass operations
In this procedure, long lengths of the small intestine are joined together so that food bypasses the absorptive areas of the small intestine. This results in food passing through the intestine without being absorbed. It is a major abdominal operation and carries several serious risks, including haemorrhoids, imbalances in fluids and minerals, protein malnutrition, liver failure, kidney stones, bone disease and a rate of death of three per cent.

Weight loss can be very high, varying from 5 to 70 kilograms (11 to 154 pounds) in the first year post-operatively. However, is it really worth the risk?

The stomach may also be bypassed or stapled so that only very small meals can be consumed, but once again there is a significant risk of serious complications.

Some surgeons have also had success in helping patients to eliminate hunger pangs and lose weight easily by dividing the stomach nerve (vagus nerve) alongside the junction of the oesophagus and stomach. This reduces the sensation of hunger pangs from the stomach.

2 Wiring of the jaws
When the jaws are surgically wired together, the patient cannot open the mouth wide enough to ingest solid food and, thus, only a liquid diet can be taken. It is quite effective, although a little macabre, and in one clinical study sixteen patients lost around twenty kilograms in the first five months. It is not without risk, however, as some damage to the teeth may occur and there is also the possibility of aspirating liquid into the lungs.

3 Liposuction
This is the technique of sucking fat out from beneath the skin through a one centimetre incision with a hollow metal rod

attached to a suction machine. It was first invented by a French gynaecologist in 1972, and the technique has been considerably refined and improved in the USA.

Liposuction is not suitable for removing large amounts of fat and indeed, the maximum amount of fat which can be removed is one and a half litres. The true role of liposuction is to remove localized accumulations of fat in such areas as the buttocks, thighs, breasts and chin, so that the contours of these areas can be improved. In other words, liposuction is designed to take away those ugly bulges but it will not help women who are obese all over.

In good hands this is a safe procedure, the only risks being infection or nerve damage which may result in areas of numb skin where the suction was performed.

4 The stomach bubble

A great deal of interest has been generated recently by the inflatable stomach bubble which has proved itself to be as effective as stomach stapling but without the associated risks.

This bubble is called the 'Garren-Edwards gastric bubble' and is a plastic cylinder which, when inflated, floats in the upper stomach and reduces appetite. See Figure 50.

The bubble has been recently approved by the US Food and Drug Administration and, to date, around 15,000 obese patients have used the bubble in the USA.

The bubble is only recommended for people who are more than 20 per cent above ideal body weight. The average weight loss is 0.7 to 1 kilogram (1 to 3 pounds) each week during the first month, which then gradually slows down, so that after having the bubble in place for six months, the average total weight loss is around 20 kilograms (44 pounds).

The bubble is simple to insert and remove. It is compressed within an insertion tube that is passed into the stomach, via the mouth, and a general anaesthetic is not required. Once in the stomach the bubble is inflated to a volume of 200 millilitres (half a pint) and measures 9 by 5 centimetres (4 by 2 inches). Normally the bubble stays in place for three to four months, and is then easily removed by pulling it out, after deflation. Another bubble

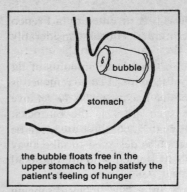

the bubble floats free in the
upper stomach to help satisfy the
patient's feeling of hunger

Figure 50

is then inserted for a further three months. It has been found that
the bubble needs to remain in the stomach for a minimum of six
months to effect a satisfactory weight loss. During these six
months, if the bubble accidentally becomes deflated, the patient
is usually quickly aware of it as hunger pangs return.

This simple bubble is very safe, especially compared to the
dangers of gastric stapling, and the only complications that have
occurred are stomach ulcers due to the edges of the cylindrical
bubble abrading the stomach lining. These ulcers are normally
only superficial. Some patients also experience nausea and cramps
in the first few days after insertion, but these symptoms usually
quickly disappear.

In the United Kingdom, use of the stomach bubble is rare and
the feeling is that it's a procedure which warrants further investigation. The success rate appears to be mixed with the small
numbers of people who have used it and there is some medical
feeling that such procedures may not be successful in the long
term because obesity is a behavioural problem.

Treatments for obesity that will not work

There are several treatments promoted by entrepreneurs who are
really only interested in making money out of the millions of
women desperate to become slim again. In particular, since the

word 'cellulite' has been on everyone's lips, miracle treatments have flourished in the marketplace. French women are especially fond of creams and brushes that they can rub fiercely into the cellulite to 'melt' it away. Alas, cellulite is no more than plain old fat and is resistant to these trendy therapies. The treatment for cellulite is the same as the treatment for obesity and consists of calorie restriction and exercise.

Some weight-reducing clinics offer massage, vibrating rubber massage belts, saunas or special high fibre tablets as part of their programmes. These methods are quite useless in lightening your weight, although they will lighten your wallet!

Beware of fad diets that claim to be a new breakthrough in breaking up fat, as these diets often concentrate on a few foods only and the patient ends up with nutritional and health problems. The only diet that works is a lean one with a lid on your total caloric allowance, so why not enjoy it with foods from all five groups and you will be healthy to boot.

In summary

The overweight person faces a real challenge and must learn to recognize the negative states of mind that lead to overeating. These negative feelings are commonly caused by boredom, stress, depression and lack of confidence. We all suffer from these things but we have to learn how to convert them into positive thoughts and actions. This can be truly character building and involves not only building a better body but also a stronger personality.

A supportive relationship with a psychiatrist, psychologist or hypnotherapist can often help an obese person to understand why she overeats and to reveal hidden conflicts in her subconscious mind. Once these conflicts are resolved, there will no longer be a need to escape to food in order to ease anxiety. The therapist should help the patient to regain self-esteem and develop techniques to avert binge eating. After all, emotional comfort is not really obtainable through food or self-pity, but rather through the attainment of realistic goals that the patient can set for herself every day.

It takes time and patience to lose weight, so just go day by day, setting yourself the goal of turning away from food towards something else. When thoughts do turn to food, don't act upon them, take those thoughts and convert them into another action – learn a new skill, write a poem, exercise, meditate or get involved with other people. There is a well-known phrase, 'get out of yourself', which means don't be self-obsessed but rather reach out to take on new challenges involving social interaction. There is no need to feel anxious and afraid, as, once you unlock the prison door of obesity, you will find that life *can* be enjoyed without dependence on food. In achieving the goal of weight loss you will need twenty-four-hour support, so get yourself a good therapist (this could be your doctor) and try to involve several friends in your programme.

300-calorie menus

Breakfast menus

Menu 1
1 glass grapefruit juice (use saccharin for sweetening)
1 rasher grilled bacon (the leaner the better)
1 poached egg and grilled tomato
1 crispbread

Menu 2
2 slices cold ham and tomato
½ round toast thinly buttered

Menu 3
1 cup cereal (Kelloggs special high protein, low carbohydrate
  cereal) plus one cup milk and saccharin
½ grapefruit

Menu 4
2 grilled kipper fillets
1 round dry toast
1 glass grapefruit juice

Menu 5
28 grams (1 ounce) cheddar or similar cheese (preferably fat free)
1 thinly buttered crispbread
1 apple

Menu 6
1 yoghurt (low fat type)
1 small slice rye bread *or*
1 crispbread thinly buttered

Menu 7
1 boiled or poached egg
1 round toast thinly buttered
1 glass orange or grapefruit juice

Menu 8
2 tablespoons porridge (made with water), a little milk and
   saccharin
4 to 6 prunes or stewed rhubarb sweetened with saccharin

Menu 9
1 large grilled sausage and grilled tomato
½ round toast thinly buttered

Menu 10
1 to 2 eggs scrambled with a little butter or margarine
1 round dry toast

Menu 11
85 grams (3 ounces) lean grilled steak and grilled tomato
1 orange

Menu 12
113 grams (4 ounces) smoked fish
1 round toast thinly buttered
small slice pawpaw

Lunch menus

Menu 1
2 tablespoons cottage pie
1 raw fruit

Menu 2
2 slices any cold meat and salad with low calorie Italian salad
   dressing
1 raw fruit

Menu 3
filled omelette (2 eggs with cheese, ham, mushrooms, and so on)
green salad

Menu 4
plain omelette (2 eggs)
green salad
1 raw fruit

Menu 5
1 grilled hamburger in a roll

Menu 6
cheese or ham roll
pickled onions
½ pint light ale or lager

Menu 7
½ round ham sandwich
1 glass milk (skimmed)

Menu 8
1 cup thickened soup
1 roll thinly buttered

Menu 9
2 plain biscuits
1 pat butter
28 grams (1 ounce) cheese (preferably fat free)
1 apple

Menu 10
2 grilled frankfurt or vienna sausages
grated carrot and pineapple salad or sauerkraut or other vegetable
1 raw fruit

Menu 11
113 grams (4 ounces) lean grilled steak and one medium grilled
      tomato
green salad
2 semi-sweet biscuits (Arrowroot)

Menu 12
cottage cheese salad (with celery, olives or pineapple if desired)
½ round bread thinly buttered

Menu 13
57 grams (2 ounces) canned tuna (without oil)
green salad
1 water ice made with a dash of fruit juice

Dinner menus

Menu 1
1 lean grilled lamb cutlet and vegetables
1 plain yoghurt (fat free)

Menu 2
2 slices roast beef and vegetables
1 boiled or mashed potato
stewed fruit sweetened with saccharin

Menu 3
85 grams (3 ounces) grilled liver, one grilled lean rasher of bacon
   and vegetables
1 boiled or mashed potato
1 tablespoon tinned fruit (tinned without sugar)

Menu 4
1 small pork chop and apple sauce
2 vegetables
1 raw fruit

Menu 5
113 grams (4 ounces) baked or steamed fish and 2 vegetables
2 tablespoons jelly

Menu 6
85 grams (3 ounces) grilled lean steak, small grilled sausage,
   grilled kidney, tomato and mushrooms

Menu 7
2 to 3 slices poultry (meat only) and vegetables
1 boiled or mashed potato
1 tablespoon ice-cream

Menu 8
2 to 3 slices poultry (meat only)
small helping of sauce or orange salad
2 vegetables
fresh fruit salad

Menu 9
1 cup stewed meat and vegetables
1 boiled or mashed potato
stewed fruit or baked apple

Menu 10
1 cup curried meat and three tablespoons rice
fresh tomato and onion salad
1 raw fruit

Menu 11
4 grilled fish fingers
2 vegetables
1 tablespoon jelly

Menu 12
2 slices boiled ham and small amount of parsley sauce
2 vegetables
fruit sweetened with saccharin

Menu 13
4 tablespoons boiled spaghetti and meat sauce
2 vegetables
no sweet course

Menu 14
1 cup mince
2 vegetables
egg custard or junket or plain yoghurt (fat free) sweetened with
  saccharin

Menu 15
steak and kidney pie (about 2/3 cup meat with small amount of pastry)
2 vegetables
1 raw fruit

Menu 16
braised or grilled kidneys
1 boiled or mashed potato and vegetables
2 plain dry biscuits and 28 grams (1 ounce) cheese (preferably fat free)

Snack menus

Menu 1
113 grams (4 ounces) salmon or 57 grams (2 ounces) tuna
1 round brown bread thinly buttered

Menu 2
1 slice dry toast and 1 slice grilled cheese (preferably fat free)

Menu 3
1 slice dry toast
3 grilled sardines (drained of oil)

Menu 4
1 slice buttered toast
1 poached egg

Menu 5
1 slice bread with one lean grilled rasher of bacon (toasted bacon sandwich)

Menu 6
1 slice dry toast
2 tablespoons baked beans

Note: Each of these snack menus contains up to 300 calories. In general, those who are on a 1000 calorie a day diet or less should not eat these in addition to their other meals, but could eat them as alternatives.

Items which may be added to any meal: Worcester, soy, horseradish and tabasco sauces, pickled onions, gherkins, piccalilli, condiments, vinegar, lemon wedges or lemon juice.

Parts of one meal should not be exchanged for parts of another and potatoes, rice, sauces and butter should be taken only as part of the meal into which they are written. Butter and other fats should not be used in preparation unless they are specified as part of the menu. Vegetables, except for potatoes, may be consumed as desired but no foods should be fried. Raw fruits are a suitable dessert and can be sweetened with saccharin if desired. Cheese and biscuits are very high in calories and should not be used as a dessert. Alcohol should be forsaken, until the desired weight is achieved, as it is a very concentrated source of calories. For example, one nip (30 millilitres) of the spirits brandy, gin, vodka, rum or whisky, is equal to 70 calories and 200 millilitres of stout is equal to 136 calories. Soft drinks are dangerous, as well as commercial fruit juices, with a 200 millilitre glass being 85 to 90 calories. Soda or mineral water should be taken in preference.

Once desirable weight has been achieved, an occasional glass of dry sherry, wine or spirits may be substituted for the sweet course of the meal. The best starters are grapefruit juice or tomato juice.

Tea or coffee with a dash of milk (sweetened with saccharin if desired) may be added to any meal.

Calorie counter

Food	Normal helping	Calories
almonds, shelled	28 grams	170
apple, one	113 grams	60
apple chutney	28 grams	60
apple dumpling	170 grams	340
apple juice	170 grams	110
apple sauce, sweetened	28 grams	100
apricots, canned, sweet	113 grams	120
apricots, dried	28 grams	50
apricots, fresh	113 grams	32
arrowroot	28 grams	100

Food	Normal helping	Calories
asparagus, 6 stalks	85 grams	15
avocado pear, whole	170 grams	150
bacon, fat, grilled	57 grams	350
bacon, lean, grilled	57 grams	135
banana, one	113 grams	88
barley, pearl, dry	28 grams	100
beans, baked	113 grams	100
beans, broad	57 grams	25
beans, butter, boiled	28 grams	25
beans, french or runner	113 grams	8
beans, haricot, dried	28 grams	70
beef, corned	113 grams	265
beef, roast, fat	113 grams	435
beef, roast, lean	113 grams	255
beef, steak, grilled	113 grams	345
beefburger, cooked	113 grams	415
beefsteak pudding	113 grams	270
beef stew	170 grams	320
beer	284 mls	115
beer, stout	284 mls	150
beetroot, boiled	57 grams	26
biscuits, chocolate	57 grams	290
biscuits, plain, 3 to 5	28 grams	125
biscuits, sweet, 3 to 5	28 grams	160
blackberries, canned	113 grams	100
blackberries, fresh	113 grams	30
blackcurrants, fresh	57 grams	15
blancmange	57 grams	70
brandy	28 grams	65
brazil nuts	28 grams	185
bread, brown or white, fresh or toasted	28 grams	70
bread and butter pudding	113 grams	185
bread sauce	28 grams	30
broccoli, fresh	113 grams	15
brussels sprouts, boiled	113 grams	20
buns, currant	57 grams	175
butter	7 grams	55

Food	Normal helping	Calories
cabbage, boiled	113 grams	8
cake, fruit	57 grams	250
cake, plain, sponge	57 grams	175
carrots, boiled or raw	57 grams	10
cauliflower	113 grams	12
celery, raw	113 grams	12
cereals, breakfast	28 grams	100
champagne	170 grams	125
cheese, cheddar	28 grams	120
cheese, cream	28 grams	230
cheese, Danish blue	28 grams	100
cheese, Dutch	28 grams	90
cheese omelette	113 grams	410
cheese straws	28 grams	170
cherries, fresh	113 grams	45
chicken, roast, meat only	113 grams	215
chocolate, milk	28 grams	165
chocolate, plain	28 grams	155
chop suey	113 grams	150
chow mein	113 grams	150
cider	284 mls	110
cocoa, half milk with sugar	1 cup	160
cocoa, powder	7 grams	30
coconut, fresh	28 grams	105
coffee, black, no sugar	1 cup	5
coffee, milk only	1 cup	25
coffee, milk and sugar	1 cup	115
corn	1 cob	145
corn, canned	½ cup	90
cornflakes	28 grams	100
cornflour	28 grams	100
crab, meat only	57 grams	75
cream, double	28 grams	130
cream, single	28 grams	60
cucumber	57 grams	5
curried meat	113 grams	190
custard with milk and sugar	57 grams	65

Food	Normal helping	Calories
dates, dried	28 grams	70
doughnut	113 grams	400
duck, roast, meat only	113 grams	355
dumpling	57 grams	120
egg, one, fried	57 grams	135
egg, one, poached or boiled	57 grams	90
eggplant	100 grams	19
endive	57 grams	5
fat, cooking	28 grams	260
figs, dried	57 grams	120
fishcakes	113 grams	250
flour, raw	28 grams	100
fruit pie	113 grams	210
fruit salad, canned	113 grams	108
fudge	28 grams	120
gin	28 grams	65
goose, roast, meat only	113 grams	220
gooseberries, dessert	113 grams	40
grapefruit, half	113 grams	50
grapes, black or white	113 grams	60
gravy, thick	1 tablespoon	50
gravy, thin	1 tablespoon	35
haddock, fresh, steamed or smoked	113 grams	110
hake, steamed	113 grams	110
ham, fat	113 grams	490
ham, lean	113 grams	250
heart, sheep, roast	113 grams	200
herring, one, grilled	113 grams	270
honey	28 grams	80
ice-cream	57 grams	110
jam	14 grams	38
jam roll, baked	113 grams	460

Food	Normal helping	Calories
jam tart	28 grams	110
jelly	113 grams	90
kidneys, ox, stewed	113 grams	180
kidneys, sheep, fried	113 grams	230
kippers	113 grams	230
lamb, chop, fat, grilled	113 grams	570
lamb, chop, lean, grilled	113 grams	310
lamb, roast leg	113 grams	330
lard	7 grams	65
leeks, boiled	113 grams	30
lemon, one	85 grams	10
lemonade	284 mls	60
lemon butter	14 grams	45
lemon butter tarts	28 grams	125
lettuce	57 grams	8
liver, fried	113 grams	340
liver, raw	113 grams	165
lobster, meat only	113 grams	135
loganberries, canned	113 grams	115
loganberries, fresh	113 grams	20
macaroni, boiled	113 grams	130
macaroni, uncooked	57 grams	205
mackerel, grilled	113 grams	230
mandarin	113 grams	30
margarine	7 grams	55
marmalade	14 grams	35
marrow, boiled	113 grams	10
mayonnaise	1 tablespoon	100
meat paste	28 grams	60
melon	227 grams	45
milk, condensed, sweetened	28 grams	100
milk, evaporated	28 grams	45
milk, skimmed	1 cup	70
milk, whole, pasteurized	1 cup	115
mincemeat, fruit	28 grams	35

Food	Normal helping	Calories
mince pie	57 grams	220
mineral water (natural)	170 grams	0
mushrooms, fried	57 grams	125
mushrooms, raw	57 grams	5
oatmeal, raw	28 grams	115
olive oil	7 grams	65
olives	28 grams	25
omelette, plain	113 grams	230
onions, boiled	113 grams	15
onions, spring, raw	57 grams	20
orange, one	170 grams	56
orange juice, canned, unsweetened	170 grams	70
oysters, raw	6	80
pancakes	57 grams	170
parsley	7 grams	0
parsnips, boiled	57 grams	30
pastry, flaky or short	57 grams	280
peaches, fresh	113 grams	44
peaches, tinned, sweetened	113 grams	100
peanut butter	28 grams	160
peanuts	28 grams	170
pears, fresh	170 grams	55
pears, tinned	170 grams	130
peas, dried	28 grams	80
peas, fresh	113 grams	60
peas, tinned	113 grams	95
pepper, green	113 grams	30
pilchards, tinned	113 grams	215
pineapple, fresh	170 grams	80
pineapple, juice	113 grams	60
pineapple, tinned	170 grams	150
plaice, steamed	113 grams	60
plums, fresh	113 grams	40
plums, tinned	113 grams	85
pork, fat	113 grams	515
pork, lean	113 grams	325

Food	Normal helping	Calories
porridge	113 grams	450
port	57 grams	90
potato crisps	57 grams	320
potatoes, boiled or baked in foil, 2 medium	113 grams	95
potatoes, chips	113 grams	270
prawns	57 grams	60
prunes, dried raw	57 grams	40
pumpkin, mashed	½ cup	50
radishes	57 grams	8
raisins, dried	57 grams	140
raspberries, fresh	113 grams	30
raspberries, tinned	113 grams	120
redcurrants, raw	113 grams	25
rhubarb, raw	113 grams	8
rice, dry	28 grams	100
rice pudding	113 grams	170
rum	28 grams	65
sago	57 grams	200
salad oil	1 tablespoon	125
salmon, fresh, steamed	113 grams	220
salmon, tinned	113 grams	155
sardines, tinned	57 grams	170
sausage roll	57 grams	285
sausages, beef, fried	57 grams	160
sausages, pork, fried	57 grams	185
scones	28 grams	105
scotch egg	113 grams	300
semolina, dry	57 grams	200
shepherd's pie	57 grams	130
sherry	57 grams	70
shrimps	57 grams	65
sole, steamed	113 grams	95
soup, clear consommé	113 grams	30
soup, creamed	113 grams	100
spaghetti, canned in tomato sauce	113 grams	70

Food	Normal helping	Calories
spaghetti, dry	57 grams	200
spinach	113 grams	30
spirits	28 grams	65
squash, boiled	170 grams	20
steak and kidney pie	113 grams	360
strawberries, fresh	113 grams	30
strawberries, tinned	113 grams	120
sugar, brown or white	14 grams	55
sweetbreads	113 grams	205
sweetcorn	113 grams	105
sweet potatoes, boiled, 2 medium	113 grams	250
sweets, boiled	28 grams	95
sweets, fruit gums	28 grams	50
sweets, pastilles	28 grams	75
sweets, peppermints	28 grams	110
sweets, toffees	28 grams	125
syrup	28 grams	85
tapioca, dry	57 grams	205
tartar sauce	1 tablespoon	70
tea, lemon, no sugar	1 cup	5
tea, milk only	1 cup	20
tea, milk and sugar	1 cup	75
toad in the hole	113 grams	330
tomato chutney	28 grams	45
tomato juice	113 grams	20
tomato sauce	28 grams	30
tomatoes, fresh	113 grams	15
tongue	113 grams	335
treacle, black	28 grams	75
trifle	113 grams	170
tripe, stewed	113 grams	115
tuna, canned	113 grams	280
turkey	113 grams	225
turnips, boiled	113 grams	10
veal, roast	113 grams	260

Food	Normal helping	Calories
waffle with syrup and cream	113 grams	260
walnuts, shelled	28 grams	155
watercress	28 grams	4
whisky	28 grams	65
wine, dry, white	113 grams	85
wine, red	113 grams	75
wine, sweet, white	113 grams	105
Worcester sauce	1 tablespoon	25
yoghurt, fat free, plain	142 grams	50
yoghurt, low fat, flavoured	142 grams	100
Yorkshire pudding	113 grams	250

A farewell note

This book has taken one year to write and I could not have done it without the thousands of women who have written to me, both as friends and patients, with their individual experiences. Through this widespread communication, I have been made aware of the special needs and problems that women face and have also gained much knowledge from the solutions that many have discovered, often on their own, in isolated conditions, by means of trial and error.

I have also been made aware that, because of inadequate community facilities, lack of communication, and professionals who have failed to take them seriously, many of these women have been forced to accept suffering and compromise. In order to be able to break out of this unsatisfactory situation and to provoke society and professionals alike into doing something practical about it, women need certain essential facts at their fingertips.

Women are hungry for knowledge concerning their physical and mental health because they realize that this will enable them to have control over their destinies. Some of the most important reasons why women should educate themselves are:

1 So that they can assert their needs and goals with confidence, free from excessive emotionalism. This will enable them to participate actively with professionals in making decisions concerning their physical and mental well-being. Women no longer want to be passive guinea pigs, accepting advice in blind faith.

2 To have access to the best of both medical worlds, namely the orthodox and the naturopathic, which will give them a balanced approach to their health.

3 To take responsibility for their own well-being by instigating and participating in self-help programmes. Although we need doctors and psychiatrists, the greatest healer is the self, and self-healing is especially good for self-esteem.

4 To feel good about themselves and be free from guilt and shame concerning ailments peculiar to women, such as the symptoms of the menopause, PMS, post-natal depression, period pains, and so on. The understanding that such disorders are not personality defects or neuroses of women, but, rather, well-defined physical disorders which respond well to specific physical treatments, can rid women of negative attitudes towards themselves.

These specific female disorders should not be used as 'emotive political footballs' to create prejudice against women. By education and the acquisition of knowledge many misconceptions concerning conditions peculiar to women can be removed.

5 To extend the quality and quantity of their life. Unless women educate themselves and act now, the world will soon be full of little old ladies, many of them ill and at least one third with osteoporosis that could have been prevented. By the year 2050, the average life span of women will be around ninety years with women outliving men by approximately six years. Will this extra life be worth it, if the quality is crippled by osteoporosis and other signs of hormone deficiency or degenerative diseases?

Hormone replacement therapy can safely be given for twenty years to prevent osteoporosis and this, together with a healthy life-style and nutritional supplements, can help women to appreciate their longer life span. These days many women are still vital and energetic at sixty and may be free, for the first time, to pursue a career, interest, love affair or travel. In order to maintain that vitality and implement these desires they need a basic foundation in preventative medicine.

6 To protect themselves against overexposure to dangerous drugs, addiction and sexist advertising by pharmaceutical companies. The advertising of sedative drugs often portrays women as being more at risk for mental illness. In other words, women's

vulnerabilities are being preyed upon by commercial forces. It is important to be aware of this.

7 To form social and political groups to promote the rights of women. Women need to be more aware of their rights as human beings and must work together politically to achieve government-funded programmes for childcare facilities, specialized women's health centres, women's shelters and legal aid for domestic violence and sexual abuse. These issues should achieve much greater media exposure to create public awareness and female unity.

As Medical Director of the Women's Health Advisory Service in Australia, I would like to add a few further thoughts. The Women's Health Advisory Service aims to help women realize their goal of improved knowledge concerning their physical and mental health. So much information is now available and new discoveries are being made every day, and yet such knowledge often remains locked in the brains of academics and ivory university towers, taking far too long to trickle down into everyday language that we can all appreciate. Women need specialized healthcare centres as they will always be different from men; equal yes, but equality is not sameness.

The twentieth century has seen the beginning of emancipation of women from the stereotyped roles in society previously dictated to them by chauvinistic governments, societies, religions and professionals. They also now have the means to control their fertility and biological functions and I hope this book, *Women's Health*, has gone some way towards equipping women with knowledge of that means, and also of how to get the very best out of their lives, both physically and mentally.

Glossary

abscess An infected cavity filled with pus.

acidity A state of excessive acid in the body.

acne An inflammatory disorder of the skin's sebaceous glands, producing pimples and lumps in the skin.

adrenal glands Two small glands situated on top of the kidneys which secrete the stress hormones, cortisone and adrenalin.

adrenalin A hormone secreted by the adrenal glands and sympathetic nervous system which causes acceleration of the heart beat, increase in blood pressure, dilation of the pupils and an increase in metabolic rate. It is classed as one of the stress hormones.

alkaline A chemical state that is opposite to an acidic state. The acid-alkaline balance of a substance is measured by its pH value. Neutral substances have a pH of seven, alkaline substances a pH greater than seven, and acidic substances, a pH less than seven.

allergy An overreaction to an environmental substance such as dust, pollens, particular foods or chemicals; a state of excessive sensitivity to a substance.

allicin The natural sulphur chemical found in raw garlic which is responsible for the beneficial effects of garlic on the blood and its capacity to fight infections.

allopathic The type of medicine which utilizes orthodox methods of drug therapy to alleviate the symptoms of disease.

amenorrhoea An abnormal suppression or absence of menstruation.

amino acids The sub-units of body proteins. They contain amino groups ($NH2$) and carboxyl groups ($COOH$). From dietary amino acids the body synthesizes its protein. Ten of the amino acids are essential dietary components as they cannot be synthesized by the body. Dietary protein is said to be first class if it contains all the ten essential amino acids. Examples of first class protein are animal and dairy products and a combination of any three of the following: nuts, grains, seeds, legumes.

amniocentesis The removal of a sample of the amniotic fluid surrounding the foetus for examination and testing to diagnose congenital diseases and the sex of the foetus.

anaemia   A deficiency of red blood cells.

anaesthetic   A drug given to remove sensation from all or part of the body, enabling surgical procedures to be performed painlessly.

analgesics   Painkilling drugs, for example, paracetamol, aspirin and phenacetin, and opiates such as morphine, heroin, pethidine and codeine.

androgenic   Having a masculine effect in the body and thus stimulating growth of hair in a male pattern, production of oil in the skin, deepening of the voice and increased muscle mass.

anorexia   Loss of appetite.

antibiotics   Various chemicals, such as penicillin, which are manufactured in nature by certain fungi or moulds, or synthetically in a laboratory, and which can effectively stop the growth of or destroy micro-organisms. They may be taken in the form of injections, tablets, creams or suppositories.

antibodies   Various proteins in the blood that are manufactured by cells of the immune system in response to the invasion of the body by bacteria, viruses, toxins and foreign proteins. The antibodies then neutralize these bacteria, viruses, and so on, thus producing some immunity against infections.

anti-inflammatory   Preventing or reversing inflammation in the body tissues.

anti-male hormone   A hormone which counteracts or blocks the effect of male hormones in the body.

anti-prostaglandins   Drugs capable of blocking the synthesis or action of the prostaglandins in the body. Examples of such drugs are aspirin, Naprosen, mefenamic acid, indomethacin and ibuprofen.

asthenic   A person with a slender, small-boned and long-limbed physique.

atherosclerosis   Degeneration of the blood vessels caused by hardening of the vessel walls and blockage with fatty plaques.

autism   A mental disorder characterized by an inability to relate to and communicate with other people.

auto-immune diseases   A group of diseases in which the immune system attacks various parts of the body, for example, the joints, fibrous tissues or blood vessels.

azoospermia   Absence of spermatozoa in the semen.

bacteria   Living micro-organisms, usually single-celled, occurring in a wide variety of forms. Most bacteria live on dead matter causing decomposition or are infectious parasites causing disease in animals and humans.

basal body temperature thermometer A thermometer capable of reading temperatures in the low range, such as when the body is at rest.

basal metabolic rate The rate at which energy is utilized by a living creature when at complete rest.

benign Non-cancerous or non-malignant.

benzodiazepines A family of sedative drugs, examples of which are Valium, Serepax and Mogadon.

beta rutosides Vitamin-like substances occurring in some foods and herbs which have a beneficial effect upon the blood vessels.

bioflavonoids Bioflavonoids, also called vitamin P, are found in plants along with vitamin C and have a beneficial effect upon the walls of the blood and lymphatic vessels.

biopsy The surgical removal of tissue for examination under a microscope.

bone mineral concentration The concentration of minerals, especially calcium, in the bones, as measured by a bone densitometer machine.

bromocriptine A drug which blocks the action of the pituitary hormone, prolactin.

caesarean section A surgical incision made through the walls of the abdomen and uterus for the purpose of delivering a baby through the incision.

calcium A mineral found throughout the body, but especially concentrated in the bones.

calcium ascorbate A complex of vitamin C and calcium.

cancer Any malignant growth, tumour or lesion characterized by rapid multiplication of abnormal cells that can invade and spread to other organs or distant body parts.

capillaries Minute blood vessels, connecting the smallest arteries to the smallest veins.

carbohydrates A group of chemical compounds, including sugars, cellulose and starches. Complex carbohydrates contain vitamins and minerals and are more slowly metabolized than refined or processed carbohydrates.

cardiovascular system The system of the blood circulation, including the heart and blood vessels.

cartilage A tough, compressible fibrous substance attached to the ends of bones where they rub against each other.

CAT scan A computerized X–ray of consecutive sections of the body.

cell The smallest structural unit of a living organism that can function independently.

cerebral cortex The outer layer of brain cells concerned with sophisticated mental and motor functions.

cervical incompetence The condition of having a weakened cervix, incapable of holding the foetus and placenta inside the uterus for the normal duration of pregnancy.

cervical os The opening of the cervical canal.

cervix The lower part of the uterus projecting down into the vagina. It is also called the mouth of the womb.

chemotherapy The treatment of cancer with specific anti-cancer drugs which stop the cancer cells from multiplying.

chicken pox An acute contagious viral disease, usually of children, characterized by a blistering rash, fever and weakness.

cholesterol A constituent of all animal fats and oils. It is found in the blood in two forms:

1 High density lipo-protein (HDL) which protects against atherosclerosis.

2 Low density lipo-protein (LDL) which promotes atherosclerosis.

chorionic villus biopsy (CVB) The removal of cells from the chorionic membrane surrounding the foetus for examination and testing to diagnose genetic diseases of the foetus.

chromosomes Threadlike structures existing in the nucleus of all cells, containing DNA, RNA and protein. They carry genes which determine and transmit hereditary characteristics.

clitoris A small pink vascular structure capable of enlargement during sexual stimulation. It is an organ of pleasure and is situated in the vulva at the point where the inner lips of the vagina merge below the pubic bone.

coitus Sexual intercourse.

coitus interruptus The technique of withdrawing the penis from the vagina just prior to ejaculation.

collagen A fibrous protein giving strength and elasticity to bone, skin, cartilage and connective tissues.

collagen diseases A group of diseases in which the immune system attacks the tissues of the body containing collagen, for example, the blood vessels, joints, ligaments and muscles. SLE, rheumatoid arthritis and dermato-myositis are collagen diseases.

congenital Existing at birth.

congestion Engorgement of blood vessels because of an increase in blood flow to a particular area or organ.

congestive dysmenorrhoea Painful menstrual bleeding due to congestion of the pelvic organs with blood.

corpus luteum The yellow-coloured tissue which is formed in the ovary from the remains of the follicle after it has released its contained egg (ovum). Corpus luteum manufactures the hormone progesterone.

cortisone One of the hormones produced by the adrenal glands. It can also be synthesized in the laboratory and has an anti-inflammatory effect.

curette The procedure of surgically scraping a body cavity to remove tissue, blood or abnormal growths. Also called curettage.

cyst A sac-like structure containing semi-solid material or fluid.

cystic fibrosis A hereditary disease of childhood affecting the mucous and sweat glands, resulting in severe disease of the pancreas and lungs and failure to thrive.

dehydrated Deficient in body fluids.

delirium tremens A condition of mental excitement, confusion, fear and clouded mental functioning, often accompanied by delusions and hallucinations, and precipitated by withdrawal from chronic alcohol abuse.

dermabrasion Surgical abrasion of the skin with sandpaper-like instruments, with the aim of flattening uneven scars and lumps.

dermatitis Inflammation of the dermis of the skin.

dermatologist A medical doctor who specializes in diseases of the skin.

dermis The deep inner layer of the skin.

diagnosis The identification of the cause or nature of a disease by examination and testing.

digital thermometer An instrument which displays body temperature in numerical figures and gives an audible signal when the maximum temperature is reached. It only takes a minute to give a reading, and is very accurate.

dilatation Enlargement, as of a hollow organ or vessel.

diuretic A substance, whether herbal or synthetic, which promotes the production of urine, thus relieving fluid retention.

DNA (deoxyribonucleic acid) A nucleic acid. It is the chief constituent of chromosomes, is able to replicate itself, and is responsible for transmitting genetic information, in the form of genes, from parents to offspring. It takes the form of a double helix of two long chains of linked proteins (nucleotides).

dopamine A chemical which is found in high concentration in the brain and which acts as a brain transmitter and helps to regulate the production of the hormone prolactin.

dowager's hump A curve in the spine occurring just below the neck because of compression of the spinal vertebrae.

dydrogesterone (duphaston) An oral form of progesterone whose chemical structure closely resembles that of natural progesterone produced in the ovaries.

dysmenorrhoea Painful menstruation or period pains.

eczema An inflammatory disorder of the skin producing itchiness, dryness, redness and discomfort.

egg follicle The roundish structure surrounding the developing egg in the ovary before ovulation occurs. It is also known as the ovarian follicle.

ego The conscious part of the mind and personality.

ejaculation Discharge of semen from the penis at orgasm.

elastin A protein that is the major component of the elastic tissue in the dermis of the skin.

electrocardiograph The recording on paper of the electrical activity of heart muscle contractions.

eliminate To get rid of or remove.

embryo The product of conception up to the beginning of the ninth week of pregnancy. *See* foetus.

endemic Existing within a particular geographic area or peculiar to persons in a particular area.

endocrinologist A medical doctor who specializes in diseases of the hormonal glands and their hormones.

endometriosis The presence of endometrium, which is normally confined inside the uterine cavity, in other parts of the pelvis and abdomen such as the ovaries, bladder and bowel.

endometrium The mucous membrane lining the uterus.

endorphins Naturally produced brain hormones that reduce pain and depression.

enzyme A protein produced by living cells which functions as a catalyst in specific biochemical reactions.

epilepsy A brain disorder characterized by sudden recurring attacks of motor, sensory or psychic malfunction, with or without unconsciousness or convulsive movements of the body.

episiotomy A surgical incision made at the vaginal opening, so as to enlarge it for the delivery of a baby.

equine Relating to or derived from a horse.

erogenous Arousing sexual desire.

erosion, cervical The replacement of normal cervical tissue on the surface of the cervix with mucus-secreting cells which give the cervix a red and irregular appearance on examination with a speculum. It is a harmless condition and in reality there is no erosion or ulcer on the cervix.

excision The process of cutting out or removing surgically.

fellatio Oral stimulation of the penis.

fibrocystic breast tissue Painful, generally lumpy, breasts with the presence of many small cysts and fibrous thickening in the breast tissues.

fibroids Non-cancerous tumours of the muscular wall of the uterus. They are also known as myomas or fibromyomas.

fibrosis The formation of excessive fibrous tissues in various organs.

fissure 1 A groove or cleft in an organ.

2 A crack or split in the skin or a mucous membrane.

foetal Of or relating to a foetus.

foetus The developing human from the end of the eighth week of pregnancy up until birth. *See* embryo.

follicle *See* egg follicle.

follicle stimulating hormone (FSH) A hormone produced in the pituitary gland which travels to the ovaries by means of the circulation and stimulates the growth and development of ovarian follicles.

free radical An electrically unbalanced atom or group of atoms capable of causing damage to the nucleus of a cell.

gene A hereditary structure situated on a chromosome in the nucleus of a cell. The genes determine specific characteristics and vital functions in a living organism, and are capable of replication.

genesis The original development of something.

genetic Relating to or produced by genes.

genitals The sexual organs.

glans The head of the penis.

gonads The sex glands, namely the ovary and the testicle.

gonorrhoea A highly infectious venereal disease caused by the bacterium *Neisseria gonorrhoea* (gonococcus).

haemophilia A hereditary disorder of blood coagulation affecting males, but transmitted by female carriers. Haemophilia produces excessive bleeding and requires multiple blood transfusions.

haemorrhoids Dilated veins inside swollen tissues of the anus.

helper inducer T4 lymphocyte A type of white blood cell belonging to the cellular immune system which must be produced in normal numbers to defend the body against cancer and infection with bacteria and viruses. The T4 lymphocytes are destroyed by the AIDS virus.

hepatitis Inflammation of the liver due to infection or toxic substances.

high density lipo-protein (HDL) *See* cholesterol.

hirsutism A condition of excessive body hair, other than on the scalp.

histamine A powerful chemical released by cells during allergic reactions.

homoeopathy A system of treatment using minute doses of remedies that, if given in large doses, would produce symptoms similar to those of the disease being treated.

hormonal glands Organs that manufacture hormones. They are also known as endocrine glands.

hormone replacement therapy The use of hormonal preparations to compensate for a loss of natural hormone production by various hormonal glands.

hormones Chemicals produced by various glands (for example, the ovaries, thyroid and adrenal glands) and then transported in the blood to exert a specific regulatory effect upon certain tissues, distant from the gland.

HTLV 111 virus The technical name for the AIDS virus.

hydrotherapy The treatment of painful joints and muscles by exercising in water.

hymen A fold of membrane that partly blocks the entrance to the vagina. The opening in the hymen may be of several forms, namely circular, crescentric or multiple, or there may not be a hymen at all. If there is no opening in the hymen, it is called imperforate.

hypochrondriac A person suffering from the imaginary conviction that he or she is or is likely to become ill.

hypomenorrhoea An abnormally small amount of menstrual blood loss.

hypothalamus A major control centre of the brain, regulating body functions such as temperature, appetite, thirst and the hormonal glands. It is situated at the base of the brain and is directly connected to the pituitary gland.

hysteria A neurosis characterized by emotional instability, increased susceptibility to suggestion, and sometimes loss of memory (amnesia). The afflicted person may develop severe physical symptoms, such as paralysis, deafness or blindness, due to emotional conflict and fear.

hysterical Suffering from or characterized by signs of hysteria.

hysterosalpingogram A special X-ray using a radio-opaque dye to outline the shape of the uterine cavity and the Fallopian tube passageways.

id The subconscious mind which contains instinctive impulses and desires.

immune system The defence system of the body which protects against infection by micro-organisms and invasion by foreign proteins. It is divided into two parts:

1 **humoral** –consisting of proteins in the blood known as immunoglobulins or antibodies which neutralize invaders.

2 **cellular** –consisting of various types of white blood cells which attack and destroy invaders. These cells are under the control of the thymus gland in the neck.

implant A chemical substance or object that is surgically implanted into a part of the body.

impotence Inability in the male to sustain an erection of the penis for effective sexual intercourse.

infertility Temporary or permanent inability to conceive or reproduce.

inflammation A state characterized by heat, swelling, redness and pain, in any tissue, as a result of trauma, infection or irritation.

inseminate To insert semen directly into the uterine cavity.

insomniac A person who has difficulty in sleeping.

intravenous drug (IV drug) A drug that is injected directly into the blood by inserting a needle into a vein.

in vitro fertilization (IVF) Fertilization of the egg by the sperm outside the body, in a laboratory environment.

iris The coloured round mobile membrane of the eye, situated in front of the lens and perforated by the pupil.

ischaemia Lack of blood supply to an organ or body part.

Kaposi's sarcoma A purplish skin cancer which commonly occurs in patients with severe AIDS infection.

laparoscopy A surgical procedure in which a thin telescopic instrument is inserted through a small puncture in the abdominal wall for the purpose of directly viewing the organs of the abdominal and pelvic cavities.

libido Sex drive.

ligaments Bands of strong fibrous tissue joining muscles to bones or bones to bones, or supporting organs and muscles.

lipids Another name for various fats in the body.

low density lipo-protein (LDL) *See* cholesterol.

luteinizing hormone (LH) A hormone which is produced in the pituitary gland and acts on the ovaries to stimulate ovulation.

lymphatic system The interconnected system of capillary vessels between all body tissues and organs through which the lymph fluid circulates and returns to the large venous blood vessels.

lymph fluid The clear watery fluid which travels through the lymphatic system. It contains mainly of white blood cells and acts to remove bacteria from the tissues.

lymph glands Small bean-shaped glands sited along the small vessels of the lymphatic system. They act as filters to trap bacteria, pus cells and cancer cells and are part of the immune system. They are also known as lymph nodes.

lymphocyte A type of white blood cell belonging to the cellular immune system.

malfunction The failure of normal function.

marginal subfertility A subtle or slight reduction in fertility; not absolute in degree.

masculine progesterone A progesterone synthesized from male hormones which may exert masculine effects in the body, such as stimulation of appetite, growth of facial hair and increase in acne and low density cholesterol.

melancholia A mental disorder characterized by depression and unhappiness.

melanin The dark-coloured pigment found in the skin, eyes and hair.

melanotic freckles Dark-coloured freckles.

membranous Made of a thin pliable layer of tissue.

menarche The first occurrence of menstruation in a woman.

menopause The permanent cessation of menstrual bleeding, known colloquially as 'the change of life'.

menorrhagia Excessively heavy bleeding during menstruation.

menstrual cycle The period of time between the beginning of one menstrual period and the beginning of the next menstrual period.

menstrual period The discharge of blood from the uterus through the vagina that occurs in non-pregnant women at approximately monthly intervals between puberty and menopause. It is also called menstrual bleeding.

metabolic rate The speed at which an individual burns up a given amount of food energy.

metabolism The system of chemical and physical processes involved in producing energy for the maintenance of life.

metrorrhagia Irregular vaginal bleeding occurring in between normal menstrual periods. The bleeding may be small or large in amount and may be a short episode or continue for days.

microsurgical techniques Surgical techniques performed on tiny structures with the aid of a microscope, using minute surgical instruments.

minerals Inorganic chemicals found in nature. Some are essential dietary nutrients, for example, zinc, magnesium, potassium, calcium, manganese, selenium, copper and phosphorus.

miscarriage The loss of pregnancy before the beginning of the twenty-first week without outside interference. *See* stillbirth.

molecule The most simple structural unit of a compound.

morbidity The state of being diseased.

mortality rate The death rate.

mucosa A mucous membrane.

mucous membrane The moist tissue lining the body cavities and passageways that open to the outside, such as the mouth, uterine cavity and vagina, the glands of which secrete mucus.

mucus A clear or opaque secretion from a mucous membrane.

multiple sclerosis A degenerative disease of the nervous system.

natural Existing in or fabricated by nature; not artificial.

naturopathy A system of healing that relies only on the use of naturally occurring substances, such as certain foods, water, juices, vitamins, minerals, herbs, homoeopathic dilutions and so on.

neurosis A disorder of the mind or emotions. It may take the form of depression, anxiety, phobias, obsessions, hysteria, panic attacks or other abnormal behaviour.

neurotic Of, relating to or afflicted by neurosis.

non-androgenic Not causing masculine effects in the body.

noradrenaline A hormone secreted by the adrenal glands and the endings of the nerves of the sympathetic nervous system. It is classed as one of the stress hormones.

nucleus The central, usually spherical, body within a cell, which contains hereditary material and controls the growth, reproduction and metabolism of the cell.

obstructive dysmenorrhoea Painful menstrual bleeding due to mechanical obstruction of blood flow from the uterus.

oedema An excessive accumulation of fluid in the tissues. It is also known as fluid retention.

oestrogen Any of several female hormones that are secreted by the ovaries and produce female sexual characteristics. Oestrogen stimulates the growth of breast tissue and endometrium. Chemical oestrogens may be prescribed in the form of tablets, injections, suppositories, creams or implants. There are various chemical types of oestrogen, namely:

Natural	Synthetic	Animal
oestradiol valerate (Progynova);	ethinyloestradiol; mestranol;	equine oestrogens (Premarin).
oestriol (Ovestin);	dienoestrol;	
piperazine oestrone sulphate;	diethylstilboestrol or stilboestrol.	
oestrone.		

oestrogenic contraceptive pill An oral contraceptive pill which is formulated in such a way that its effects will be mainly caused by the hormone oestrogen, in preference to progesterone. This means it will have a stronger effect on the breasts and endometrium and will be beneficial in reducing acne and breakthrough bleeding. An oestrogenic pill is also better tolerated by women with PMS.

oligomenorrhoea Abnormally infrequent menstrual periods.

oligospermia A deficiency in the number of spermatozoa in the semen.

oral 1 Of or relating to the mouth.

2 Involving the mouth.

3 Denoting a drug to be taken by mouth.

orthodox medicine Conventional medicine, adhering to the traditional use of drugs, hormones and sophisticated modern methods of diagnosis and investigation.

orthodox sleep Sleep during which no dreaming occurs, and in which the brain is in a state of very low activity. *See* paradoxical sleep.

ortho-molecular psychiatry The use of nutritional supplements to balance chemicals in the brain in order to overcome mental and emotional illness.

osteoporosis A deficiency of the mineral, calcium, in the bones.

ovaries The female sex glands or gonads which produce the female hormones, oestrogen and progesterone.

ovulation The release of the egg from the ovary.

palpate To feel something with the fingertips.

palpitations Rapid or irregular beating of the heart.

panacea A remedy to cure all evils and diseases.

Pap smear A test in which cells are gently scraped from the inner cervix and smeared onto a glass slide for examination under a microscope. It is a screening test for cancer of the cervix. It is also called a Papanicolaou test.

paradoxical reaction An unusual, contradictory or inexplicable reaction to a drug.

paradoxical sleep Sleep characterized by rapid eye movement (REM) and during which dreaming occurs. *See* orthodox sleep.

paranoia A psychosis characterized by delusions of persecution.

pharmacology The science of drugs, incorporating their chemical structure, uses and beneficial and adverse effects.

phenylalanine A natural amino acid. When given in supplemental doses it slows down the breakdown of the brain's endorphins.

phenylketonuria A hereditary disorder of protein metabolism which can lead to intellectual retardation if a special diet, avoiding the amino acid, phenylalanine, is not instituted from birth.

photodye A coloured substance which when exposed to certain wavelengths of light becomes capable of inducing chemical changes in body cells.

physiology All the vital processes and functioning of the various parts and organs of living organisms.

pituitary gland A mushroom-shaped gland connected by a stalk to the base of the brain. The pituitary gland manufactures many different hormones, which in turn control other hormonal glands, such as the thyroid, adrenal glands, ovaries, testicles and breasts.

platelets Irregularly shaped particles, smaller than blood cells, which circulate in the blood and may promote the formation of clots.

polyunsaturated fats Fats and oils containing long chains of carbon atoms with many double carbon-carbon linkages. Polyunsaturated fats are beneficial for the circulation and immune system. Sources of polyunsatured fats are raw seeds (sunflower, sesame, blackcurrant and linseed), primrose oil, most cold pressed vegetable oils, cod liver oil, mackerel and fresh fish from the cold deep oceans, marine lipid oils.

potassium An important dietary material, found mainly inside body cells.

potassium-sparing diuretic A drug which promotes the production of urine, without promoting a loss of potassium from the body cells.

potency The concentration or dilution of a medicinal substance.

premature menopause The cessation of menstrual periods before the age of forty-five years.

premenopausal Of or relating to the years immediately preceding the cessation of menstrual periods.

progesterone A female hormone produced in the ovary by the corpus luteum after ovulation has occurred. It prepares the lining of the uterus to accept the fertilized egg. Progesterone may be taken in the form of tablets, injections, supppositories or implants. It occurs in two chemical forms, natural and synthetic, and it can be non-androgenic or androgenic:

| Natural progesterone (not available in tablet form). | Synthetic – non-androgenic medroxyprogesterone acetate (Depo Provera); dydrogesterone; ethynodiol diacetate; hydroxyprogesterone; norethynodrel; desogestrel. | Synthetic – androgenic norgestrel; levonorgestrel (Micronor); norethisterone (slightly androgenic); lynoestrol. |

prolactin A hormone produced by the pituitary gland. It is normally produced in large amounts during lactation and stimulates milk production in the breasts.

prolactinoma A tumour which occurs in the pituitary gland and secretes large amounts of the hormone, prolactin.

prolapse The falling down of an organ because of weakened muscular and fibrous tissue support. The most common organs to prolapse are the uterus, bladder and bowel.

prostaglandin F2 alpha A particular type of prostaglandin involved in uterine contractions and period pains.

prostaglandins Chemicals manufactured in most body cells from fatty acids. They exert a hormone-like effect which influences circulation, muscular contractions and inflammation.

psyche The mind as a functional entity.

psychological Of or relating to the mind or emotions.

psychosexual Of or relating to the psychological aspects of sex or the mental processes relating to it.

psychosis Any severe mental disorder in which there is deterioration of intellectual and social functioning, as well as withdrawal from reality. There may or may not be associated brain damage.

psychosomatic Of or relating to physical symptoms that are totally or partially due to a psychological cause; for example, high blood pressure, tension headaches and so on.

psychotic illness A mental illness having the characteristics of a psychosis.

pus Thick yellow-green fluid formed in infected tissue.

pyruvic acid An intermediate product formed in the metabolism of carbohydrates and proteins.

radiation, ionizing 1 X-rays used in medical diagnosis or radiotherapy against cancer.
2 Contaminating emissions from nuclear power plants or the atomic bomb.

rapid eye movement (REM) Continual movement of the eyes behind the closed eyelids, as when dreaming takes place. *See* paradoxical sleep.

replication The act of duplicating or reproducing.

rupture To break open or burst.

saturated fats Fats having all available valency bonds filled. Sources of saturated fats are animal fats and dairy products. Saturated fats increase low density cholesterol in the blood which, if excessive, will promote atherosclerosis.

schizophrenia A psychotic mental illness characterized by withdrawal from reality, emotional imbalance and intellectual confusion, and often accompanied by delusions and hallucinations.

sedative A drug or herbal substance which has a calming and tranquillizing effect.

senile dementia The deterioration of mental functioning due to degeneration and shrinking of the brain, as a result of old age.

serotonin A powerful brain chemical which exerts a controlling influence on sleep, mood, libido and appetite.

serum hepatitis Inflammation of the liver due to infection with a virus called the hepatitis B virus.

shingles An infection with the chicken-pox virus characterized by blistering and crusting skin eruptions along the routes of the spinal nerves, on one side of the body.

side effect An indirect or secondary effect; especially, an undesirable effect produced by a drug or treatment.

steroid effect An effect similar to that produced by steroid hormones, but produced by substances other than steroids; especially, an effect that causes inflammation, pain and swelling.

steroids Any of numerous naturally occurring compounds such as bile acids, sterols and many hormones. The best known steroid hormone is cortisone.

stillbirth The birth of a dead child, when the pregnancy has continued for more than twenty weeks. *See* miscarriage.

stroke A brain haemorrhage.

subconscious mind The deeper part of the mind of which an individual is usually unaware. Its contents can sometimes be made conscious through the techniques of hypnosis or psychoanalysis.

suppressive effect The effect of stopping an expression of symptoms and signs of a disease, as opposed to curing it.

swab 1 A small piece of absorbent material attached to the end of a stick, used for cleansing, applying medicine or removing specimens of mucus for examination.
2 The specimen so removed.

sympathetic nervous system That part of the autonomic (automatic) nervous system which prepares the body for stress and energy expenditure. When activated, it causes the blood pressure and pulse rate to rise, increases sweating and blood flow to organs and muscles and causes the release of stress hormones.

syndrome A group of signs and symptoms that collectively characterize a disease.

synthetic oestrogens Oestrogens which are metabolized or broken down in the body by means of a mechanism which is different from that used in the metabolism of oestrogens manufactured in the ovaries or natural oestrogens.

testosterone The major male hormone. It produces masculine effects in the body, such as increased body hair, increased appetite, increased libido and deepening of the voice.

therapy The remedial treatment given for a disease or disability.

thrombophlebitis Inflammation of a vein after a blood clot has formed in it.

thyroid gland The endocrine gland situated in the front of the neck which produces the hormone thyroxine. Thyroxine regulates the metabolic route of the body.

topical cream A cream applied directly to the skin.

toxic lymphatic system A lymphatic system that is overburdened with toxins and waste products from the metabolism.

toxin A harmful, irritating, destructive and, in extreme cases, poisonous substance.

triglyceride A natural fat occurring in the blood, which, if excessive, predisposes to atherosclerosis.

trimester A period of three months; especially, a period of three months during a pregnancy. Pregnancy has three trimesters, totalling nine months.

tryptophan An essential dietary amino acid which is converted in the brain into serotonin.

tumour An abnormal growth which may be cancerous or benign.

ultrasound test The procedure of passing high frequency sound waves through various parts of the body to display the shape and size of different structures, such as the unborn child, the pelvic and abdominal organs, the heart and so on.

vaccine A substance consisting of weakened or killed disease-causing micro-organisms, such as bacteria or viruses, which when introduced into the body stimulates the production of antibodies. These confer protection (immunity) against the natural form of the infectious micro-organism.

varicose veins Veins that are excessively dilated, knotted and tortuous.

venereal disease (VD) Any of several contagious diseases, for example, gonorrhoea and herpes, contracted through sexual intercourse or sexual activity.

virostatic Of or relating to a substance which can stop the replication and growth of infectious viruses.

virus A submicroscopic infectious organism consisting of a central core of nucleic acid (genetic material) surrounded by a protein coat. It can only replicate itself inside a living cell.

vitamin B complex The group of B vitamins, namely B1 thiamine, B2 riboflavine, B3 niacin, B5 pantothenic acid, B6 pyridoxine and B12 cyanocobalamin. Other components of the B group are biotin, folic acid, lipoic acid and inositol. B complex vitamins are found in yeast, liver, eggs and fresh vegetables.

withdrawal syndrome The unpleasant and distressing symptoms that may occur when an addictive drug or a drug that has been taken for a long time is withdrawn from a patient.

Appendix A handy guide to treatments for common disorders

Disorder	Symptoms	Diet Include often	Avoid	Helpful natural supplements	Helpful drugs and hormones
Painful periods	The menstrual blood loss is accompanied by lower abdominal pain. There may also be backache, pain in the thighs, vomiting and diarrhoea.	Fresh fruit and vegetables, dolomite powder, raw vegetable juices, primrose oil, fish, raw seeds, liver.	Fatty meats, excess saturated fats, excess salt, processed meats.	**Minerals:** Magnesium, calcium, potassium. **Herbals:** crampbark, cimicifuga, chamomile, ruscus aculeatus, aesculus, hamamelis, ranunculaceae, beta-hydroxy-bioflavonoids, rutosides, uva ursi, juniper, buchu, evening primrose oil. Chiropractic and regular yoga may be helpful.	Anti-prostaglandin drugs, e.g., aspirin. The oral contraceptive pill (OCP). Progesterone tablets. Codeine phosphate. Doxylamine succinate.
PMS	Depression, anxiety, mood changes, breast pain, fluid retention, weight gain, low blood sugar, skin problems and headaches.	Raw salads and fruit, fish, raw seeds and nuts, cold pressed vegetable oils, whole grain products (unless allergic), water. Raw garlic or alternatively garlic, four to six capsules daily with food.	Fried foods, sugar, salt, alcohol, cigarettes, excessive dairy products.	Kelp, vitamin E, vitamins B6, B1, B3, C, zinc, manganese, magnesium, iron phosphate, chromium, potassium. **Herbals:** Uva ursi, parsley, juniper, crampbark, valerian, chamomile. Breast cream containing the herb phytolacca may be massaged into the breasts.	Progesterone in the form of: tablets (Duphaston); implants; injections (Proluton). Some brands of the OCP. A doctor's consultation will be necessary for these drugs. OCP's containing masculine progesterone should be avoided.

Meno-pause	Short-term: Hot flushes, sweating, insomnia, itching skin, fatigue, poor memory, depression, vaginal dryness and soreness, painful intercourse, loss of libido. Long-term: Osteoporosis (deficiency of calcium in the bones). Atherosclerosis (hardening of the arteries).	Cold pressed vegetable oils, linseed oil, primrose oil, raw seeds and nuts, fish, raw salads, raw vegetable juices, skim milk, low fat yoghurt, garlic, fish oil supplements, lecithin.	Fried foods, alcohol, antacids containing aluminium, fatty meats, cream, fatty cheeses, cigarettes.	**Vitamins:** A, E, B6, B1, D. **Minerals:** calcium silica, zinc, manganese. **Herbals:** smilax, cimicifuga, passiflora, viburnum opulus, garlic.	Hormone replacement therapy using natural oestrogens such as Ogen, Progynova, oestradiol. Oestrogen can be administered as injections, tablets, skin implants or vaginal creams. A progesterone tablet should be added to balance the oestrogen. If you have high blood pressure, anxiety and hot flushes, a beta-blocker drug can be effective.
Skin problems	Acne.	Raw vegetable juices, water, fruit, whole grains, lean meats, fish, fresh fruit and salads.	Fatty foods, nuts, chocolate and lollies, processed foods, soft drinks, cigarettes.	**Garlic** two capsules three times daily with food. **Zinc chelate** one tablet three times daily with food. **Pure C powder** (pure calcium ascorbate) ¼ tsp: three times daily. Water soluble **tea tree oil** topically.	In severe cases, antibiotics, e.g., tetracycline. There is a new drug for extreme cases, synthetic vitamin A, called Roaccutane, available from dermatologists only. In hormonal cases, a tailor-made OCP can be excellent. Avoid masculine progesterones. The anti-androgen drug called

Disorder	Symptoms	Diet Include often	Avoid	Helpful natural supplements	Helpful drugs and hormones
					Cyproterone is extremely effective.
					If acne and greasy skin are associated with excessive facial hair, new treatments available are Aldactone and Cyproterone.
	Herpes – genital and facial.	Raw foods, raw vegetable juices, liver, lecithin, whole grains, fish.	Alcohol, cigarettes.	**Zinc chelate** 50mg, twice daily with food. **Amino acids: lysine,** DL phenylalanine. **Pure C powder** (pure calcium ascorbate) 1/4 tsp. three times daily.	A topical solution of idoxuridine can be applied every two hours to early blisters. A new drug Acyclovir is sometimes used in severe cases, but long-term effects are unknown.
	Dermatitis, eczema and fungal infections, e.g., thrush, tinea, pityriasis (fungal infections may be increased by the OCP and cortisone drugs).	Fresh salads, vegetable juices, grains, nuts, seeds, legumes, fish, cod liver oil capsules, cold pressed vegetable oils, garlic and carrot juice.	Alcohol, cigarettes, refined carbohydrates, yeast foods, sweet foods and sugar, artificial chemicals, preservatives and processed foods.	**Zinc chelate** one tablet with every meal. **Garlic** two capsules with every meal. **Vitamin C** 1000mg, three times daily. To be taken orally: evening primrose oil capsules (Omega 6) two, three times	Antifungal tablets, e.g., Nystatin, Amphotericin, Griseofulvin, Nizoral (can have side effects on the liver). Antifungal creams, e.g., Canesten, Gynodaktarin, Tea Tree. Cortisone creams can be helpful in dermatitis but

	Symptoms	Recommended foods	Avoid	Supplements	Treatments
				daily. Fish oil capsules (Omega 3) one, three times daily. Apply fresh gel from living **aloe vera** plant to areas of sun damaged skin.	should be used sparingly as they cause thinning of the skin.
Vaginal infections	Vaginal discharge and odour, irritation, itch, burning on passing urine.	Fresh fruit and vegetables, raw vegetable juices, yoghurt, garlic, water, whole grains.	Yeast, sugar, alcohol.	**Zinc chelate** one tablet three times daily with food. **Garlic** two capsules three times daily with food. **Pure C powder** (pure calcium ascorbate) 1/4 tsp. three times daily. **Acidophilus powder** 1 tsp. in 1 litre of water to make a vaginal douche.	Nystatin cream and tablets, Flagyl tablets, Sultrin vaginal cream, Tea Tree oil cream or pessaries. Always have a swab and culture done by your doctor for every infection. A new oral tablet for difficult cases of thrush is Nizoral.
Arthritis, rheumatic disorders	Pain in the articular joints. This may be in the spine, shoulders, elbows, wrists, hands, hips, knees, ankles, feet. There may be associated swelling, heat, stiffness and	Raw vegetable juices, four to five glasses daily. Salads, whole grains, cold pressed vegetable oils, raw seeds, e.g., sunflower, sesame, linseed. Fish. Everyone is an individual and it	Fried foods, excess alcohol, white flour and white sugar, junk foods, salt.	**Anti-inflammatory herbs:** devil's claw, yucca, white willow bark. **Enzymes:** trypsin, papain, bromelain. **Vitamins:** bioflavonoids, vitamin C, B1, B6, B12, A and E. **Minerals:** calcium orotate,	Codeine phosphate, paracetamol. High dose soluble aspirin. Anti-prostaglandin drugs, e.g., Indocid, Naprosyn, Voltaro. In severe cases, cortisone or gold tablets may be given.

Disorder	Symptoms	Diet Include often	Avoid	Helpful natural supplements	Helpful drugs and hormones
	'cracking' in the joints.	may be necessary to experiment a little, e.g., some people can take dairy products, while in others they may induce a flare-up of inflammation. Some people with excess acidity do better on a vegetarian diet, but fish is usually beneficial.		manganese chelate, green lipped muscle extract, zinc, silica, magnesium. **Amino acid:** DL phenylalanine. **Homoeopathics:** rhus tox, arnica, hypericum. To be taken orally: Fish oil capsules (Omega 3) two, three times daily with meals. Evening primrose oil capsules (Omega 6) one, three times daily with meals.	
Circulatory problems	Varicose veins, haemorrhoids, thrombophlebitis, clots, cold hands and feet, leg cramps, wounds on legs that are slow to heal, swollen aching legs with fluid retention,	Raw vegetable juices, citrus fruit, carrots, rosehip, whole grains, raw bran, salads, apple cider vinegar, cold pressed vegetable oils, fish (fresh), marine lipid extract.	Salt, fried foods, fatty foods, processed meats, full fat dairy products, cigarettes, excessive alcohol.	**Garlic** two capsules three to four times daily with food.	Aspirin. Warfarin, hospital use only. Heparin, hospital use only. Vasodilators, especially calcium blockers and nitrates, and a new drug called Trental.

hardening of the arteries (atherosclerosis), angina, chilblains.				
Hypertension (high blood pressure).	Raw vegetable juices, citrus fruit, carrots, rosehip, whole grains, raw bran, salads, apple cider vinegar, cold pressed vegetable oils, fish (fresh), marine lipid extract.	Salt, fried foods, fatty foods, processed meats, alcohol.	**Garlic** six capsules daily. **Pure C powder** (pure calcium ascorbate) ¼ tsp. three times daily in juices. People with high blood pressure should only take vitamin E under doctor's supervision. **Herbals:** Beta-hydroxy rutosides, nicotinic acid, bioflavonoids, ruscus aculeatus, aesculus, hamamelis, ranunculaceae. **Minerals:** potassium and magnesium. Natural vitamin E, vitamin C, 4000mg daily. Fish oil capsules (Omega 3) one, three times daily.	Diuretics, vaso-dilators, e.g., Minipress, especially calcium blockers and beta-blockers. Also, Ace inhibitors. Please see your doctor regularly for measurement of your blood pressure, as people with high blood pressure may not have any symptoms.

Disorder	Symptoms	Diet Include often	Avoid	Helpful natural supplements	Helpful drugs and hormones
Chronic headaches	These may be due to migraine, allergy, inflammation, neuralgia. They may be worse premenstrually or during menopause due to hormonal imbalance.	Raw vegetable juices, salads, brown rice, grains, seeds, legumes, raw bran, fish, three to four glasses water daily. Exercise regularly. Try yoga, massage, acupuncture, chiropractic.	Fried foods, sugar, candy, processed foods, excess salt, alcohol, cigarettes, coffee, strong tea. Migraine sufferers should not eat foods containing tyramine, e.g., red wine, beer, chocolate, lima and Italian beans, cheddar cheese, chicken liver, raisins, avocados, plums, nuts and monosodium glutamate.	**Herbals:** humulus, belladonna, gelsemium, white willow bark, yucca, evening primrose oil capsules, fever few, camomile, homoeopathics iris versicolor, viola oderata, sanguinaria. Vitamins B1, B6 and B12. Primrose oil capsules. **Amino acid:** DL phenylalanine can be tried as a preventative on a regular basis as it can have a natural analgesic effect. Vitamins B1, B2, B3, B6, B12, C, E. Zinc chelate. Magnesium.	Codeine phosphate, soluble aspirin. Cafergot and other ergotamine preparations for migraines. If the headaches are worse premenstrually, hormonal therapy may be necessary using a low dose contraceptive pill or small doses of oestrogen during the contraceptive pill break.
Side effects of the oral contraceptive pill	Headaches.	Salads, juices, fruit.	Salt, wine, mature cheese.		Use lower dose OCP.
	Acne, greasy hair.	Water, juices, salads, fruit, rice, bran.	Fatty foods, sugar, nuts.	Garlic four capsules daily with food.	Avoid OCPs containing the progesterones 'norgestrel' or 'levonorgestrel'.

Skin pigmentation.		Sunlight.	Apply **aloe vera gel** to dark patches.	Use mini pill. Avoid oestrogen.
Fluid retention, weight gain.	Salads, juices, bran, rice, fresh fish.	Salt, sugar.	A homoeopathic preparation containing beta-hydroxy-rutosides, nicotinic acid, bioflavonoids, calcium ascorbate and the herbs ruscus aculeatus, aesculus, hamamelis, ranunculaceae. Dosage: two tablets three times daily. A homoeopathic preparation containing kelp, natural vitamin E, zinc chelate, manganese chelate, magnesium phosphate, vitamin B6, nicotinamide, vitamin B1 (thiamine), chromium chelate, iron phosphate, potassium chloride and the herbs uva ursi, parsley, juniper, crampbark. Dosage: one tablet daily.	Use low dose pill. Aldactone with a thiazide diuretic.
Breast pain.	Salads, water, juices, garlic, fish, raw seeds and nuts.	Alcohol, fatty meats, processed meats, salts, dairy products.	**Garlic** six capsules daily.	Use low dose pill, especially one low in oestrogen.

NOTE: If you notice severe migraine headaches with visual changes or pain and swelling in the legs – see your doctor immediately as the pill should be discontinued.

Disorder	Symptoms	Diet Include often	Avoid	Helpful natural supplements	Helpful drugs and hormones
Stress syn- dromes	Anxiety-tension, insomnia, chronic fatigue, eating dis- orders, depression.	Raw fruits, especially citrus variety, raw vegetable salads and juices, foods high in calcium, e.g., sardines, fish, dairy (preferably low fat variety). Foods high in magnesium and zinc: nuts, soya beans, beetroot, alfalfa, figs, peaches, almonds, whole grains, sunflower and sesame seeds, brown rice, bran, wheatgerm, brewers yeast, eggs, onions, oysters and herrings.	Refined carbohydrates, high fat diet, fried food, sugar, excess alcohol, cigarettes, caffeine.	**Amino acids: tryptophan, tyrosine, phenylalanine.** Vitamin B complex. Vitamin C. **Minerals: potassium, magnesium, calcium. Vitamin C powder.** Amino acids, tyrosine and phenylanine, two or three times daily on an empty stomach. B complex. **Herbal teas camomile,** passionflower, hops, golden seal, passiflora.	Benzodiazepines, e.g., Valium, Serepax, Ativan, if possible to be used only for a period of several months. Anti-depressant drugs, e.g., tryptanol, Sinequan.

Index

Index compiled by Peva Keane.